Obstetrics and Gynecology for Practitioners

Obstetrics and Gynecology for Practitioners

Edited by Larry Stone

hayle
medical

New York

Hayle Medical,
750 Third Avenue, 9th Floor,
New York, NY 10017, USA

Visit us on the World Wide Web at:
www.haylemedical.com

ISBN: 978-1-63241-508-0

Cataloging-in-Publication Data

Obstetrics and gynecology for practitioners / edited by Larry Stone.
    p. cm.
Includes bibliographical references and index.
ISBN 978-1-63241-508-0
1. Obstetrics. 2. Gynecology. 3. Obstetrics--Practice. 4. Gynecology--Practice. I. Stone, Larry.
RG526 .O27 2018
618.2--dc23

Table of Contents

Preface

This book has been a concerted effort by a group of academicians, researchers and scientists, who have contributed their research works for the realization of the book. This book has materialized in the wake of emerging advancements and innovations in this field. Therefore, the need of the hour was to compile all the required researches and disseminate the knowledge to a broad spectrum of people comprising of students, researchers and specialists of the field.

Obstetrics and gynecology is a field of medical science that concerns itself with the study of childbirth, pregnancy, and also with the detailed study of female reproductive health and reproductive parts of the body. It has many sub-branches namely menopausal and geriatric gynecology, female pelvic medicine and reconstructive surgery, contraception and abortion, reproductive endocrinology and infertility, etc. The topics included in this book on obstetrics and gynecology, are of utmost significance and bound to provide incredible insights to readers. It will serve as a reference to a broad spectrum of readers.

At the end of the preface, I would like to thank the authors for their brilliant chapters and the publisher for guiding us all-through the making of the book till its final stage. Also, I would like to thank my family for providing the support and encouragement throughout my academic career and research projects.

Editor

Maternal Tenofovir Disoproxil Fumarate Use in Pregnancy and Growth Outcomes among HIV-Exposed Uninfected Infants in Kenya

Jillian Pintye,[1,2] **Agnes Langat,**[3] **Benson Singa,**[4] **John Kinuthia,**[1,5] **Beryne Odeny,**[1]
Abraham Katana,[3] **Lucy Nganga,**[3] **Grace John-Stewart,**[1,6,7] **and Christine J. McGrath**[1,8]

[1]*Department of Global Health, University of Washington, Seattle, WA 98104, USA*
[2]*Department of Nursing, University of Washington, Seattle, WA 98195, USA*
[3]*United States Centers for Disease Control and Prevention (CDC), Nairobi 00202, Kenya*
[4]*Center for Microbiology Research and Center for Clinical Research, Kenya Medical Research Institute,
Nairobi 00202, Kenya*
[5]*Department of Obstetrics & Gynecology, Kenyatta National Hospital, Nairobi 00202, Kenya*
[6]*Department of Medicine, University of Washington, Seattle, WA 98195, USA*
[7]*Department of Epidemiology, University of Washington, Seattle, WA 98195, USA*
[8]*University of Texas Medical Branch, Galveston, TX 77555, USA*

Correspondence should be addressed to Christine J. McGrath; mcgrathc@uw.edu

Academic Editor: Faustino R. Perez-Lopez

Background. Tenofovir disoproxil fumarate (TDF) is commonly used in antiretroviral treatment (ART) and preexposure prophylaxis regimens. We evaluated the relationship of prenatal TDF use and growth outcomes among Kenyan HIV-exposed uninfected (HEU) infants. *Materials and Methods.* We included PCR-confirmed HEU infants enrolled in a cross-sectional survey of mother-infant pairs conducted between July and December 2013 in Kenya. Maternal ART regimen during pregnancy was determined by self-report and clinic records. Six-week and 9-month z-scores for weight-for-age (WAZ), weight-for-length (WLZ), length-for-age (LAZ), and head circumference-for-age (HCAZ) were compared among HEU infants with and without TDF exposure using t-tests and multivariate linear regression models. *Results.* Among 277 mothers who received ART during pregnancy, 63% initiated ART before pregnancy, of which 89 (32%) used TDF. No differences in birth weight (3.0 kg versus 3.1 kg, $p = 0.21$) or gestational age (38 weeks versus 38 weeks, $p = 0.16$) were detected between TDF-exposed and TDF-unexposed infants. At 6 weeks, unadjusted mean WAZ was lower among TDF-exposed infants (-0.8 versus -0.4, $p = 0.03$), with a trend towards association in adjusted analyses ($p = 0.06$). There were no associations between prenatal TDF use and WLZ, LAZ, and HCAZ in 6-week or 9-month infant cohorts. *Conclusion.* Maternal TDF use did not adversely affect infant growth compared to other regimens.

1. Introduction

Tenofovir disoproxil fumarate- (TDF-) containing combination antiretroviral therapy (ART) is currently considered a first-line regimen for HIV treatment and prevention of mother-to-child transmission (PMTCT) Option B/B+ by the World Health Organization (WHO) [1]. TDF and the fixed-dose combination of emtricitabine (FTC) 200 mg and TDF 300 mg are also recommended by WHO for antiretroviral

preexposure prophylaxis (PrEP) in key populations, including women in HIV-serodiscordant couples who may wish to conceive [2]. TDF is considered a Pregnancy Category B drug, which means that no adequate evidence of risk in humans has been established by the United States Food and Drug Administration (FDA) [3]. The FDA recommends TDF as an alternative nucleotide analogue reverse transcriptase inhibitor (NRTI) for HIV-infected antiretroviral-naïve pregnant women due to limited data on TDF safety during pregnancy [4]. Animal studies in macaques have found adverse effects of high-dose TDF during pregnancy on bone mineralization and intrauterine growth measured at birth, but these effects were not observed at lower doses, which are more consistent with human TDF use [5–8]. As ART and PMTCT Option B/B+ programs expand and PrEP accessibility scales up, the likelihood of pregnant women using TDF will increase and obtaining safety information on TDF use during pregnancy will have important public health implications [9].

Several studies [10–20] and one systematic review [9] reported that prenatal TDF use for HIV treatment generally appears to be safe for pregnancy outcomes. Additionally, the most recent report from the Antiretroviral Pregnancy Registry showed no evidence of increased birth defects among 1,982 infants born to HIV-infected women in the United States who took TDF during their first trimester [21]. Limited data are available on the safety of TDF use for PrEP in pregnancy, though small studies suggest no difference in birth outcomes between mothers with and without short-term prenatal PrEP use [22, 23]. However, few studies have assessed the effects of prolonged prenatal TDF use on postnatal infant growth and bone health, and these have mixed results [14, 18, 19, 24, 25]. Only one small study evaluated prolonged prenatal TDF use and infant growth outcomes in a sub-Saharan African cohort indicating a need for additional data from this setting [26]. Data from HIV-exposed uninfected (HEU) infants could be particularly useful when assessing safety of prenatal TDF use for PrEP. We aimed to evaluate the relationship of prenatal TDF use and growth outcomes among HEU infants born to mothers who used combination ART for PMTCT or HIV treatment during pregnancy in Kenya.

2. Materials and Methods

2.1. Study Design and Participants. Data, from participants enrolled in two cross-sectional surveys evaluating the national PMTCT program and maternal-child health (MCH) indicators in Kenya conducted between June and December 2013, were analyzed for this study. The first survey used probability proportionate to size sampling to select 121 MCH clinics in seven of the eight geographical regions in Kenya from which all mother-infant pairs were sampled to participate during a 5-day period per clinic. The second survey sampled only HIV-infected women attending 30 MCH clinics in Nyanza province during a fixed 10-day period. In total, 140 clinics were sampled as some clinics were selected for both surveys. Women were eligible to be included in the survey if they were willing and able to provide informed consent and their infant was attending clinic to receive week 6 or month 9 immunizations. Infants were excluded if they were brought to the clinic by someone other than their biological mother or informed consent from their mother was not provided.

At enrollment into both surveys, a nurse administered the study questionnaire and obtained anthropometric measurements of the mother and infant. Mothers were identified as HIV-infected through self-report. HIV status during pregnancy and timing of HIV diagnosis were confirmed using MCH booklets, a form of clinical records used in Kenya

which documents MCH and HIV services received in pre-/postnatal care. All mothers identified as HIV-infected were offered infant HIV testing and a dried blood spot (DBS) sample was taken for HIV DNA PCR testing after consent. All infants with PCR-confirmed HIV-negative serostatus and complete anthropometric measurements born to HIV-positive mothers with documented use of 3-drug combination ART during pregnancy were included in this analysis.

2.2. Data Collection. Study questionnaires obtained information on maternal sociodemographics, sexual behaviors, and medical history. Data on infant birth and medical characteristics was also collected. Maternal body mass index (kilograms/meters^2) was calculated from height and weight measurements ascertained by study nurses at questionnaire administration. MCH booklets confirmed clinical data self-reported on questionnaires. Data were abstracted from MCH booklets if mothers were not sure of ART regimen used during pregnancy, WHO clinical stage, last CD4 count, infant birth weight, or gestational age at birth. Trimester of ART initiation was calculated using the date of ART initiation and infant birth date, as documented in MCH booklets. All mothers with confirmed ART initiation prior to pregnancy were considered to have first trimester ART use. Maternal prenatal TDF use was defined as a documented use of TDF-containing ART regimen for any amount of time during pregnancy.

2.3. Outcome Measures. Trained study nurses obtained standardized anthropometric measurements from each infant, including length in centimeters (cm), weight in kilograms (kg), and head circumference in cm [27]. z-scores for weight-for-age (WAZ), weight-for-length (WLZ), length-for-age (LAZ), and head circumference-for-age (HCAZ) were calculated using the WHO Child Growth Standards in WHO Anthro software [27, 28].

2.4. Statistical Methods. All HIV-infected mother-HEU infant pairs with information on prenatal 3-drug combination ART regimen type and anthropometric measurements were included in this analysis; HIV-infected mothers without information on ART regimen type and verification from their MCH booklets were excluded. Separate analyses were conducted for infants attending 6-week and 9-month immunization visits. Chi-squared tests for proportions and Kruskal-Wallis tests for continuous measures were used to detect differences in sociodemographic and medical characteristics among mother-infant pairs with and without prenatal TDF use. Growth outcomes among HEU infants with and without maternal prenatal TDF use were compared using t-tests and multivariate linear regression for continuous measures of weight (kg), length (cm), head circumference (cm), WAZ, WLZ, LAZ, and HCZ. Characteristics associated with growth faltering, defined as WAZ, WLZ, LAZ, and HCZ < −2 standard deviations (SD), were assessed using Chi-squared tests and multivariate logistic regression. All linear and logistic regression models accounted for clustering at the clinic level.

We determined *a priori* to adjust our statistical models for maternal age, education level, BMI, time since HIV diagnosis, and infant breastfeeding and gestational age at birth due to the known associations of these factors with TDF use or infant growth outcomes [29–32]. Additionally, we identified several demographic, behavioral, and medical characteristics to assess as potential confounders: WHO clinical stage, number of living children, marital status, marriage type (monogamous versus polygamous), enrollment site in Nyanza (a culturally distinct region with high HIV prevalence), ever having received CD4 testing, last CD4 count (cell/μL) during pregnancy, and trimester of first combination ART regimen use during pregnancy and protease inhibitor- (PI-) containing ART regimen (versus no PI). Additional potential confounders were included in the final models if they substantially changed the logistic regression model odds ratio or linear regression coefficient (>10% change). Multivariate risk scores were used to simultaneously adjust for maternal age, maternal education level, breastfeeding, gestational age at birth, time since maternal HIV diagnosis, maternal WHO clinical stage, timing of ART initiation (before or during pregnancy), and trimester of first use of 3-drug combination ART regimen during pregnancy and PI-containing ART regimen in final models. Multivariate risk scores were used to impute missing data for adjustment in multivariate models. The validity and details regarding this approach have been described elsewhere [33, 34]. These scores were included in the final models as quintiles.

To examine our statistical models with the most precision for first trimester 3-drug combination ART exposure, we restricted our dataset to only mother-infant pairs with documented ART initiation prior to pregnancy. Current WHO Child Growth Standards calculate age and sex-adjusted z-scores based on infants born >37 weeks of gestation and therefore potential nondifferential z-score misclassification may occur in preterm infants (gestational age <37 weeks) [35]. To examine the robustness of our multivariate regression models without the effect of prematurity, we repeated the primary analysis restricted to infants born >37 weeks of gestation. We also repeated the primary analysis using indicator variables for missing values to account for the potential categorical effect of missing data. Data were analyzed using STATA 13.1/MP for Windows (Stata Corporation, College Station, TX).

2.5. Ethical Considerations. The study was approved by the institutional review boards of the 3 collaborating institutions including the Kenya Medical Research Institute, the University of Washington, and the US Centers for Disease Control and Prevention.

3. Results

3.1. Enrollment Characteristics. A total of 277 HIV-infected mothers and their HEU infants (56% of all HEU infants in both surveys) had documented 3-drug combination ART use during pregnancy that met criteria for inclusion in this analysis; 155 (56%) attend 6-week infant immunizations; 122 (44%) attend 9-month infant immunizations. Most

mothers were married (84%), the median age was 29 years (interquartile range (IQR) 25–34), and the median time since HIV diagnosis was 8 years (IQR 5–8). Over half of the mothers (64%) initiated 3-drug combination ART before pregnancy and 89 (32%) used a TDF-containing regimen at any time during pregnancy. Among mothers that did not use TDF-containing regimens, the most common combination ART was zidovudine, lamivudine, and nevirapine (AZT/3TC/NVP) (78%) followed by stavudine, lamivudine, and nevirapine (d24/3TC/NVP) (8%). Tenofovir, lamivudine, and nevirapine (TDF/3TC/NVP) and tenofovir, lamivudine, and efavirenz (TDF/3TC/EFV) were the most common regimens among mothers who used TDF-containing ART (65% and 26%, resp.). Mothers with and without prenatal TDF use had similar sociodemographic characteristics (Table 1). Compared to mothers without prenatal TDF use ($n = 188$), mothers with prenatal TDF use ($n = 89$) were more likely to receive PIs (26% versus 7%, $p < 0.001$), were more likely to be WHO clinical stage III (14% versus 6%, $p = 0.030$), and had modestly lower median BMI (22 versus 23, $p = 0.031$). There was no difference in median time since ART initiation between mothers with and without TDF use that initiated 3-drug combination ART prior to pregnancy (42 versus 36 months, $p = 0.654$). Similarly, mothers with and without TDF use that initiated 3-drug combination ART in pregnancy ($n = 76$) did not have a significant difference in median time since ART initiation (6 versus 9 months, $p = 0.809$).

Most infants were currently breastfeeding (87%) and half (51%) were male. Mean gestational age at birth was similar for infants with and without mothers that used TDF during pregnancy (37.8 weeks versus 38.1, $p = 0.337$). We did not detect differences in mean birth weight (3.0 kg versus 3.2 kg, $p = 0.14$) or prevalence of low birth weight <2.5 kg (10% versus 7%, $p = 0.449$) among infants with and without prenatal TDF exposure.

3.2. Growth Outcomes among HEU Infants Attending 6-Week Visits. We detected a modest difference in mean weight (4.3 kg versus 4.7 kg, $p = 0.015$, Table 2) and WAZ (-0.8 versus -0.4, $p = 0.033$) between infants attending 6-week visits with *in utero* TDF exposure compared to infants without exposure to TDF. There was no detectable difference between prenatal TDF use and WAZ < -2 SD among infants attending 6-week visits (12% versus 7%, $p = 0.288$). There were no detectable differences for WLZ (0.3 versus 0.6, $p = 0.462$), WLZ < -2 SD (10% versus 16%, $p = 0.317$), length (52.8 cm versus 53.0 cm, $p = 0.766$), LAZ (-1.2 versus -1.2, $p = 0.951$), and LAZ < -2 SD (37% versus 38%, $p = 0.976$). There were also no differences in head circumference among HEU infants attending 6-week visits with and without prenatal TDF exposure.

After adjustment for maternal age, maternal education, breastfeeding, gestational age at birth, time since maternal HIV diagnosis, maternal WHO clinical stage, timing of ART initiation (before or during pregnancy), and trimester of first combination ART regimen use during pregnancy and PI-containing ART, we found no association between maternal prenatal TDF use and weight, length, and HC among infants attending 6-week visits (Table 3): WAZ (adjusted coefficient

TABLE 1: Distribution of demographic and medical characteristics by any maternal prenatal TDF use, among HEU infants exposed for combination ART[1].

	Median (IQR) or N (percentage)					
	Mother-infant pairs at 6-week visit ($n = 155$)			Mother-infant pairs at 9-month visit ($n = 122$)		
	Maternal TDF use during pregnancy[2]			Maternal TDF use during pregnancy[2]		
	Yes ($n = 51$)	No ($n = 104$)	p value[3]	Yes ($n = 38$)	No ($n = 84$)	p value[3]
	Maternal demographic characteristics					
Age (years)	28 (24–33)	28 (25–33)	0.730	30 (26–35)	31 (25–34)	0.930
Education completed (years)	8 (7–11)	8 (7–10)	0.430	8 (8–11)	8 (7–12)	0.901
Number of children	3 (2–4)	3 (2–4)	0.109	4 (2–4)	3 (2–4)	0.460
Married/cohabiting	45 (88%)	85 (82%)	0.301	32 (84%)	71 (85%)	0.965
Monogamous marriage (versus polygamous)	36 (86%)	67 (80%)	0.415	25 (81%)	56 (80%)	0.940
Enrollment site in Nyanza (versus outside Nyanza)	40 (78%)	67 (64%)	0.076	28 (74%)	63 (75%)	0.877
	Maternal medical characteristics					
Time since first HIV diagnosis (years)	8 (5–8)	8 (4–8)	0.862	8 (6–8)	8 (7-8)	0.838
Initiated ART before pregnancy (versus during pregnancy)	30 (60%)	69 (75%)	0.063	30 (79%)	47 (65%)	0.137
Ever received CD4 testing	45 (94%)	97 (97%)	0.348	38 (100%)	81 (96%)	0.238
Last CD4 (cell/μL) during pregnancy	365 (268–520)	395 (273–553)	0.589	481 (326–600)	550 (368–741)	0.144
Maternal WHO clinical stage						
Stage 1	16 (32%)	25 (24%)	0.311	14 (37%)	29 (35%)	0.804
Stage 2	8 (16%)	20 (19%)	0.608	8 (21%)	15 (18%)	0.676
Stage 3	8 (16%)	10 (10%)	0.257	4 (11%)	1 (1%)	**0.016***
Unknown	18 (36%)	48 (47%)	0.214	12 (32%)	39 (46%)	0.124
PI-containing maternal ART regimen	16 (31%)	7 (7%)	**<0.001***	7 (18%)	7 (8%)	0.105
Trimester of first combo ART use						
1st trimester[4]	39 (89%)	82 (94%)	0.253	33 (97%)	58 (94%)	0.459
2nd trimester	3 (7%)	2 (2%)	0202	0 (0%)	1 (2%)	0.457
3rd trimester	2 (5%)	3 (3%)	0.416	1 (3%)	3 (5%)	0.682
Body mass index (kg/m^2)	23 (20–25)	23 (21–25)	0.193	21 (20–24)	23 (20–25)	**0.005***
	Infant characteristics					
Gestational age at birth (weeks)	38 (36–39)	38 (36–40)	0.562	38 (37–39)	38 (37–40)	0.121
Birth weight (kilograms)	3.0 (2.7–3.5)	3.1 (2.8–3.5)	0.338	3.3 (2.5–3.5)	3.1 (2.8–3.7)	0.363
Infant male sex	35 (49%)	59 (57%)	0.365	23 (61%)	35 (42%)	0.053
Currently breastfeeding	49 (98%)	99 (99%)	0.615	31 (84%)	57 (68%)	0.070

*$p < 0.05$.
[1]Missing data not shown.
[2]Maternal TDF use during pregnancy defined as any reported TDF-containing regimen used at any time during pregnancy among mothers that used combination ART.
[3]Chi-squared test for proportions or Kruskal-Wallis test for continuous measures.
[4]Including women that initiated ART before pregnancy.

TABLE 2: Distribution of mean weight, length, and head circumference (HC) anthropometric measurements and age and sex-adjusted z-scores among HEU infants attending 6-week and 9-month immunization visits, by maternal TDF use in pregnancy.

Anthropometric measure	Infants attending 6-week visit Mean (95% CI) or N (%)				Infants attending 9-month visit Mean (95% CI) or N (%)			
	Total ($n = 155$)	No maternal TDF use during pregnancy ($n = 104$)	Any maternal TDF use during pregnancy[1] ($n = 51$)	p value[2]	Total ($n = 122$)	No maternal TDF use during pregnancy ($n = 84$)	Any maternal TDF use during pregnancy[1] ($n = 38$)	p value[2]
Weight								
Absolute weight (kg)	4.6 (4.4, 4.7)	4.7 (4.5, 4.8)	4.3 (4.1, 4.6)	**0.015***	8.3 (8.1, 8.5)	8.4 (8.1, 8.7)	8.1 (7.7, 8.6)	0.302
Absolute WAZ	−0.5 (−0.7, −0.3)	−0.4 (−0.6, −0.1)	−0.8 (−1.2, −0.5)	**0.033***	−0.4 (−0.6, −0.1)	−0.3 (−0.6, 0.0)	−0.6 (−1.2, 0.0)	0.306
WAZ < −2 SD	13 (8%)	7 (7%)	6 (12%)	0.288	17 (14%)	10 (12%)	7 (18%)	0.336
Absolute WLZ	0.5 (0.1, 0.9)	0.6 (0.1, 1.1)	0.3 (−0.3, 0.9)	0.462	0.3 (−0.1, 0.7)	0.4 (−0.2, 0.9)	0.1 (−0.5, 0.8)	0.597
WLZ < −2 SD	21 (14%)	16 (16%)	5 (10%)	0.317	12 (10%)	7 (9%)	5 (13%)	0.432
Length								
Absolute length (cm)	52.9 (51.2, 53.7)	53.0 (52.0, 54.0)	52.8 (51.6, 53.9)	0.766	68.1 (66.9, 69.2)	68.2 (66.7, 69.7)	67.7 (66.3, 69.2)	0.710
Absolute LAZ	−1.2 (−1.5, −0.8)	−1.2 (−1.6, −0.7)	−1.2 (−1.7, −0.6)	0.951	−1.0 (−1.5, −0.5)	−1.0 (−1.7, −0.3)	−1.1 (−1.9, −0.3)	0.797
LAZ < −2 SD	58 (37%)	39 (38%)	19 (37%)	0.976	36 (30%)	22 (26%)	14 (37%)	0.232
Head circumference (HC)								
Absolute HC (cm)	38.7 (38.3, 39.0)	38.7 (38.3, 39.1)	38.5 (37.9, 39.1)	0.596	44.0 (43.6, 44.4)	44.0 (43.5, 44.5)	44.0 (43.2, 44.8)	0.995
Absolute HCZ	0.7 (0.4, 1.0)	0.7 (0.4, 1.1)	0.7 (0.2, 1.2)	0.892	−0.3 (−0.7, 0.0)	−0.3 (−0.7, 0.1)	−0.4 (−1.1, 0.4)	0.873
HCZ < −2 SD	4 (3%)	2 (2%)	2 (4%)	0.461	22 (18%)	14 (17%)	8 (21%)	0.560

SD = standard deviation.
* $p < 0.05$.
[1] Maternal TDF use defined as any reported TDF-containing ART regimen used for any amount of time during pregnancy among mothers that used combination ART while pregnant.
[2] Chi-squared test for proportions or 2-sample t-test for means.

TABLE 3: Association of age and sex-adjusted z-scores for weight, weight-for-length, length, and head circumference (HC) among HEU infants and maternal TDF use in pregnancy, by 6-week and 9-month immunization visits[1].

| Growth outcome | Infants attending 6-week immunization visit | | | | Infants attending 9-month immunization visit | | | |
| | Univariate[2] | | Multivariate[2,3] | | Univariate[2] | | Multivariate[2,3] | |
	Coeff. or OR (crude) (95% CI)	p value	Coeff. or OR (adj) (95% CI)	p value	Coeff. or OR (crude) (95% CI)	p value	Coeff. or OR (adj.) (95% CI)	p value
Weight								
Absolute WAZ	−0.46 (−0.93, 0.01)	0.056	−0.46 (−0.93, 0.01)	0.057	−0.31 (0.96, 0.34)	0.341	−0.31 (−0.97, 0.35)	0.349
WAZ < −2 SD	1.84 (0.55, 6.23)	0.322	1.86 (0.54, 6.35)	0.321	1.67 (0.59, 4.72)	0.333	1.60 (0.56, 4.56)	0.378
Absolute WLZ	−0.31 (−1.15, 0.53)	0.461	−0.30 (−1.16, 0.56)	0.483	−0.24 (−1.19, 0.71)	0.608	−0.22 (−1.19, 0.76)	0.655
WLZ < −2 SD	0.58 (0.18, 1.93)	0.377	0.59 (0.17, 1.93)	0.374	1.62 (0.46, 5.71)	0.450	1.63 (0.45, 5.94)	0.452
Length								
Absolute LAZ	0.02 (−0.81, 0.86)	0.954	−0.00 (−0.83, 0.83)	0.992	−0.15 (−1.17, 0.88)	0.775	−0.35 (−1.40, 0.71)	0.514
LAZ < −2 SD	0.99 (0.49, 1.99)	0.977	1.03 (0.51, 2.06)	0.941	1.64 (0.70, 3.88)	0.255	1.89 (0.80, 4.46)	0.147
Head circumference								
Absolute HCZ	−0.04 (−0.77, 0.69)	0.911	−0.02 (−0.76, 0.71)	0.948	−0.06 (−1.07, 0.95)	0.905	−0.07 (−1.04, 0.90)	0.888
HCZ < −2 SD	2.08 (0.27, 15.9)	0.480	2.07 (0.27, 16.06)	0.483	1.33 (0.33, 5.38)	0.686	1.33 (0.33, 5.29)	0.684

SD = Standard deviation.

[1] Maternal TDF use defined as any reported TDF-containing ARV regimen used at any time during pregnancy for any amount of time among mothers that used combination ART for HIV treatment or PMTCT while pregnant.

[2] Logistic regression models for binary outcomes and linear regression for continuous outcomes.

[3] Adjusted for maternal age, maternal education level, breastfeeding, gestational age at birth, time since maternal HIV diagnosis, maternal WHO clinical stage, timing of ART initiation (before or during pregnancy), trimester of first combo ART regimen use during pregnancy, and PI-containing ART regimen.

(adj. coeff.) = −0.46, 95% confidence interval (CI): −0.93, 0.01, p = 0.057); WLZ (adj. coeff. = −0.30, 95% CI: −1.16, 0.56, p = 0.483); LAZ (adj. coeff. = −0.0, 95% CI: −0.83, 0.83, p = 0.992); HCZ (adj. coeff. = −0.02, 95% CI: −0.76, 0.71, p = 0.948). We also found no association between z-scores < −2 SD and maternal prenatal TDF use for WAZ (adjusted odds ratio (aOR) = 1.9, 95% CI: 0.5, 6.4, p = 0.321), WLZ (aOR = 0.6, 95% CI: 0.2, 1.9, p = 0.374), LAZ (aOR = 1.0, 95% CI: 0.5, 2.1, p = 0.941), or HCZ (aOR = 2.1, 95% CI: 0.3, 16.1, p = 0.483). Because maternal BMI and maternal WHO stage were collinear, a separate multivariate model was constructed including all covariates except for WHO stage. The association between maternal prenatal TDF use and WAZ remained non-significant (adj. coeff. = −0.4, 95% CI: −0.9, 0.2, p = 0.192).

3.3. Growth Outcomes among HEU Infants Attending 9-Month Visit.

Among infants receiving 9-month immunizations, we did not detect differences for any measure of weight between HEU infants with or without mothers that used TDF during pregnancy (Table 3): weight (8.1 kg versus 8.4 kg, p = 0.302); WAZ (−0.6 versus −0.3, p = 0.306); WAZ < −2 SD (18% versus 12%, p = 0.336); WLZ (0.1 versus 0.4, p = 0.597); and WLZ < −2 SD (13% versus 9%, p = 0.431). Similarly, we did not detect differences between length or head circumference.

Among infants attending 9-month visits, we found no association between weight, length, or HC growth indicators and whether or not mothers had used TDF during pregnancy after adjustment (Table 3): WAZ (adjusted coefficient [adj. coeff.] = −0.31, 95% CI: −0.97, 0.35, p = 0.349); WLZ (adj. coeff. = −0.22, 95% CI: −1.19, 0.76, p = 0.655); LAZ (adj. coeff. = −0.35, 95% CI: −1.40, 0.71, p = 0.514);

HC (adj. coeff. = −0.07, 95% CI: −1.04, 0.90, p = 0.888). Similarly, we did not find any association between z-scores < −2 SD and maternal prenatal TDF use for WAZ (aOR = 1.6, 95% CI: 0.6, 4.6, p = 0.378), WLZ (aOR = 1.6, 95% CI: 0.5, 5.9, p = 0.452), LAZ (aOR = 1.9, 95% CI: 0.8, 4.5, p = 0.147), or HCZ (aOR = 1.3, 95% CI: 0.3, 5.3, p = 0.684). When substituting maternal BMI for maternal WHO stage, the association between maternal prenatal TDF use and WAZ remained non-significant (adj. coeff. = −0.4, 95% CI: −1.2, 0.4, p = 0.319).

3.4. Sensitivity Analyses.

When restricting our dataset to only mother-infant pairs with documented 3-drug combination ART initiation prior to pregnancy (n = 176), we found that maternal prenatal TDF use was associated with a trend for lower absolute WAZ (crude coeff. = −0.59, 95% CI: −1.17, 0.02, p = 0.044), similar to our primary results. In adjusted models, we did not detect significant associations between maternal prenatal TDF use and any growth indicator, though our power to detect associations was reduced. To reduce the effect of potentially misclassified z-scores for preterm infants, we repeated the primary analysis excluding HEU infants from the overall study population born ≤37 weeks of gestation (n = 63). Among HEU infants attending 6-week visits born >37 weeks of gestation (n = 91), we detected a modest difference in mean weight (4.4 kg versus 4.8 kg, p = 0.011) and mean WAZ (−0.3 versus −0.8, p = 0.021) between those born to mothers with and without prenatal TDF use. After adjustment, maternal prenatal TDF use was not associated with WAZ (adj. coeff. = −0.5, 95% CI: −0.9, 0.04, p = 0.072) or WAZ < −2 SD (aOR = 2.0, 95% CI: 0.4, 10.2, p = 0.418) among HEU infants born >37 weeks of gestation. Results for length, HC, WLZ, LAZ, and HCZ excluding infants born <37 weeks of gestation did not have appreciable differences with those of the full study population for infants attending 6-week or 9-month visits (data not shown). Results using indicator variables for missing values to account for the potential categorical effect of missing data were similar to our primary results (data not shown).

4. Discussion

Given the increasing use of TDF for HIV treatment and biomedical prevention strategies in sub-Saharan Africa, further evaluation on postnatal effects of prenatal TDF use in this setting is crucial. While data on PrEP use in pregnancy accumulates, current data available from HEU infants born to mothers on TDF-containing ART regimens may potentially contribute to the growing safety profile of prolonged maternal prenatal TDF use on infant growth outcomes. In this study of HEU infants in Kenya, we found marginal differences in weight and WAZ between infants attending 6-week visits born to mothers with and without TDF use during pregnancy. After adjustment for sociodemographic and medical characteristics, prenatal TDF use was associated with a trend for modest decrease in weight or WAZ. We found no association of prenatal TDF use with length, WLZ, LAZ, HC, or HCZ among infants attending 6-week or 9-month visits. Our data contribute to the limited number of studies investigating safety of TDF on postnatal growth outcomes among sub-Saharan African HEU populations [26].

Growth indicators, specifically height and HAZ, may provide important information on prenatal TDF use and infant bone health in settings where bone mineralization tests are not readily available. Similar to Gibb et al. (2012), which examined a population ($n = 182$) of PCR-confirmed negative HEU infants in Uganda and Zimbabwe, we did not find differences in height or HAZ among infants with and without maternal TDF during pregnancy [26]. A larger cohort study ($n = 2029$) in the United States detected slightly lower infant length at 12 months of age between infants with and without in utero TDF exposure (LAZ −0.17 versus −0.03, $p = 0.04$). The long-term clinical relevance of this modest difference is not well understood.

WHO Child Growth Standards, commonly used in clinical settings of Kenya and other sub-Saharan African countries, relate observed growth parameters (height, weight, HC, and middle upper arm circumference) to those expected in normal children according to percentiles using z-scores [27]. However, current WHO Child Growth Standards are calibrated for infants born >37 weeks and do not account for growth trajectories of preterm infants which differ from term infants [28, 35]. This may lead to misclassification of growth faltering among infants born ≤37 weeks. Other studies investigating safety of TDF use during pregnancy have used alternative growth charts that account for gestational age at birth [24, 25]. However, these methods have not been validated in sub-Saharan Africa where WHO Child Growth Standards are typically used. To our knowledge, this is the first study evaluating prenatal TDF use and growth outcomes among HEU in Africa to incorporate the potential effect

of prematurity on postnatal growth outcomes. A systematic review and meta-analysis reported that 12% of infants in sub-Saharan Africa are born preterm [36]. In our study, which included only infants born to HIV-infected mothers, ~24% of infants were born ≤37 weeks of gestation, similar to other studies of HIV-exposed infants in sub-Saharan Africa [37, 38]. Future evaluations of prenatal TDF use on infant growth outcomes in this setting should make analytic considerations for z-scores of preterm infants when accurate gestational age at birth information is available. Forthcoming international growth standards for weight, length, and head circumference by gestational age and sex developed by the INTERGROWTH-21st Project may be particularly useful for evaluating postnatal growth in settings with high prevalence of birth ≤37 weeks of gestation in Africa [39].

Our study has limitations that should be noted. The relatively small sample size may have limited our power to detect statistical differences and associations, though most studies examining prenatal TDF use and growth outcomes have included fewer infants [14, 18, 19, 26]. As roll out of TDF as a first-line PMTCT Option B/B+ scales up and longitudinal data becomes available, larger prospective studies will remain important in evaluating the safety of prenatal TDF use. TDF exposure was determined by self-report and clinical records in our study. This limited our ability to precisely investigate the association between timing of in utero TDF exposure, fetal development, and subsequent growth outcomes. Data from future prospective studies that follow ART or TDF naïve women that initiate TDF use during pregnancy will be especially valuable as timing of TDF exposure as it relates to fetal bone development is not well understood.

5. Conclusions

Our findings add to previous studies, indicating that prenatal TDF use appears to be safe compared to non-TDF-containing ART regimens. More specifically, our study contributes to the very limited data available on safety of TDF use and growth outcomes in Africa where TDF-containing regimens are expanding for HIV treatment and PMTCT. PrEP for HIV-uninfected women during pregnancy may have additional benefit in Africa where maternal seroconversion during pregnancy and breastfeeding contributes significantly to the pediatric HIV burden [40]. Further research on long-term effects of maternal prenatal TDF use, particularly from mothers using PrEP in pregnancy, is vital as TDF use rapidly scales up.

Disclaimer

The findings and conclusions in this paper are those of the authors and do not necessarily represent the official position of the U.S. Centers for Disease Control and Prevention/Government of Kenya.

Conflict of Interests

The authors declare that no conflict of interests exists.

Acknowledgments

The authors thank all the study participants for their contributions and the staff at all participating institutions for their support. The study team acknowledges the Director of KEMRI for support. They thank Dr. Joachim Voss, Associate Professor, University of Washington School of Nursing, for his careful review of early drafts. They also acknowledge Collaborative HIV Impact on MCH Evaluation (CHIME) Study Team. The study was funded by the President's Emergency Plan for AIDS Relief (PEPFAR) and Centers for Disease Control and Prevention (COAG#U2GPS002047). Jillian Pintye was supported by a NIH Training Grant T32AI07140, Christine J. McGrath was supported by the University of Washington STD/AIDS Research Training Fellowship (NIH NRSA T32AI007140), and Grace John-Stewart was supported by a NIH K24 Grant (HD054314). The CHIME Team was supported by the University of Washington's Global Center for Integrated Health of Women Adolescents and Children (Global WACh) and Center for AIDS Research (CFAR) (P30 AI027757).

References

[1] World Health Organization, *Consolidated Guidelines on the Use of Antiretroviral Drugs for Treating and Preventing HIV Infection*, WHO, Geneva, Switzerland, 2013.

[2] World Health Organization, *Consolidated Guidelines on HIV Prevention, Diagnosis, Treatment and Care for Key Populations*, WHO Library Cataloguing-in-Publication Data, Geneva, Switzerland, 2014.

[3] National Institutes of Health, "Recommendations for use of antiretroviral drugs in pregnant hiv-1-infected women for maternal health and interventions to reduce perinatal hiv transmission in the united states," 2012.

[4] Panel on Treatment of HIV-Infected Pregnant Women and Prevention of Perinatal Transmission, *Recommendations for Use of Antiretroviral Drugs in Pregnant HIV-1-Infected Women for Maternal Health and Interventions to Reduce Perinatal HIV Transmission in the United States*, 2012.

[5] A. F. Tarantal, A. Castillo, J. E. Ekert, N. Bischofberger, and R. B. Martin, "Fetal and maternal outcome after administration of tenofovir to gravid rhesus monkeys (*Macaca mulatta*)," *Journal of Acquired Immune Deficiency Syndromes*, vol. 29, no. 3, pp. 207–220, 2002.

[6] K. K. Van Rompay, L. L. Brignolo, D. J. Meyer et al., "Biological effects of short-term or prolonged administration of 9-[2-(phosphonomethoxy)propyl]adenine (tenofovir) to newborn and infant rhesus macaques," *Antimicrobial Agents and Chemotherapy*, vol. 48, no. 5, pp. 1469–1487, 2004.

[7] K. K. A. Van Rompay, L. Durand-Gasselin, L. L. Brignolo et al., "Chronic administration of tenofovir to rhesus macaques from infancy through adulthood and pregnancy: summary of pharmacokinetics and biological and virological effects," *Antimicrobial Agents and Chemotherapy*, vol. 52, no. 9, pp. 3144–3160, 2008.

[8] A. B. Castillo, A. F. Tarantal, M. R. Watnik, and R. Bruce Martin, "Tenofovir treatment at 30 mg/kg/day can inhibit cortical bone mineralization in growing rhesus monkeys (*Macaca mulatta*)," *Journal of Orthopaedic Research*, vol. 20, no. 6, pp. 1185–1189, 2002.

[9] L. Wang, A. P. Kourtis, S. Ellington, J. Legardy-Williams, and M. Bulterys, "Safety of tenofovir during pregnancy for the mother and fetus: a systematic review," *Clinical Infectious Diseases*, vol. 57, no. 12, pp. 1773–1781, 2013.

[10] B. H. Chi, M. Sinkala, F. Mbewe et al., "Single-dose tenofovir and emtricitabine for reduction of viral resistance to non-nucleoside reverse transcriptase inhibitor drugs in women given intrapartum nevirapine for perinatal HIV prevention: an open-label randomised trial," *The Lancet*, vol. 370, no. 9600, pp. 1698–1705, 2007.

[11] E. Arrivé, M.-L. Chaix, E. Nerrienet et al., "Tolerance and viral resistance after single-dose nevirapine with tenofovir and emtricitabine to prevent vertical transmission of HIV-1," *AIDS*, vol. 23, no. 7, pp. 825–833, 2009.

[12] E. Arrive, M. L. Chaix, E. Nerrienet et al., "Maternal and neonatal tenofovir and emtricitabine to prevent vertical transmission of HIV-1: tolerance and resistance," *AIDS*, vol. 24, no. 16, pp. 2481–2488, 2010.

[13] P. M. Flynn, M. Mirochnick, D. E. Shapiro et al., "Pharmacokinetics and safety of single-dose tenofovir disoproxil fumarate and emtricitabine in HIV-1-infected pregnant women and their infants," *Antimicrobial Agents and Chemotherapy*, vol. 55, no. 12, pp. 5914–5922, 2011.

[14] E. Kinai, S. Hosokawa, H. Gomibuchi, H. Gatanaga, Y. Kikuchi, and S. Oka, "Blunted fetal growth by tenofovir in late pregnancy," *AIDS*, vol. 26, no. 16, pp. 2119–2120, 2012.

[15] C. Q. Pan, L.-J. Mi, C. Bunchorntavakul et al., "Tenofovir disoproxil fumarate for prevention of vertical transmission of hepatitis b virus infection by highly viremic pregnant women: a case series," *Digestive Diseases and Sciences*, vol. 57, no. 9, pp. 2423–2429, 2012.

[16] R. Beigi, L. Noguchi, T. Parsons et al., "Pharmacokinetics and placental transfer of single-dose tenofovir 1% vaginal gel in term pregnancy," *Journal of Infectious Diseases*, vol. 204, no. 10, pp. 1527–1531, 2011.

[17] F. Sabbatini, F. Prati, V. Borghi, A. Bedini, R. Esposito, and C. Mussini, "Congenital pyelectasis in children born from mothers on tenofovir containing therapy during pregnancy: report of two cases," *Infection*, vol. 35, no. 6, pp. 474–476, 2007.

[18] D. Nurutdinova, N. F. Onen, E. Hayes, K. Mondy, and E. T. Overton, "Adverse effects of tenofovir use in HIV-infected pregnant women and their infants," *Annals of Pharmacotherapy*, vol. 42, no. 11, pp. 1581–1585, 2008.

[19] A. Viganò, S. Mora, V. Giacomet et al., "In utero exposure to tenofovir disoproxil fumarate does not impair growth and bone health in HIV-uninfected children born to HIV-infected mothers," *Antiviral Therapy*, vol. 16, no. 8, pp. 1259–1266, 2011.

[20] A. P. H. Colbers, D. A. Hawkins, A. Gingelmaier et al., "The pharmacokinetics, safety and efficacy of tenofovir and emtricitabine in HIV-1-infected pregnant women," *AIDS*, vol. 27, no. 5, pp. 739–748, 2013.

[21] Antiretroviral Pregnancy Registry Steering Committee, *Antiretroviral Pregnancy Registry International Interim Report for 1 January 1989 through 31 July 2013*, Registry Coordinating Center, Wilmington, NC, USA, 2013.

[22] N. R. Mugo, T. Hong, C. Celum et al., "Pregnancy incidence and outcomes among women receiving preexposure prophylaxis for HIV prevention: a randomized clinical trial," *The Journal of the American Medical Association*, vol. 312, no. 4, pp. 362–371, 2014.

[23] P. L. Vernazza, I. Graf, U. Sonnenberg-Schwan, M. Geit, and A. Meurer, "Preexposure prophylaxis and timed intercourse for

HIV-discordant couples willing to conceive a child," *AIDS*, vol. 25, no. 16, pp. 2005–2008, 2011.

[24] C. E. Ransom, Y. Huo, K. Patel et al., "Infant growth outcomes after maternal tenofovir disoproxil fumarate use during pregnancy," *Journal of Acquired Immune Deficiency Syndromes*, vol. 64, no. 4, pp. 374–381, 2013.

[25] G. K. Siberry, P. L. Williams, H. Mendez et al., "Safety of tenofovir use during pregnancy: early growth outcomes in HIV-exposed uninfected infants," *AIDS*, vol. 26, no. 9, pp. 1151–1159, 2012.

[26] D. M. Gibb, H. Kizito, E. C. Russell et al., "Pregnancy and infant outcomes among HIV-infected women taking long-term art with and without tenofovir in the DART trial," *PLoS Medicine*, vol. 9, no. 5, Article ID e1001217, 2012.

[27] World Health Organization, *WHO Child Growth Standards and the Identification of Severe Acute Malnutrition in Infants and Children: A Joint Statement by the World Health Organization and the United Nations Children's Fund*, World Health Organization, Geneva, Switzerland, 2009.

[28] M. B. Duggan, "Anthropometry as a tool for measuring malnutrition: impact of the new WHO growth standards and reference," *Annals of Tropical Paediatrics*, vol. 30, no. 1, pp. 1–17, 2010.

[29] S. Keino, G. Plasqui, G. Ettyang, and B. van den Borne, "Determinants of stunting and overweight among young children and adolescents in sub-Saharan Africa," *Food and Nutrition Bulletin*, vol. 35, no. 2, pp. 167–178, 2014.

[30] R. E. Black, C. G. Victora, S. P. Walker et al., "Maternal and child undernutrition and overweight in low-income and middle-income countries," *The Lancet*, vol. 382, no. 9890, pp. 427–451, 2013.

[31] S. Isanaka, C. Duggan, and W. W. Fawzi, "Patterns of postnatal growth in HIV-infected and HIV-exposed children," *Nutrition Reviews*, vol. 67, no. 6, pp. 343–359, 2009.

[32] H. S. Kruger, "Maternal anthropometry and pregnancy outcomes: a proposal for the monitoring of pregnancy weight gain in outpatient clinics in South Africa," *Curationis*, vol. 28, no. 4, pp. 40–49, 2005.

[33] M. Tadrous, J. J. Gagne, T. Stürmer, and S. M. Cadarette, "Disease risk score as a confounder summary method: systematic review and recommendations," *Pharmacoepidemiology and Drug Safety*, vol. 22, no. 2, pp. 122–129, 2013.

[34] D. Strauss, "On miettinen's multivariate confounder score," *Journal of Clinical Epidemiology*, vol. 51, no. 3, pp. 233–236, 1998.

[35] J. Villar, H. E. Knight, M. de Onis et al., "Conceptual issues related to the construction of prescriptive standards for the evaluation of postnatal growth of preterm infants," *Archives of Disease in Childhood*, vol. 95, no. 12, pp. 1034–1038, 2010.

[36] S. Beck, D. Wojdyla, L. Say et al., "The worldwide incidence of preterm birth: a systematic review of maternal mortality and morbidity," *Bulletin of the World Health Organization*, vol. 88, no. 1, pp. 31–38, 2010.

[37] J. Y. Chen, H. J. Ribaudo, S. Souda et al., "Highly active antiretroviral therapy and adverse birth outcomes among HIV-infected women in botswana," *Journal of Infectious Diseases*, vol. 206, no. 11, pp. 1695–1705, 2012.

[38] K. van der Merwe, R. Hoffman, V. Black, M. Chersich, A. Coovadia, and H. Rees, "Birth outcomes in South African women receiving highly active antiretroviral therapy: a retrospective observational study," *Journal of the International AIDS Society*, vol. 14, no. 1, article 42, 2011.

[39] J. Villar, L. Cheikh Ismail, C. G. Victora et al., "International standards for newborn weight, length, and head circumference by gestational age and sex: the newborn cross-sectional study of the intergrowth-21st project," *The Lancet*, vol. 384, no. 9946, pp. 857–868, 2014.

[40] L. F. Johnson, K. Stinson, M.-L. Newell et al., "The contribution of maternal HIV seroconversion during late pregnancy and breastfeeding to mother-to-child transmission of HIV," *Journal of Acquired Immune Deficiency Syndromes*, vol. 59, no. 4, pp. 417–425, 2012.

Clinical Characteristics Associated with Antibiotic Treatment Failure for Tuboovarian Abscesses

Huma Farid,[1,2] **Trevin C. Lau,**[2,3] **Anatte E. Karmon,**[2,3,4] **and Aaron K. Styer**[2,3,4]

[1]*Department of Obstetrics and Gynecology, Beth Israel Deaconess Medical Center, Boston, MA 02215, USA*
[2]*Department of Obstetrics, Gynecology and Reproductive Biology, Harvard Medical School, Boston, MA 02115, USA*
[3]*Vincent Department of Obstetrics and Gynecology, Massachusetts General Hospital, Boston, MA 02114, USA*
[4]*Vincent Reproductive Medicine and IVF, Massachusetts General Hospital, Boston, MA 02114, USA*

Correspondence should be addressed to Huma Farid; hfarid@bidmc.harvard.edu

Academic Editor: Gilbert Donders

Objective. Although parenteral antibiotic treatment is a standard approach for tuboovarian abscesses, a significant proportion of patients fail therapy and require interventional radiology (IR) guided drainage. The objective of this study is to assess if specific clinical factors are associated with antibiotic treatment failure. *Study Design*. Retrospective medical record review of patients hospitalized for tuboovarian abscesses from 2001 through 2012 was performed. Clinical characteristics were compared for patients who underwent successful parenteral antibiotic treatment, failed antibiotic treatment necessitating subsequent IR drainage, initial drainage with concurrent antibiotics, and surgery. *Results*. One hundred thirteen patients admitted for inpatient treatment were identified. Sixty-one (54%) patients were treated with antibiotics alone. Within this group, 24.6% failed antibiotic treatment and required drainage. Mean white blood cell count (K/μL) (18.7 ± 5.94 versus 13.9 ± 5.12) ($p = 0.003$), mean maximum diameter of tuboovarian abscess (cm) (6.8 ± 2.9 versus 5.2 ± 2.0) ($p = 0.03$), and length of stay (days) (9.47 ± 7.43 versus 4.59 ± 2.4) ($p = 0.002$) were significantly greater for patients who failed antibiotic treatment. *Conclusions*. Admission white blood cell count greater than 16 K/μL and abscess size greater than 5.18 cm are associated with antibiotic treatment failure. These factors may provide guidance for initial selection of IR guided drainage.

1. Introduction

Tuboovarian abscesses (TOAs) are a common complication of pelvic inflammatory disease (PID) and affect approximately 10–15% of women with PID [1]. Previously, it was assumed that *Chlamydia trachomatis* and *Neisseria gonorrhea* infections were the primary causative agents of TOA [2]. However, it is now known that this disease process is often polymicrobial. In most cases, TOAs represent a significant complication of an ascending lower genital tract infection which evolves to PID and involves the uterus and adnexal structures. TOAs may also be caused by inflammatory bowel disease, appendicitis, or diverticulitis, with direct local spread of bacteria to the fallopian tubes from the gastrointestinal tract [3]. Following upper genital tract involvement, a significant inflammatory response ensues, resulting in local tissue necrosis, proliferation of anaerobic organisms, and abscess formation within the fallopian tube and ovary [4].

Historically, the treatment of TOAs involved a total abdominal hysterectomy with bilateral salpingo-oophorectomy, resulting in significant morbidity and infertility [4]. With the advent of antibiotics targeting anaerobes and gram negative aerobes, broad-spectrum intravenous (IV) antibiotics became the first-line treatment for TOAs, with treatment success ranging from 75% to 85% in some case series [1, 5]. However, due to the variable rates of success with antibiotic therapy alone, minimally invasive drainage techniques have been developed and utilized over the past three decades either as a secondary treatment option or as the initial treatment approach.

Percutaneous drainage of abdominal abscesses of all etiologies was described by Johnson et al. in 1981, after the group had been performing percutaneous drainage guided by either CT or ultrasound since 1976 for abscesses, with a success rate of 89% [6]. In 1986, Worthen and Gunning applied this technique to TOAs and reported success rates ranging from 77%

to 94% [7]. Subsequent studies confirmed success rates for transvaginal ultrasound-guided drainage of TOAs ranging from 78% to 100% [2, 8–10]. Levenson et al. reported a success rate of 95% with CT-guided or ultrasound-guided drainage of 57 TOAs in 49 patients. These investigators found that TOAs of gynecologic etiology were more likely to be treated successfully with interventional radiology (IR) guided drainage than those caused by appendicitis, Crohn's disease, diverticulitis, or other gastrointestinal diseases [10].

Despite the success rates of IR abscess drainage and the inconsistent success rate of exclusive parenteral antibiotic treatment, the Centers for Disease Control and Prevention (CDC) recommends antibiotic therapy as the first-line treatment for TOAs [11]. Although a proportion of patients will fail parenteral antibiotic treatment for TOA and require abscess drainage, there are no standardized guidelines to direct clinicians as to when either antibiotics or IR drainage treatment is the most appropriate initial option. It is ideal to expand our understanding of pretreatment risk factors for antibiotic treatment failure and the subsequent clinical course following treatment failure. To this end, the objectives of this study were to assess if specific clinical characteristics are associated with antibiotic treatment failure and to investigate how treatment failure impacts outcome (length of stay).

2. Methods

This study was approved by the Partners Healthcare Institutional Review Board (IRB number 2012-P-001483/1). A retrospective electronic medical record review of women admitted for the inpatient care of TOA at the Massachusetts General Hospital (MGH) from January 1, 2001, through December 31, 2012, was performed. Potential subjects were identified with the use of ICD-9 codes for PID (614.9), acute salpingitis and oophoritis (614.0, 614.3), acute pelvic peritonitis (614.5), and TOA (614.2). A broad range of ICD-9 codes were used in order to capture all patients who might have been admitted with a TOA. One thousand ninety-three electronic and hardcopy charts were reviewed to confirm eligibility. Inclusion criteria included the following: confirmation of TOA by imaging and clinical criteria according to CDC criteria (abdominal or pelvic pain and one or more of the following: cervical motion tenderness, uterine tenderness, or adnexal tenderness [12]) and inpatient admission greater than 24 hours to our institution for treatment. Women who declined admission or did not have a TOA confirmed by clinical criteria and imaging were excluded.

Patient records were reviewed for demographics, medical and surgical history, and treatment undertaken for TOA. All subjects underwent radiographic imaging, which included combined real-time pelvic and abdominal ultrasound, computed topography (CT), or magnetic resonance imaging (MRI). The majority of subjects had multiple imaging modalities performed prior to final diagnosis per clinician discretion. The largest dimension (cm) of the TOA from the radiology reports was used. Subjects were categorized into four groups based upon treatment course: IV antibiotic treatment only (MED), failed IV antibiotic treatment requiring subsequent interventional radiology drainage (IRD) during the initial hospitalization, initial IR drainage with concurrent IV antibiotics (MED/IRD), and initial surgical intervention (SURG). Management of patients was decided upon by the evaluating clinical team, and the decision to treat patients medically or surgically was based on clinical status and the discretion of the medical team. There is currently no standard of care, which is what prompted the study.

The primary dependent variable was the rate of treatment failure, and the primary independent variables were clinical characteristics associated with treatment failure. Treatment failure was defined as persistent pain and/or fever following initial IV antibiotics for 48–72 hours necessitating IR drainage. The secondary dependent variable was mean length of stay (days) among respective treatment groups. Patients who were successfully managed with IV antibiotics (MED) were designated as the reference treatment group to which the other groups were compared. Continuous and categorical variables were analyzed within treatment groups. Chi-square tests were performed for categorical variables, and t test analyses were performed for continuous variables with the use of EpiCalc 2000 (version 1.02, Brixton Health, Llanidloes, UK, 1998), with p-values < 0.05 designating statistical significance. Demographic, clinical, and reproductive characteristics were compared for patients among all treatment groups. Descriptive variables were expressed as means and proportions and analyzed with univariate analyses. A multivariate logistic regression model was fit to evaluate the independent relationships between failed antibiotic therapy and age, maximum TOA dimension, and white blood cell count (WBC) at the time of admission (SAS version 9.3, SAS institute, Inc., Cary, North Carolina).

3. Results

Of the 1,093 charts reviewed, 113 patients met inclusion criteria, and the remainder did not have a TOA by imaging criteria. Sixty-one (54%) patients initially underwent treatment with antibiotics alone. Within this group, 24.6% failed treatment with antibiotics alone and required IR drainage (IRD). Demographic characteristics are provided in Table 1 and were similar across all groups. The mean age for the entire study population at the time of admission was 40.4 ± 13.1 years of age (yo) (range: 16 to 75 yo). Thirty-six percent of patients were nulliparous, and 63% were Caucasian. Six percent were HIV positive, and 6% had multiple concurrent partners.

Admission clinical characteristics were analyzed for the entire cohort. Subjects reported a mean of 4.78 ± 4.62 days of abdominal/pelvic pain prior to presentation, although women in the SURG group had the fewest days of abdominal/pelvic pain prior to admission, with a mean of 2.6 ± 2.16 days of pain ($p = 0.003$). Forty-three percent of patients demonstrated cervical motion tenderness on pelvic exam. Upon presentation, the mean oral temperature was 100.2 ± 1.97°F, and the mean white blood cell count was 15.4 ± 5.38 K/μL. Upon admission, 73% were tested for gonorrhea and chlamydia; none were positive for N. gonorrhoeae and 7% tested positive for C. trachomatis. The majority of patients (112/113) underwent an imaging modality: 74% underwent

TABLE 1: Demographic characteristics by treatment group.

Demographics	MED (N = 46)	MED/IRD (N = 26)	IRD (N = 15)	SURG (N = 26)	All patients (N = 113)
Age (years) (mean ± SD)	38 (11.33)	37 (11.91)	45 (20)	46 (10.49)	40.4 (13.1)
Nulliparous	18 (41%)	18 (72%)	3 (23%)	9 (35%)	39 (36%)
Caucasian	18 (40%)	19 (73%)	9 (60%)	17 (74%)	79 (63%)
African American	8 (18%)	2 (8%)	2 (13%)	4 (17%)	16 (13%)
Hispanic	15 (33%)	5 (19%)	3 (20%)	0 (0%)	23 (18%)
Prior gonorrhea/chlamydia infection	8 (21%)	2 (9%)	1 (8%)	0 (0%)	11 (13%)
Current contraception use	17 (49%)	12 (57%)	3 (38%)	12 (63%)	66 (59%)
History of Bilateral Tubal Ligation (BTL)	0 (0%)	4 (19%)	1 (13%)	2 (11%)	16 (19%)

MED: intravenous antibiotic treatment only.
MED/IRD: initial interventional radiology drainage with concurrent intravenous antibiotics.
IRD: failed intravenous antibiotic treatment requiring subsequent interventional radiology drainage.
SURG: initial surgical intervention.

TABLE 2: Admission clinical characteristics by treatment group.

	MED* N = 46	MED/IRD N = 26 (p)	IRD N = 15 (p)	SURG N = 26 (p)
Duration of pain prior to presentation (days) (mean ± SD)	5.49 (4.87)	5.2 (5.68) 0.82	4.25 (2.7) 0.4	2.6 (2.16) **0.03
Presence of cervical motion tenderness (CMT)	22 (58%)	8 (44%) 0.26	1 (20%) 0.13	0 (0%) **0.01
Admission temperature (F) (mean ± SD)	100.6 (1.84)	99.7 (2.02) 0.08	100 (2.03) 0.3	99.9 (2.13) 0.2
Mean white blood cell count (WBC), K/μL (SD)	13.9 (5.12)	15 (3.97) 0.3	18.7 (5.94) **0.003	16.5 (5.82) **0.05
Unilateral abscess	30 (71%)	19 (76%) 0.28	12 (80%) 0.38	20 (80%) 0.31
Largest dimension of TOA (cm) (SD)	5.18 (2.05)	7.42 (3.22) **0.02	6.78 (2.95) **0.03	7.85 (3.96) **0.001

*MED is reference group for comparisons.
**$p < 0.05$ denotes statistical significance.
MED: intravenous antibiotic treatment only.
MED/IRD: initial interventional radiology drainage with concurrent intravenous antibiotics.
IRD: failed intravenous antibiotic treatment requiring subsequent interventional radiology drainage.
SURG: initial surgical intervention.

transvaginal/abdominal ultrasounds, 75% underwent CT, and 6% underwent MRI. Sixty-five percent of subjects underwent two imaging modalities, most commonly pelvic ultrasound (PUS) and CT. Mean TOA size was 6.31 ± 3.0 cm. Twenty-six percent of patients had bilateral TOAs, and the mean dimension of the largest TOA in bilateral cases was 7.56 cm ± 3.62 cm. Forty-four percent were determined to have a gynecologic etiology of their TOAs, and the rest of the TOAs were due to a gastrointestinal etiology. The frequency of etiology was similar among all treatment groups, with the exception of appendicitis, which was found more commonly in the SURG group (44%, $p = 0.006$).

Symptoms upon presentation, frequency of unilateral abscess, and admission temperature were similar between patient groups. However, when these clinical characteristics were further analyzed by treatment group, there were significant differences in clinical characteristics, specifically white blood cell count and TOA size (Table 2).

Subjects in the IRD group had the greatest admission mean WBC (18.7 K/μL ± 5.94 K/μL) of the entire study population ($p = 0.03$). There was a statistically significant difference in mean WBC between the MED and IRD groups (13.9 K/μL versus 18.7 K/μL, $p = 0.003$) and between the MED/IRD and IRD groups (15.0 K/μL versus 18.7 K/μL, $p = 0.026$). Admission WBC greater than 16.0 K/μL increased the odds of failing antibiotic treatment (odds ratio: 22.0; 95% CI 2.3–201.2, p trend: 0.006 (Table 3)).

Subjects in the SURG group also had the largest mean dimension of TOA (7.85 ± 3.96 cm, $p = 0.001$). Compared to the IRD group, subjects in the MED group had smaller mean maximum diameter of TOA (5.18 cm (SD 2.05) versus 6.78 cm (SD 2.95), $p = 0.03$). Logistic regression demonstrated

TABLE 3: Assessment of the likelihood of antibiotic treatment failure.

Variable	Odds ratio (95% confidence interval)	p-value
Age	1.1 (1.0–1.1)	0.0590
Maximum dimension of TOA	1.5 (1.1–2.0)	**0.0169
WBC tertile		0.0049
WBC < 13	Reference group	—
WBC ≥ 13 and <16	8.0 (0.9–74.5)	0.0684
WBC ≥ 16	22.0 (2.4–201.2)	**0.0063

**denotes p-value < 0.05.

that maximum dimension of TOA greater than 5.2 cm was predictive of antibiotic failure (odds ratio: 1.5; 95% CI 1.1–2.0, p-value = 0.0169). Age was not associated with the likelihood of antibiotic treatment failure (Table 3).

The mean inpatient length of stay (LOS) across the entire cohort of patients was 5.8 days ± 4.2 days. Compared to subjects in the MED group, women in IRD and SURG groups had the greatest inpatient LOS (9.47 days, p = 0.002, and 6.77 days, p = 0.006, resp.) as seen in Table 4. Subjects in the IRD group had the longest LOS of all women in the entire cohort. Compared to women who underwent initial IR drainage and concurrent IV antibiotics (MED/IRD), LOS in the IRD group was 4 days longer (4.85 days versus 9.47 days, p = 0.008). Women in the IRD group underwent IR drainage 2.5 days later than women in MED/IRD group (3.2 days versus 0.58 days, p = 0.001).

The four most common antibiotic regimens were as follows: gentamicin/clindamycin (14%), second generation cephalosporins/doxycycline/flagyl (11%), fluoroquinolone/flagyl (11%), and aminopenicillin/fluoroquinolone/flagyl (11%). The frequency of use of antibiotic regimens was similar among all the treatments (data not shown). Only one patient in the MED group and one patient in the MED/IRD group had positive blood cultures. Thirty-seven percent of patients had positive microbiology cultures. There was no statistically significant difference in the frequency of specific abscess organisms that were isolated among groups who either underwent IR drainage or had surgery. In the SURG group, 20% of patients' microbiology cultures were positive for E. coli, and 13% were positive for Gram Positive Cocci (GPC) along with Peptostreptococcus. In the MED/IRD group the microbiology data was notable for 27% of patients with the combination GPC, Gram Negative Rods (GNR), and Gram Positive Rods (GPR) and 18% with E. coli. In the IRD group, 38% of patients' microbiology data were positive for E. coli (although 40% of patients had other bacteria in addition to E. coli growing in the culture), and 23% were positive for GNR. An association between microbiology culture data and risk of treatment failure was not observed (data not shown).

4. Discussion

The current CDC clinical guidelines recommend medical management as the initial treatment approach for TOAs in

women who are hemodynamically stable with abscess size less than 9 cm and no signs or symptoms of abscess rupture [12]. However, studies have demonstrated that antibiotics have maximum success rates of approximately 85% [1] and mean success rates approaching 70% [4]. Minimally invasive techniques of TOA drainage are an alternative to antibiotic treatment alone, and when compared directly with IV antibiotics alone, some investigators have demonstrated that drainage may be the more successful treatment. Despite the lower than expected success rates of medical treatment and the widespread availability of IR, it still remains unclear who may benefit most from exclusive medical treatment versus concurrent medical treatment and image-guided drainage as the initial treatment approach. This lack of consensus lies in a limited ability to identify patients who may be at greatest risk for antibiotic failure at the time of initial presentation. As a result, this study was conducted to assess if specific admission clinical parameters are associated with antibiotic treatment failure and to assess if outcomes are affected following failure of initial antibiotic treatment.

This study demonstrated that WBC greater than 16 K/μL and TOA size greater than 5.18 cm were predictive of treatment failure when IV antibiotics were exclusively used as the initial treatment for TOA. Interestingly, subjects who failed antibiotic treatment and required IR drainage had the highest WBC count of the entire cohort, whereas subjects who were treated successfully with IV antibiotics had the lowest WBC count (Table 2). These findings suggest that white blood cell count may be a useful parameter to help guide treatment choice. However, there may be limitations to using leukocytosis as a marker of the severity of infection in cases with bacteremia or other inflammatory illnesses or comorbidities.

Worthen and Gunning recommend transvaginal ultrasound-guided drainage of TOAs in conjunction with antibiotics as the first-line treatment for TOAs of any size [7]. DeWitt et al. described that patients with a mean TOA size of ≤6.3 cm were successfully treated with medical management alone [13]. In contrast to that study, this analysis found that the upper limit of mean abscess size was 5.18 cm for successful antibiotic treatment, and the success of antibiotic therapy was not impacted by antibiotic regimen. We realize that there may be significant variation in the size of greatest dimension depending on the specific imaging modality. In this study, a majority of patients had either a pelvic CT or MRI to confirm initial ultrasound measurements, and this may have been contributory to variability in measuring TOA abscess dimensions. Interestingly, the percentage of patients with bilateral TOAs in the MED/IRD group and the percentage of patients with bilateral TOAs in IRD group were similar (Table 3). Based upon the findings of this study, concurrent antibiotic and abscess drainage may be considered as an ideal treatment for the case when TOA is greater than 5 cm. However, we appreciate that several factors such as patient comorbidities, patient or clinician preference, and the availability of interventional drainage resources may also impact the decision to proceed with concurrent drainage at the time of admission.

TABLE 4: Outcomes by treatment group.

	MED* (N = 46)	MED/IRD (N = 26) (p)	IRD (N = 15) (p)	SURG (N = 26) (p)
Length of stay (days) (mean ± SD)	4.59 (2.4)	4.85 (3.02) 0.6	9.47 (7.43) **0.002	6.77 (4.13) **0.006
Duration of inpatient antibiotics (days) (mean ± SD)	4.47 (7.19)	3.54 (2.75) 0.53	7.77 (6.21) 0.14	5.71 (4.09) 0.51
Duration of outpatient antibiotics (days) (mean ± SD)	13.7 (3.84)	13.3 (4.03) 0.79	12.2 (2.8) 0.24	11.2 (3.3) **0.04

* MED is reference group for comparisons.
** $p < 0.05$ denotes statistical significance.
MED: intravenous antibiotic treatment only.
MED/IRD: initial interventional radiology drainage with concurrent intravenous antibiotics.
IRD: failed intravenous antibiotic treatment requiring subsequent interventional radiology drainage.
SURG: initial surgical intervention.

Greenstein et al. examined the treatment outcomes of 122 patients with TOAs, 65.6% of whom were treated successfully with antibiotics alone and 34.4% of whom failed antibiotic therapy and required operative intervention. The vast majority of operative interventions were surgical, and only 2 patients underwent IR drainage. They reported that increasing WBC count, TOA size, older age, and increasing parity were significant predictors of failure of antibiotic therapy. Mean TOA size treated successfully with antibiotics was 4.4 cm compared to 7.3 cm in the surgical group. Mean white blood cell counts for patients in the surgical group were 15.91 K/μL compared to 12.36 K/μL in the medical treatment group [14]. Our findings are consistent with this study, although we found that abscesses up to 5.18 cm could be treated successfully with antibiotics alone. A significant point of difference is that Greenstein et al.'s study did not include any patients who underwent IR drainage prior to antibiotic treatment and only 2 who underwent IR drainage after antibiotic failure. In contrast, our study included 41 patients who underwent IR drainage initially or after failed antibiotic treatment. As a result, the findings of our study may be more applicable to institutions with available resources and expertise with IR drainage. Since our study analyzed each treatment group separately, this study was able to assess the demographic and clinical differences between the patients who were treated successfully with IR drainage compared to those who failed antibiotic treatment. The results of our study demonstrated that the IRD group and MED/IRD group were similar in clinical characteristics. However, since the patients in the IRD group required IR drainage, it seems that this group of patients was incorrectly identified as lower risk when they were assigned to antibiotic therapy alone. In contrast to Greenstein et al., who recommended trial of IV antibiotics in all patients, the findings of our study support concurrent antibiotics and IR drainage as the initial treatment approach when TOA is greater than 5 cm.

Multiple studies have demonstrated excellent success rates for IR drainage. Perez-Medina et al. randomized 40 women with unilateral TOAs less than 10 cm in maximal diameter to IV antibiotics or IV antibiotics and transvaginal ultrasound-guided drainage. They discovered that 90% were treated successfully with drainage and antibiotics compared with 65% of patients with antibiotics alone [15]. Goharkhay et al. found similar results when comparing women managed with IV antibiotics alone or with drainage and antibiotics. In their study sample, all eight patients who underwent drainage and concomitant antibiotics had complete resolution of their symptoms, while 50% of patients who received only IV antibiotics failed treatment and required either drainage or surgery [16]. Gjelland et al. reported a similar success rate of 93.4% with transvaginal ultrasound-guided drainage of TOAs in 302 women who received concurrent IV antibiotics [17]. These studies support our findings that IR drainage may be considered a first-line treatment option in select patients.

Length of stay is of particular interest in this emerging era of cost-effective health care. This study observed an association of increased LOS with antibiotic treatment failure. Subjects in the IRD group had the longest LOS, whereas those in the MED and MED/IRD groups had the shortest lengths of stay (Table 4). Perez-Medina et al. reported that patients undergoing drainage were discharged 5 days sooner than patients treated with antibiotics alone [15]. However, our study only observed a greater LOS in patients who failed antibiotic therapy. The increase in length of stay may have resulted from the fact that treatment failure with antibiotics was not recognized until after several days of hospitalization, as patients in the IRD group did not undergo drainage for a mean of 3.2 days. This practice correlates with previous recommendations that patients be treated with at least 48 to 72 hours of antibiotic treatment prior to transitioning to an alternative treatment. These findings highlight the significance of this study's aim to identify characteristics of those who are at increased risk of antibiotic failure and who may benefit from concurrent abscess drainage and a potential reduction of overall morbidity and LOS. Ideally, if utilized in patients identified as high risk for antibiotic treatment failure, IR drainage may minimize the risk of an extended LOS and reduce excessive inpatient care costs.

There were several limitations to consider in this study. There were a limited number of patients who failed antibiotic therapy and ultimately underwent abscess drainage. While we were able to observe statistically significant differences in several clinical characteristics of patients and in the primary outcome (length of stay), the study was likely underpowered to demonstrate additional characteristics associated with antibiotic treatment failure. Additional limitations included the single institution retrospective cohort design of this study, which may limit the generalizability of the results. A notable strength of this study was the comparison of outcomes among several types of TOA management: medical, drainage with interventional radiology, and surgical ones. Since all aspects of patient care were rendered from a single institution, there was greater consistency in management decisions and similar technique and protocols in drainage during the study period. Although our study did not suggest that antibiotic failure corresponded with any specific antibiotic regimen, this would be of interest for future investigation to assess if a specific antibiotic regimen modifies the risk of medical treatment failure in specific subsets of patients.

A significant point to consider is that the clinical presentation for TOA can be variable, and it may be quite challenging to identify which patients may be at increased risk of antibiotic treatment failure. The decision regarding initial treatment for patients with TOAs may be impacted by several clinical factors during initial presentation and not by a limited number of discrete laboratory values at the time of admission. Interestingly, patients in the MED and IRD groups had similar demographic and admission clinical characteristics (Tables 1 and 2) with the notable exception of differences in WBC count and TOA size. Based upon our findings, the IRD group seems to have been incorrectly identified as low risk. Moreover, the use of admission clinical characteristics may serve to identify those subsets of patients at greater risk for antibiotic treatment failure.

In summary, this study provides additional insight into clinical characteristics which may identify patients who are at risk to fail conservative parenteral antibiotic therapy and who may benefit from concurrent abscess drainage with antibiotic treatment. In select patients, concurrent abscess drainage may represent the most optimal treatment option. Previous studies have demonstrated the efficacy and safety of TOA drainage, and the findings of this study support the feasibility of initial drainage of patients with specific thresholds of TOA size and leukocytosis. Additional larger observational studies will be necessary to provide further guidance and standardization of treatment for TOA.

Disclosure

The findings of this paper were presented at the annual American Congress of Obstetrics and Gynecology meeting on May 3–5, 2015, in San Francisco, CA.

Conflict of Interests

The authors report no conflict of interests.

References

[1] S. G. McNeeley, S. L. Hendrix, M. M. Mazzoni et al., "Medically sound, cost-effective treatment for pelvic inflammatory disease and tuboovarian abscess," *American Journal of Obstetrics and Gynecology*, vol. 178, no. 6, pp. 1272–1278, 1998.

[2] S. Granberg, K. Gjelland, and E. Ekerhovd, "The management of pelvic abscess," *Best Practice & Research: Clinical Obstetrics and Gynaecology*, vol. 23, no. 5, pp. 667–678, 2009.

[3] R. L. Sweet, "Soft tissue infection and pelvic ascess," in *Infectious Diseases of the Female Genital Tract*, R. L. Sweet and R. S. Gibbs, Eds., pp. 95–112, Lippincott Williams & Wilkins, Philadelphia, Pa, USA, 5th edition, 2009.

[4] R. Mirhashemi, W. M. J. Schoell, R. Estape, R. Angioli, and H. E. Averette, "Trends in the management of pelvic abscesses," *Journal of the American College of Surgeons*, vol. 188, no. 5, pp. 567–672, 1999.

[5] S. D. Reed, D. V. Landers, and R. L. Sweet, "Antibiotic treatment of tuboovarian abscess: comparison of broad-spectrum β-lactam agents versus clindamycin-containing regimens," *American Journal of Obstetrics and Gynecology*, vol. 164, no. 6, part 1, pp. 1556–1562, 1991.

[6] W. C. Johnson, S. G. Gerzof, A. H. Robbins, and D. C. Nabseth, "Treatment of abdominal abscesses: comparative evaluation of operative drainage versus percutaneous catheter drainage guided by computed tomography or ultrasound," *Annals of Surgery*, vol. 194, no. 4, pp. 510–519, 1981.

[7] N. J. Worthen and J. E. Gunning, "Percutaneous drainage of pelvic abscesses: management of the tubo-ovarian abscess," *Journal of Ultrasound in Medicine*, vol. 5, no. 10, pp. 551–556, 1986.

[8] R. T. Tyrrel, F. B. Murphy, and M. E. Bernardino, "Tubo-ovarian abscesses: CT-guided percutaneous drainage," *Radiology*, vol. 175, no. 1, pp. 87–89, 1990.

[9] J. L. Nosher, H. K. Winchman, and G. S. Needell, "Transvaginal pelvic abscess drainage with US guidance," *Radiology*, vol. 165, no. 3, pp. 872–873, 1987.

[10] R. B. Levenson, K. M. Pearson, A. Saokar, S. I. Lee, P. R. Mueller, and P. F. Hahn, "Image-guided drainage of tuboovarian abscesses of gastrointestinal or genitourinary origin: a retrospective analysis," *Journal of Vascular and Interventional Radiology*, vol. 22, no. 5, pp. 678–686, 2011.

[11] Centers for Disease Control and Prevention, "Pelvic Inflammatory Disease. Sexually Transmitted Diseases Treat-ment Guidelines," 2010, http://www.cdc.gov/std/treatment/2010/pid.htm.

[12] K. Workowski, S. Berman, and Centers for Disease Control and Prevention (CDC), "Sexually transmitted diseases treatment guidelines," *Morbidity and Mortality Weekly Report*, vol. 59, no. 12, pp. 1–110, 2010.

[13] J. DeWitt, A. Reining, J. E. Allsworth, and J. F. Peipert, "Tubovarian abscesses: is size associated with duration of hospitalization & complications?" *Obstetrics and Gynecology International*, vol. 2010, Article ID 847041, 5 pages, 2010.

[14] Y. Greenstein, A. J. Shah, O. Vragovic et al., "Tuboovarian abscess. Factors associated with operative intervention after failed antibiotic therapy," *Journal of Reproductive Medicine*, vol. 58, no. 3-4, pp. 101–106, 2013.

[15] T. Perez-Medina, M. A. Huertas, and J. M. Bajo, "Early ultrasound-guided transvaginal drainage of tubo-ovarian abscesses: a randomized study," *Ultrasound in Obstetrics and Gynecology*, vol. 7, no. 6, pp. 435–438, 1996.

[16] N. Goharkhay, U. Verma, and F. Maggiorotto, "Comparison of CT- or ultrasound-guided drainage with concomitant intravenous antibiotics vs. intravenous antibiotics alone in the

management of tubo-ovarian abscesses," *Ultrasound in Obstetrics and Gynecology*, vol. 29, no. 1, pp. 65–69, 2007.

[17] K. Gjelland, E. Ekerhovd, and S. Granberg, "Transvaginal ultrasound-guided aspiration for treatment of tubo-ovarian abscess: a study of 302 cases," *American Journal of Obstetrics & Gynecology*, vol. 193, no. 4, pp. 1323–1330, 2005.

3

A Comparison of Colorimetric Assessment of Vaginal pH with Nugent Score for the Detection of Bacterial Vaginosis

Matthew K. Hoffman,[1] Mrutyunjaya B. Bellad,[2] Umesh S. Charantimath,[2]
Avinash Kavi,[2] Jyoti M. Nagmoti,[2] Mahantesh B. Nagmoti,[2] Ashalata A. Mallapur,[3]
Geetanjali M. Katageri,[3] Umesh Y. Ramadurg,[3] Sheshidhar G. Bannale,[3]
Amit P. Revankar,[2] M. S. Ganachari,[2] Richard J. Derman,[4] and Shivaprasad S. Goudar[2]

[1]Department of Obstetrics & Gynecology, Christiana Care Health System, Newark, DE, USA
[2]KLE University Jawaharlal Nehru Medical College, Belgaum, Karnataka, India
[3]S. Nijalingappa Medical College and HSK Hospital and Research Centre, Bagalkot, Karnataka, India
[4]Thomas Jefferson University, Philadelphia, PA, USA

Correspondence should be addressed to Matthew K. Hoffman; mhoffman@christianacare.org

Academic Editor: Bryan Larsen

Background. A Nugent score > 7 has been defined as the gold standard for the diagnosis for bacterial vaginosis (BV), though it is resource intensive and impractical as point of care testing. We sought to determine if colorimetric assessment of vaginal pH can accurately predict the occurrence of BV. *Methods.* We performed a planned subanalysis of 1,216 pregnant women between 13 0/7 and 19 6/7 weeks who underwent vaginal examination as part of a randomized controlled trial. Using a standardized technique, specimens were obtained for colorimetric assessment and two separate slides for Gram staining. These slides were subsequently evaluated by two independent blinded microbiologists for Nugent scoring. *Results.* Interrater reliability of the interpretation of the Nugent score was excellent (intraclass correlation-individual 0.93 (95 CI 0.92 to 0.94) and average 0.96 (95% CI 0.95 to 0.97)). The sensitivity of an elevated pH > 5 for a Nugent score > 7 was 21.9% while the specificity was 84.5%. The positive predictive value in our population was 33.7% with a negative predictive value of 75.0%. *Conclusion.* Though the Nugent score is internally accurate, the prediction of BV using vaginal pH alone has poor sensitivity and specificity.

1. Background

Bacterial vaginosis (BV) remains the most common form of vaginitis affecting women globally [1] and has been linked to several poor outcomes including preterm birth [2] and posthysterectomy infection [3]. Nonetheless, 29% of US women are noted to meet diagnostic criteria of BV, though the majority are clinically asymptomatic [4]. Recently, genetic microbiome studies have demonstrated that the occurrence of BV represents an absence of acid forming morphotypes of lactobacillus [5]. This lack of lactobacilli is frequently accompanied by an overgrowth of *Gardnerella vaginalis* forming an infected biofilm and creating a permissive environment for the overgrowth of numerous anaerobic Gram negative rods [6]. Nonetheless, the vaginal microbiome, as defined by Nugent scoring, is noted to vary dramatically by region of the world [7].

Several prior studies have suggested that vaginal pH alone may be an accurate marker for the detection of BV [8–10]. These high correlations have not been witnessed in other studies. It is thus important to establish the accuracy of vaginal pH to detect BV in an area where the resource intensive approaches to Gram stain and light microscopy may not be readily available. We thus sought to determine the ability of vaginal pH to detect BV as defined by the Nugent score amongst pregnant women in a low middle income setting in southern India.

2. Methods

Prior to the initiation of the study, Institutional Review Board approval was obtained from both participating institutions (Jawaharlal Nehru Medical College, Belgaum, India, and Christiana Care Health Services, Newark, Delaware). This trial was a planned substudy of a prospective individually randomized trial of pregnant women with an elevated vaginal pH (≥5.0) who would be treated with Clindamycin or placebo (ClinicalTrials.Gov NCT01800825, ICTR CTRI/2013/07/003799). Pregnant women between the gestational ages of 13 0/7 and 19 6/7 weeks were invited to participate in the trial. To be included women were to have a singleton gestation with no anomalies by history. Women were likewise excluded if they had a history of taking antibiotics in the last 14 days, had a history of vaginal bleeding in the last 3 days, had a symptomatic vaginal discharge, or were unable to consent (age < 18 years with no provisions for family/husband consent). Consistent with the guidelines of the ethics review committee, before each examination, a woman provided consent in her local language under the direct observation of trained field staff.

Our primary outcome was the presence of BV as defined as a Nugent score of 7 or greater [11]. Though competing definitions for BV exist, such as Amsel's criteria, the Nugent scoring system was chosen as it has been acknowledged as the gold standard [11, 12].

Prior to field initiation, certified Auxiliary Nurse Midwives (ANMs) were trained in a standardized methodology for both obtaining slides for Gram stain and vaginal pH using a video and direct observation by a central team member. Using a standardized speculum exam, specimens were taken from the lateral vaginal sidewalls. Gram stains were obtained using 2 separate acrylic swabs and then immediately plated on a clean glass slide that was allowed to air dry. These slides were transported to a central reading area where they underwent Gram stain. Nugent score was then read by two independent pathologists in accordance with accepted techniques [11]. Women who had a Nugent score of 7 or greater were deemed to have bacterial vaginosis. In cases wherein the two pathologists disagreed and with one scoring below 7, the higher score was chosen to define the presence or absence of bacterial vaginosis.

Vaginal pH was determined by directly placing a small portion of pH paper in the same location that the vaginal swab for the Gram stain was obtained from and it remained until being saturated with vaginal fluid. The pH was then evaluated after the pH paper had been allowed to dry after 60 seconds. PH paper was universally obtained from Micro-Essential Laboratories (Hydrion 345 S/R Dispenser; Brooklyn, NY) and is able to discriminate pH in 0.5 moles per liter increments between 3.0 and 5.5. These were recorded and read independently of the Gram stains.

Statistical analysis consisted of performing an intraclass correlation (two-way mixed effect model) between the two

TABLE 1: Demographics.

Variable		95% CI
Age in years	23.7	22.7 to 24.7
Gravidity	2.5	1.9 to 3.1
Parity	1.4	1.3 to 1.5
Height in cm	151.2	150.6 to 151.8
Weight in kg	46.0	45.2 to 46.9
Years in school	8.8	8.5 to 9.2
Respiratory disease	1.57%	
Cardiac disease	0.94%	
Diabetes	0.31%	
Other diseases	0.63%	

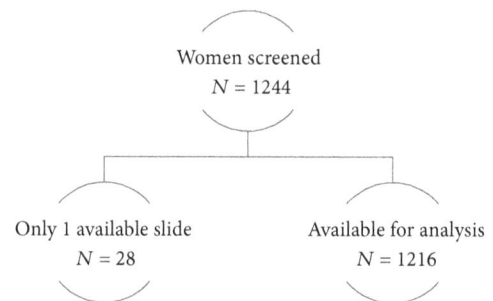

FIGURE 1

scoring microbiologists for both Nugent score and the occurrence of BV (Nugent score ≥ 7). Comparison of the presence of BV defined by an elevated vaginal pH (≥5) versus BV defined by Nugent score was likewise compared using a pairwise correlation. Summary statistics were performed using simple univariate modelling. All statistical analysis were performed using STATA 14.0 (College Station TX).

3. Results

A total of 6,473 women underwent screening in the parent study; 26.7% (N = 1,728) were found to have a vaginal pH ≥ 5. Of this cohort, a total of 1,244 women underwent screening with both a vaginal Gram stain and a vaginal pH, of which 1,216 (97.6%) met the entrance requirement (see Figure 1). Twenty-eight women were eliminated due to the lack of a second slide. Demographics of the participants are presented in Table 1. Our participants can best be summated as a young healthy but underweight cohort. This cohort is consistent with participants of our prior studies and the general population [13].

As determined by a Nugent score of 7 or greater, 17.4% of our participants had bacterial vaginosis. With reference to the Nugent score, there was a very high correlation between the two pathologists both between each other and the mean value. The intraclass correlation between raters was 0.929 (95% CI 0.920 to 0.936) and between the average was 0.963 (95% CI 0.959 to 0.967) (P value < 0.001). This suggests that Nugent score is a highly accurate and consistent test.

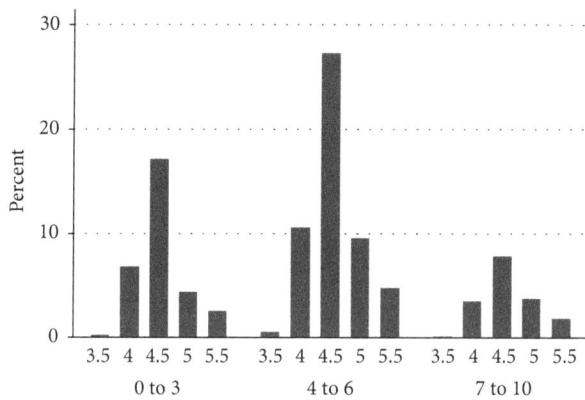

FIGURE 2: % distribution by pH and Nugent grouping.

In contrast, vaginal pH fared poorly as a predictor of bacterial vaginosis defined as a Nugent score of 7 or greater. This is graphically illustrated in Figure 2, wherein the distribution of vaginal pH values is shown by Nugent groups (0 to 3, 4 to 6, and 7 to 10). In this graph one can see that the frequency of vaginal pH values appears to be normally distributed, not skewed with the higher pH values in the 7 to 10 group. The pairwise correlation between a $pH \geq 5$ and an elevated Nugent score was 0.66 (P value of 0.021). The sensitivity of an elevated $pH \geq 5$ by Nugent score was 21.7% while the specificity was 84.1%. The positive predictive value in our population was 31.1% with a negative predictive value of 76.4%.

4. Discussion

The clinical diagnosis of bacterial vaginosis has long been made using Amsel's criteria (elevated vaginal pH, presence of clue cells, milky discharge, and positive whiff test) or Nugent's criteria [14]. Through microbiotics, we have come to understand that bacterial vaginosis is a complex entity characterized largely as the absence of acid forming lactobacillus and a concomitant proliferation of other anaerobic bacteria [5]. This lack of acidity allows the proliferation of other organisms (microbial dysbiosis) which may be causative of underlying disease [15]. As lactobacilli play a key role in acidifying the vagina, it is not surprising that vaginal pH remains part of Amsel's criteria in making the clinical diagnosis of bacterial vaginosis.

Though we were able to demonstrate that an elevated vaginal pH is significantly associated with bacterial vaginosis as defined by Nugent's criteria, our measurement of vaginal pH had poor sensitivity and specificity compared to other publications. Amongst our participants, only 21.7% of women with an elevated vaginal pH (defined as vaginal pH or greater than or equal to 5.0.) had bacterial vaginosis. This finding is much more consistent with other reports that have found vaginal pH to be a relatively poor predictor of BV [8, 10]. This may in part be explained by the fact that vaginal microbiome of southern India may be markedly different than that in other countries [7].

Though broadly accepted as the gold standard, it is important to remember that the Nugent score reflects the relative ratios of large Gram positive rods (lactobacillus), small Gram variable rods, and curved Gram variable rods [11]. Whether these findings are diagnostic of BV and are associated with both disease and poor obstetrical outcomes in rural India where the microbiome may be different is unclear [7]. Further complicating the issue, recent genomic studies have demonstrated that "healthy" women who lack appreciable colonies of lactobacilli are relatively common [16, 17]. These women appear to have other bacteria that are capable of acidifying the vagina, promoting microbial health. In such women, Nugent's criteria may not be an appropriate marker of the health of the vaginal microbiome.

Perhaps more important than how the diagnosis of bacterial vaginosis is derived is that an elevated vaginal pH represents an atypical vaginal microbiome free of acid forming organisms. Such an environment has been shown to provide permissive growth of pathological organisms like mycoplasma amongst others [18]. Several investigations have been able to link an elevated vaginal pH without either an elevated Nugent score or the other portions of Amsel's criteria with poor outcomes including preterm birth and preterm premature rupture of membranes [19–21]. It is for this reason that we will be exploring our obstetrical outcomes by vaginal pH in this unique cohort.

Competing Interests

None of the authors are aware of any financial relationships that would have influenced the conduct, analysis, or outcomes of this study.

Acknowledgments

This study was supported by the Thrasher Research Fund (Award no. 10326), Salt Lake City, Utah.

References

[1] L. O. Eckert, "Clinical practice. Acute vulvovaginitis," *The New England Journal of Medicine*, vol. 355, no. 12, pp. 1244–1252, 2006.

[2] M. A. Klebanoff, S. L. Hillier, R. P. Nugent et al., "Is bacterial vaginosis a stronger risk factor for preterm birth when it is diagnosed earlier in gestation?" *American Journal of Obstetrics and Gynecology*, vol. 192, no. 2, pp. 470–477, 2005.

[3] S. L. Hillier, R. P. Nugent, D. A. Eschenbach et al., "Association between bacterial vaginosis and preterm delivery of a low-birth-weight infant. The Vaginal Infections and Prematurity Study Group," *The New England Journal of Medicine*, vol. 333, no. 26, pp. 1737–1742, 1995.

[4] J. E. Allsworth and J. F. Peipert, "Prevalence of bacterial vaginosis: 2001–2004 national health and nutrition examination survey data," *Obstetrics & Gynecology*, vol. 109, no. 1, pp. 114–120, 2007.

[5] R. F. Lamont, J. D. Sobel, R. A. Akins et al., "The vaginal microbiome: new information about genital tract flora using molecular based techniques," *BJOG: An International Journal of Obstetrics and Gynaecology*, vol. 118, no. 5, pp. 533–549, 2011.

[6] L. Hardy, V. Jespers, N. Dahchour et al., "Unravelling the bacterial vaginosis-associated biofilm: a multiplex *Gardnerella Vaginalis* and *Atopobium vaginae* fluorescence in situ hybridization assay using peptide nucleic acid probes," *PLOS ONE*, vol. 10, no. 8, Article ID e0136658, 2015.

[7] J. E. Tolosa, S. Chaithongwongwatthana, S. Daly et al., "The International Infections in Pregnancy (IIP) study: variations in the prevalence of bacterial vaginosis and distribution of morphotypes in vaginal smears among pregnant women," *American Journal of Obstetrics and Gynecology*, vol. 195, no. 5, pp. 1198–1204, 2006.

[8] Z. Mengistie, Y. Woldeamanuel, D. Asrat, and M. Yigeremu, "Comparison of clinical and gram stain diagnosis methods of bacterial vaginosis among pregnant women in Ethiopia," *Journal of Clinical and Diagnostic Research*, vol. 7, no. 12, pp. 2701–2703, 2013.

[9] J. S. Huppert, E. A. Hesse, M. C. Bernard, J. R. Bates, C. A. Gaydos, and J. A. Kahn, "Accuracy and trust of self-testing for bacterial vaginosis," *Journal of Adolescent Health*, vol. 51, no. 4, pp. 400–405, 2012.

[10] R. Hemalatha, B. A. Ramalaxmi, E. Swetha, N. Balakrishna, and P. Mastromarino, "Evaluation of vaginal pH for detection of bacterial vaginosis," *Indian Journal of Medical Research*, vol. 138, no. 3, pp. 354–359, 2013, http://www.pubmedcentral.nih.gov/artid=3818598&tool=pmcentrez&rendertype=abstract.

[11] R. P. Nugent, M. A. Krohn, and S. L. Hillier, "Reliability of diagnosing bacterial vaginosis is improved by a standardized method of gram stain interpretation," *Journal of Clinical Microbiology*, vol. 29, no. 2, pp. 297–301, 1991.

[12] "Sexually transmitted diseases treatment guidelines, 2015," *Morbidity and Mortality Weekly Report (MMWR)*, vol. 64, no. 3, pp. 1–137, 2015, https://www.cdc.gov/std/tg2015/tg-2015-print.pdf.

[13] E. M. McClure, C. L. Bose, A. Garces et al., "Global network for women's and children's health research: a system for low-resource areas to determine probable causes of stillbirth, neonatal, and maternal death," *Maternal Health, Neonatology and Perinatology*, vol. 1, no. 1, 2015.

[14] A. G. Rouse, K. M. Gil, and K. Davis, "Diagnosis of bacterial vaginosis in the pregnant patient in an acute care setting," *Archives of Gynecology and Obstetrics*, vol. 279, no. 4, pp. 545–549, 2009.

[15] R. M. Brotman, M. A. Klebanoff, T. R. Nansel et al., "Bacterial vaginosis assessed by gram stain and diminished colonization resistance to incident gonococcal, chlamydial, and trichomonal genital infection," *Journal of Infectious Diseases*, vol. 202, no. 12, pp. 1907–1915, 2010.

[16] X. Zhou, C. J. Brown, Z. Abdo et al., "Differences in the composition of vaginal microbial communities found in healthy Caucasian and black women," *The ISME Journal*, vol. 1, no. 2, pp. 121–133, 2007.

[17] K. C. Anukam, E. O. Osazuwa, I. Ahonkhai, and G. Reid, "Lactobacillus vaginal microbiota of women attending a reproductive health care service in Benin City, Nigeria," *Sexually Transmitted Diseases*, vol. 33, no. 1, pp. 59–62, 2006.

[18] P. J. Meis, M. Klebanoff, E. Thom et al., "Prevention of recurrent preterm delivery by 17 alpha-hydroxyprogesterone caproate," *The New England Journal of Medicine*, vol. 348, no. 24, pp. 2379–2385, 2003.

[19] W. W. Andrews, J. C. Hauth, and R. L. Goldenberg, "Infection and preterm birth," *American Journal of Perinatology*, vol. 17, no. 7, pp. 357–366, 2000.

[20] G. G. Donders, K. Van Calsteren, G. Bellen et al., "Predictive value for preterm birth of abnormal vaginal flora, bacterial vaginosis and aerobic vaginitis during the first trimester of pregnancy," *BJOG: An International Journal of Obstetrics and Gynaecology*, vol. 116, no. 10, pp. 1315–1324, 2009.

[21] J. C. Hauth, C. MacPherson, J. Carey et al., "Early pregnancy threshold vaginal pH and Gram stain scores predictive of subsequent preterm birth in asymptomatic women," *American Journal of Obstetrics and Gynecology*, vol. 188, no. 3, pp. 831–835, 2003.

4

Hepatitis B, HIV, and Syphilis Seroprevalence in Pregnant Women and Blood Donors in Cameroon

Jodie Dionne-Odom,[1] Rahel Mbah,[2] Nicole J. Rembert,[1]
Samuel Tancho,[2] Gregory E. Halle-Ekane,[3] Comfort Enah,[1] Thomas K. Welty,[2]
Pius M. Tih,[2] and Alan T. N. Tita[1]

[1]University of Alabama at Birmingham, Birmingham, AL 35294, USA
[2]Cameroon Baptist Convention Health Services (CBCHS), P.O. Box 1, Nkwen, Bamenda, Cameroon
[3]University of Buea, P.O. Box 12, Buea, Cameroon

Correspondence should be addressed to Jodie Dionne-Odom; jdionne@uabmc.edu

Academic Editor: Flor Munoz

Objectives. We estimated seroprevalence and correlates of selected infections in pregnant women and blood donors in a resource-limited setting. *Methods.* We performed a cross-sectional analysis of laboratory seroprevalence data from pregnant women and voluntary blood donors from facilities in Cameroon in 2014. Rapid tests were performed to detect hepatitis B surface antigen, syphilis treponemal antibodies, and HIV-1/2 antibodies. Blood donations were also tested for hepatitis C and malaria. *Results.* The seroprevalence rates and ranges among 7069 pregnant women were hepatitis B 4.4% (1.1–9.6%), HIV 6% (3.0–10.2%), and syphilis 1.7% (1.3–3.8%) with significant variability among the sites. Correlates of infection in pregnancy in adjusted regression models included urban residence for hepatitis B (aOR 2.9, CI 1.6–5.4) and HIV (aOR 3.5, CI 1.9–6.7). Blood donor seroprevalence rates and ranges were hepatitis B 6.8% (5.0–8.8%), HIV 2.2% (1.4–2.8%), syphilis 4% (3.3–4.5%), malaria 1.9%, and hepatitis C 1.7% (0.5–2.5%). *Conclusions.* Hepatitis B, HIV, and syphilis infections are common among pregnant women and blood donors in Cameroon with higher rates in urban areas. Future interventions to reduce vertical transmission should include universal screening for these infections early in pregnancy and provision of effective prevention tools including the birth dose of univalent hepatitis B vaccine.

1. Introduction

Many pregnant women in sub-Saharan Africa are infected with or exposed to pathogens that can be transmitted vertically. These include HIV, hepatitis B virus (HBV), hepatitis C virus (HCV), malaria, and syphilis. The usual mechanism for perinatal transmission of HBV, HCV, and HIV is exposure to infected maternal blood and fluids at the time of delivery. Vertical transmission of syphilis is transplacental and it occurs in 60–90% of pregnant women with early disseminated disease [1]. Pregnancy is also associated with an increased susceptibility to certain infections, including HIV and malaria [2–4].

Screening for infections during antenatal care is important since many infections are asymptomatic yet treatable. Screening practices are standardized in high-income countries, but access to antenatal care testing is more limited in low- and middle-income countries (LMIC) where infection rates are elevated [5]. Many women in LMIC also present later for antenatal care, leaving less time for intervention when infection is detected. In sub-Saharan Africa, access to screening during pregnancy has improved over the past decade, particularly as HIV prevention programs have been scaled up [6, 7]. Antenatal screening for HIV and syphilis is now commonly performed, but screening for hepatitis B is not routine. Since HBV remains an endemic infection in many countries, the World Health Organization (WHO) recommends the administration of birth dose of univalent hepatitis B vaccine to all newborns to help reduce vertical transmission and routine antenatal screening guidelines are being developed [8, 9]. Pregnant women in low-income countries also have a heightened risk of acquiring infection due to an unsafe blood supply. The prevalence of anemia in pregnancy is as high as 70% in sub-Saharan Africa and postpartum hemorrhage is the major cause of global maternal mortality [10, 11]. Blood transfusion during pregnancy and the peripartum period can be necessary, but it comes with a risk of transfusion-transmitted infection. Infection rates in the locally available blood supply may be elevated, but WHO recommended screening for bloodborne pathogens is not universally performed [12].

The Cameroon Health Initiative at the University of Alabama at Birmingham (CHI UAB) is a collaborative partnership with US and Cameroon-based investigators to improve maternal and infant health outcomes with infection as one major focus area. In order to obtain baseline information to guide future interventions, we sought to estimate the prevalence and correlates of HBV, HIV, HCV, malaria, and syphilis infection among pregnant women and blood donors at multiple program sites in Cameroon.

2. Methods

We performed a cross-sectional seroprevalence study using laboratory data collected from the antenatal clinic (ANC) (HBV, HIV, and syphilis testing) and blood donor registries (HBV, HIV, syphilis, HCV, and malaria testing) in 2014 at four large hospital facilities in geographically distinct areas of Cameroon.

2.1. Study Population and Setting. The Cameroon Baptist Convention Health Services (CBCHS) is a nongovernmental health care organization that has been active for more than 70 years with over 80 facilities in 6 of the 10 regions of the country. The study was implemented at 4 of the major facilities in 3 regions of Western Cameroon: Banso Baptist Hospital (Banso), Mbingo Baptist Hospital (Mbingo), Baptist Hospital Mutengene (Mutengene), and Mboppi Baptist Hospital in Douala (Mboppi). Pregnant women underwent routine screening for hepatitis B, syphilis, and HIV at their initial antenatal care visit or at the time of delivery. For HIV testing, an opt-out verbal consent has been standard practice since 2000 and screening acceptance rates now approach 100%. The cost of laboratory testing is included in the ANC registration fee which is approximately $15 and HIV testing is provided free of charge.

Blood donors from the same four facilities underwent verbal consent and routine clinical screening for hepatitis B, hepatitis C, syphilis, and HIV infections. Malaria screening was only performed at one facility site (Banso). Any positive screening test result led to disqualification of the donated blood sample. The system for blood donation relies on voluntary donations and donors are frequently relatives or friends of the recipient. Donors do not receive compensation and screening is performed free of charge. The cost of testing is transferred to the recipient of the blood and one unit of blood costs $30.

2.2. Clinical Tests. The hepatitis B testing used for pregnant women and blood donors was a hepatitis B surface antigen (HBsAg) immunoassay rapid test with a reported sensitivity of 98% and a 15-minute turnaround time (ABON, Alere) [13]. For HIV screening, the Determine HIV-1/2 rapid antibody test was used for both blood donors and antenatal patients (Abbott Laboratories, Chicago, Illinois, now Alere). It is a lateral flow assay with a 15-minute turnaround time. The Determine HIV-1/2 rapid test used has demonstrated 100% sensitivity and 99.8% specificity in pregnancy [14]. A second rapid HIV test (the First Response HIV Card Test) was performed on antenatal patients who had a positive Determine test. The sensitivity of the First Response HIV Card Test is 99.8% and the specificity is 100% [15, 16]. If the Determine test was positive but the First Response test was negative, repeat testing was recommended in one month using the First Response test. Positive HIV results for this analysis reflect those with two positive rapid antibody tests. All blood donors were tested with both HIV antibody tests. The HIV tests were chosen based on WHO recommendations, but there is no current WHO or CDC recommendation to use a particular antibody test for hepatitis B and hepatitis C screening.

A rapid test was also used for syphilis screening in pregnant women and blood donors. The Syphilis Ultrarapid Test Strip (ABON, Alere) has 20-minute turnaround time. It is a chromatographic treponemal antibody immunoassay and the sensitivity of similar treponemal tests has been documented at 96–100% compared to a gold standard of TPPA [17]. Nontreponemal testing was not performed to help distinguish active from prior syphilis infection.

Hepatitis C antibody testing was performed for blood donors (DFI Healthmate HCV Ab, South Korea). This test is a 3rd generation EIA with reported 98% sensitivity [18]. Malaria testing was performed on blood donation samples at one facility (Banso). The testing used was a rapid test called Care Start pLDH which detects *P. falciparum* (Pf) specific lactate dehydrogenase (Pf-pLDH) and an antigen common to all four plasmodium species (pan-pLDH). The sensitivity of this test is 94.7% for Pf compared to PCR testing although the sensitivity for non-Pf species is lower (74% for *P. vivax*, 32% for *P. malariae*, and 25% for *P. ovale*) [19]. Over 90% of the malaria in Cameroon is caused by *P. falciparum* [20].

2.3. Data Management and Statistical Analysis. The laboratory screening registers were reviewed and deidentified data were abstracted for analysis. Individual-level results for each infection were collected for analysis from three sites (Banso, Mbingo, and Mutengene), and aggregated data was available from the 4th site (Mboppi). In addition, age and location of residence (categorized into urban, suburban, and rural) were collected.

Statistical analysis was performed using SAS 9.3. The primary outcomes of interest were the prevalence of each of the infections in pregnant women and in blood donors. The Kruskal-Wallis test was used to compare the median age of pregnant women and blood donors at each site. The Chi square test was used to compare categorical variables. We estimated the prevalence and 95% CI of each infection in women and compared the prevalence across facilities. Individual-level patient data was merged from the three sites where it was available and demographics were examined as potential factors associated with infection prevalence.

TABLE 1: Demographics of pregnant women and voluntary blood donors*, n (%).

(a)

Pregnant women	Mbingo n = 1230	Mutengene n = 871	Banso n = 726	Total n = 2827	p value**
Age, median (range)	26 (14–55)	27 (15–44)	26 (14–53)	26 (4–55)	0.177
Residence					
Urban	123 (35.0)	735 (84.4)	56 (7.7)	914 (46.9)	
Suburban	87 (24.8)	136 (15.6)	398 (54.8)	621 (31.9)	<0.0001
Rural	141 (40.2)	—	272 (37.5)	413 (21.2)	

(b)

Blood donors	n = 1305	n = 889	n = 1170	n = 3364	p value**
Age, median (range)	30 (15–75)	34 (17–56)	32 (17–63)	33 (15–75)	<0.0001
Gender					
Male	920 (70.6)	807 (90.8)	878 (75.2)	2605 (77.5)	<0.0001
Female	384 (29.4)	82 (9.2)	290 (24.8)	756 (22.5)	
Residence (n = 2999)					
Urban	480 (51)	596 (67)	61 (5.2)	1138 (38.0)	
Suburban	116 (12.3)	293 (33)	839 (71.8)	1248 (41.6)	<0.0001
Rural	345 (36.7)	—	268 (23)	613 (20.4)	
Marital status (n = 2069)					
Married	69 (56)	507 (57)	693 (65.6)	1269 (61.3)	0.0002
Single*	55 (44)	382 (43)	363 (34.4)	800 (38.7)	
Blood type					
A	226 (17.4)	109 (12.3)	243 (20.8)	578 (17.2)	
B	282 (21.7)	82 (9.2)	211 (18.1)	575 (17.1)	<0.0001
AB	27 (2.1)	7 (0.8)	42 (3.6)	76 (2.3)	
O	767 (58.9)	689 (77.7)	672 (57.5)	2128 (63.4)	
Rh status					
Positive	1251 (95.9)	875 (98.4)	1129 (96.6)	3255 (96.8)	0.0033
Negative	54 (4.1)	14 (1.6)	40 (3.4)	108 (3.2)	

*Demographics were available at 3 of the 4 study sites.
**p value is to test the overall difference in seroprevalence for each categorical variable (χ^2 test) or the median difference of the continuous variable.

Logistic regression modeling was performed for pregnant women and blood donors separately. Marital status was not included in the blood donor modeling due to missing data. Cramer's V was used to assess the correlation between facilities and location of residence. Due to the moderate correlation of these two variables, location of residence (urban/suburban/rural) was chosen as the covariate for the logistic regression models instead of the facility.

2.4. Ethics. A waiver of consent was obtained from the CBCHS in-country institutional review board and an exemption was granted by the Institutional Review Board at the University of Alabama at Birmingham.

3. Results

At four CBCHS facilities in Cameroon, 7069 pregnant women and 4225 blood donors were screened for infection

in 2014. Demographic data were available for 2827 ANC clients and 3364 blood donors from three of the four sites (Table 1). For pregnant women, the median age was 26 years and this did not differ across facilities (range 26-27 years; $p = 0.177$) whereas the residency location (urban/rural) differed significantly ($p < 0.001$). Women screened in Mutengene lived predominantly in urban settings while those in Banso were mostly from suburban and rural locales. Blood donors were significantly older than pregnant women (median age 33) and their median age differed across facilities (range 30-34 years; p value < 0.0001). The majority of blood donors were male (77.5%) and married (61.3%), had blood type O (63.4%), and had a positive Rh status (96.8%). These characteristics differed across sites.

The seroprevalence and 95% CI of the infections in pregnant women and donors by facility are shown in Table 2. Overall, the rates in pregnant women were 4.4% for hepatitis B, 6% for HIV, and 1.7% for syphilis. Among blood donors,

TABLE 2: Results of screening tests in pregnant women and blood donors[*], n (%) (95% CI).

(a)

Pregnant women	Mboppi (n = 4242)	Mbingo (n = 1230)	Mutengene (n = 871)	Banso (n = 726)	p value	Total (n = 7069)
Hepatitis B	184 (4.3) (3.7, 5.0)	14 (1.1) (0.6, 1.9)	84 (9.6) (7.7, 11.8)	26 (3.6) (2.3, 5.2)	<0.0001	308 (4.4) (3.9, 4.9)
HIV	252 (5.9) (5.3, 6.7)	56 (4.6) (3.5, 5.9)	89 (10.2) (8.3, 12.4)	22 (3.0) (1.9, 4.6)	<0.0001	413 (6.0) (5.3, 6.4)
Syphilis	57 (1.3) (1.0, 1.7)	17 (1.4) (0.8, 2.2)	33 (3.8) (2.6, 5.3)	15 (2.1) (1.2, 3.4)	<0.0001	122 (1.7) (1.4, 2.1)

(b)

Blood donors	(n = 861)	(n = 1305)	(n = 889)	(n = 1170)	p value	(n = 4225)
Hepatitis B	50 (5.8) (4.3, 4.6)	115 (8.8) (7.3, 10.5)	64 (7.2) (5.6, 9.1)	58 (5.0) (3.8, 6.4)	0.001	287 (6.8) (6.1, 7.6)
HIV	24 (2.8) (1.8, 4.1)	30 (2.3) (1.6, 3.3)	24 (2.7) (1.7, 4.0)	16 (1.4) (0.7, 2.2)	0.11	94 (2.2) (1.8, 2.7)
Syphilis	39 (4.5) (3.2, 6.1)	43 (3.3) (1.7, 3.4)	40 (4.5) (3.2, 6.1)	46 (3.9) (2.9, 5.2)	0.40	168 (4.0) (3.4, 4.6)
Hepatitis C	20 (2.3) (1.4, 3.6)	32 (2.5) (2.4, 4.4)	4 (0.5) (0.01, 1.2)	15 (1.3) (0.7, 2.1)	0.001	71 (1.7) (1.3, 2.1)
Malaria	N/A	N/A	N/A	22 (1.9)	N/A	22/1170 (1.9) (1.2, 2.8)

[*] Infections are not mutually exclusive; coinfection data is discussed in Section 3.

TABLE 3: Predictors of hepatitis B, HIV, and syphilis infection in pregnant women.

Variable	Hepatitis B infection		HIV infection		Syphilis infection	
	Unadjusted OR (95% CI)	Adjusted OR (95% CI) n = 1904	Unadjusted OR (95% CI)	Adjusted OR (95% CI) n = 1904	Unadjusted OR (95% CI)	Adjusted OR (95% CI) n = 1904
Age	(n = 2758)		(n = 2758)		(n = 2758)	
Continuous	1.00 (0.98, 1.03)	1.00 (0.97, 1.04)	1.03 (1.01, 1.06)[*]	1.04 (1.01, 1.07)[*]	1.00 (0.96, 1.04)	1.01 (0.96, 1.05)
Location	(n = 1948)		(n = 1948)		(n = 1948)	
Urban	3.1 (1.7, 5.7)[*]	2.9 (1.6, 5.4)[*]	3.7 (2.0, 7.0)[*]	3.5 (1.9, 6.7)[*]	1.5 (0.7, 3.2)	1.6 (0.7, 3.6)
Suburban	1.3 (0.7, 2.7)	1.3 (0.7, 2.7)	2.1 (1.1, 4.2)[*]	2.1 (1.1, 4.3)[*]	1.0 (0.4, 2.3)	1.1 (0.4, 2.6)
Rural	REF	REF	REF	REF	REF	REF

[*] Indicating statistical significance. REF: reference.

seroprevalence was 6.8% for hepatitis B, 2.2% for HIV, and 4% for syphilis. Additional testing among blood donors showed that 1.7% had antibodies for hepatitis C and 1.9% had malaria. Furthermore, the prevalence rates in pregnant women varied significantly across facilities ranging from 1.1 to 9.6% for hepatitis B, from 3 to 10.2% for HIV, and from 1.3 to 3.8% for syphilis. The range among blood donors was 5.0–8.8% for hepatitis B, 1.4–2.8% for HIV, 3.3–4.5% for syphilis, and 0.5–2.5% for HCV. Pregnant women seen in Mutengene and Mboppi had a higher prevalence of HBV and HIV compared to women seen at Mbingo and Banso facilities. Blood donors did not show a consistent pattern of uniformly high or low prevalence at specific facilities.

Coinfection with more than one pathogen was detected in 2.9% of the pregnant women in Mutengene (13 HIV/HBV, 6 HIV/syphilis, 3 HBV/syphilis, and 3 HIV/HBV/syphilis).

Rates of coinfection at Banso and Mbingo were very low at 0.3 and 0.2%, respectively. Among blood donors at the Mutengene facility, 1.8% had coinfection (8 HBV/syphilis, 7 HIV/HBV, and 1 HIV/syphilis) and the coinfection rate was 1% at Mbingo and 0.7% at Banso. Coinfection rates were not available from Mboppi.

Table 3 shows crude and adjusted odds ratios and 95% confidence intervals resulting from logistic regression analyses of hepatitis B, HIV, and syphilis infection as outcome variables among pregnant women. Pregnant women from urban locations were more likely to have hepatitis B (aOR 2.9, CI 1.6–5.4) and HIV (aOR 3.5, CI 1.9–6.7), compared to women from rural areas. Older age (aOR 1.04, CI 1.01–1.07) was also significantly associated with HIV status. The unadjusted model for blood donors showed lower rates of HIV in older donors and lower rates of hepatitis C infection

TABLE 4: Predictors of hepatitis B, C, HIV, and syphilis in blood donors.

Variable	Hepatitis B infection		Hepatitis C infection		HIV infection		Syphilis infection	
	Unadjusted OR (95% CI)	Adjusted OR (95% CI) ($n = 2988$)	Unadjusted OR (95% CI)	Adjusted OR (95% CI) ($n = 2988$)	Unadjusted OR (95% CI)	Adjusted OR (95% CI) ($n = 2986$)	Unadjusted OR (95% CI)	Adjusted OR (95% CI) ($n = 2987$)
Age	($n = 3352$)		($n = 3352$)		($n = 3351$)		($n = 3351$)	
Continuous	1.00 (0.98, 1.01)	1.0 (0.98, 1.02)	1.03 (1.0, 1.06)	1.00 (0.98, 1.02)	0.96 (0.94, 0.99)*	0.97 (0.94, 1.005)	1.03 (1.01, 1.05)*	1.02 (1.002, 1.05)*
Location	($n = 2999$)				($n = 2997$)		($n = 2998$)	
Urban	1.4 (1.0, 2.1)	1.4 (0.9, 2.1)	0.6 (0.3, 1.4)	1.4 (0.9, 2.1)	1.4 (0.6, 2.8)	1.3 (0.6, 2.8)	1.2 (0.7, 2.1)	1.2 (0.7, 2.0)
Suburban	1.0 (0.7, 1.5)	1.0 (0.6, 1.4)	0.4 (0.2, 0.9)*	1.2 (0.8, 1.9)	1.1 (0.5, 2.3)	1.1 (0.5, 2.3)	1.3 (0.8, 2.2)	1.3 (0.7, 2.2)
Rural	REF	REF	REF	REF	REF	REF	REF	REF
Gender	($n = 3361$)		($n = 3361$)		($n = 3359$)		($n = 3360$)	
M	REF	REF	REF	REF	REF	REF	REF	REF
F	1.0 (0.7, 1.3)	0.9 (0.6, 1.3)	1.1 (0.6, 2.0)	0.8 (0.6, 1.2)	0.6 (0.3, 1.2)	0.5 (0.2, 1.2)	0.8 (0.5, 1.2)	0.8 (0.5, 1.3)

*Indicating statistical significance. REF: reference.

for donors from suburban areas. Older age among blood donors was the only factor significantly associated with risk of syphilis in the adjusted model (aOR 1.02, CI 1.002–1.05) (Table 4).

4. Discussion

Infections in pregnancy remain common in Cameroon with 2014 seroprevalence rates as high as 9.6% for hepatitis B, 10.2% for HIV, and 3.8% for syphilis. Fortunately, vertical transmission of HBV, HIV, and syphilis can be prevented with currently available tools if the infection is detected in time. As evidence of how challenging it is to reduce infection rates, rates of HBV and HIV infection in pregnancy were also elevated 20 years ago (HBV 5.4%, HIV 3.5%) [21]. Rates of syphilis among pregnant women in Cameroon have improved from 15.8% to 4% over the past 20 years with increased access to syphilis screening and treatment programs [21–23]. Infection with hepatitis C is less common with a seroprevalence among blood donors in this study that matches a recent HCV seroprevalence study in health care workers (1.7%) [24]. Fortunately, this is significantly lower than the seroprevalence of 56% noted in an older Cameroon cohort (>60 years old). The HCV prevalence in the older group has been attributed to exposure to unclean needles during medical interventions in the early 20th century [25]. Very low rates of IV drug abuse in Cameroon and the infrequency of heterosexual transmission of HCV likely contributed to this cohort effect with a much lower prevalence noted in younger age groups [26, 27].

Our findings also show wide variability in infection rates depending on the facility site in Cameroon, particularly for hepatitis B (1.1–9.6%) and HIV (3.0–10.2%). This highlights the presence of subpopulations of pregnant women who warrant targeted testing and prevention efforts. Rates of infection were elevated at the sites which capture a higher population of urban pregnant women. Douala is the largest

city in Cameroon and pregnant women seen at Mboppi Hospital in Douala had the second highest rates of HBV (4.3%) and HIV (5.9%). This finding is consistent with other studies, although there may be confounding explanatory factors (such as number of sexual partners) which were not captured in this analysis. Pregnant women seen in Mutengene also had significantly higher rates of HBV, HIV, and syphilis in the multivariate analysis and the highest rates of coinfection, particularly for HBV and HIV. Mutengene is a semiurban town with a population of 40,000 which is located at the junction of two major roadways. Many of the patients seen at the facility are itinerant or travel from long distances to receive medical care. Infection rates among blood donors at Mutengene were comparable to the infection rates seen in pregnant women, although HIV prevalence was lower (2.7%). Since most blood donors were male, the lower HIV prevalence noted in blood donors compared to pregnant women mirrors national HIV epidemiology in Cameroon where the prevalence of infection in males (2.9%) is about half of the rate documented among females (5.6%) [28].

Most of sub-Saharan Africa is endemic for HBV infection (defined as HBsAg + >8%). Antenatal HBV screening has become routine practice at the larger CBCHS facilities but is not standard practice nationwide. The importance of screening for hepatitis B in pregnancy is highlighted by the fact that vertical transmission rates are 70–90% in women with chronic hepatitis B and a positive hepatitis B e antigen (HBeAg) and 10–40% if the HBeAg is negative. Chronic HBV infection develops in 90% of infected neonates, compared to 5–10% of infected immunocompetent adults. Vertical transmission of hepatitis B is preventable in 95% of cases if the exposed infant receives prophylaxis with birth dose univalent HBV vaccine followed by completion of the series. The birth dose vaccine is not part of the national vaccine plan in Cameroon or in many other countries in sub-Saharan Africa which instead prioritize HBV-containing pentavalent vaccine starting at 6 weeks of age. The pentavalent vaccine may not prevent vertical transmission of HBV. If vertical transmission is common, addition of the univalent HBV birth dose vaccine to the current vaccine program would be one effective way to reduce pediatric HBV infection rates [29, 30]. Neonatal BCG vaccine is administered routinely in most sub-Saharan countries and univalent HPV vaccine can be administered at the same time as soon as possible after birth.

The prevalence of HIV at CBCHS antenatal clinics in Cameroon has steadily decreased from 10.5% in 2004 to 3.4% in 2014 [31]. The 2011 Cameroon Demographic and Health Survey showed that women of childbearing age in the two largest urban cities had an HIV prevalence of 7.7%, compared to 4.6% among women from rural areas, highlighting the significance of regional variation [32]. Our findings support these trends but underscore the need for sustained efforts in high risk areas despite encouraging national trends [32]. The reduction in HIV prevalence in Cameroon has occurred in the setting of a robust Prevention of Mother to Child HIV Transmission (PMTCT) program with funding from the Elizabeth Glaser Pediatric AIDS Foundation and the US President's Emergency Plan for AIDS Relief (PEPFAR).

WHO launched a global initiative in 2007 to eliminate congenital syphilis. They recommended screening for syphilis at the initial antenatal clinic visit with a goal of 95% and a follow-up screening test during the third trimester [33]. Despite these efforts, syphilis rates are increasing, antenatal screening is not universal, and adverse infection outcomes occur in an estimated 206,000 pregnancies each year in sub-Saharan Africa [34]. These outcomes include stillbirth, neonatal death, low birth weight, and congenital syphilis. Fortunately, treatment with penicillin remains highly effective, affordable, and well tolerated. Our findings suggest the importance of screening for syphilis.

In this study, infections with bloodborne pathogens were commonly documented among routine voluntary blood donors. These rates are aligned with prior studies; at one hospital in urban Cameroon, nearly 15% of the donated blood screened positive for infections with HIV, HBV, HCV, or *T. pallidum* [35, 36]. Transfusion in this setting poses a real risk of infection for women who require blood products during pregnancy or in the postpartum setting and 276 pregnant women in Cameroon received blood transfusions at one of the four facilities in 2014. Another concern is the potential for transmission of bloodborne pathogens associated with fetal risk for which testing is not performed (i.e., CMV or toxoplasmosis). Although routine screening for malaria in donated blood products was only performed at one of the four sites, this should be routinely performed since malaria is endemic in Cameroon and pregnant women are more susceptible to this infection and its consequences [37, 38].

Another issue common to sub-Saharan Africa is the source of the blood products used for transfusion. One large study of blood donors in Cameroon showed that most donors (64%) were family members of the patient [39]. One of the four key components of the WHO blood safety plan is to improve donor recruitment and collection by restricting collection to products from low-risk donors. This specifically excludes friends and family members. The ideal donors are voluntary, nonremunerated, and recruited through a centralized system, such as blood centers which are independent from hospital facilities [12]. Major challenges persist related to the safety and expense of blood product transfusion in sub-Saharan Africa and the current supply only meets 40% of the estimated need [40].

The strengths of our study include the size of the cohort and the ability to compare contemporaneous ANC seroprevalence data with voluntary blood donors at four large clinical sites. In terms of study limitations, only certain demographic information was available for pregnant women and individual-level data was not available for one of the testing sites. Also, although the characteristics of the tests used were excellent, viral load testing for HBV or HIV, nontreponemal testing for syphilis to identify active infection, and microscopy to confirm malaria infection were not performed. This may have led to an overestimation of syphilis infection rates and an underestimation of malaria infection rates.

5. Conclusions

Antenatal care provides an excellent opportunity to screen women for infections which are common and treatable and can be transmitted vertically. Hepatitis B, HIV, and syphilis infections remain common in pregnant women and blood donors in Cameroon and the prevalence rates vary by site. Timely access to quality testing and treatment can prevent vertical transmission, but ongoing attention to blood safety is also needed. Policy changes at the national and international levels would go further to ensure that early access to antenatal testing and treatment or prevention is widely available in sub-Saharan Africa where disease prevalence is high.

Competing Interests

The authors declare that there is no conflict of interests regarding the publication of this paper.

Authors' Contributions

Jodie Dionne-Odom, Gregory E. Halle-Ekane, Thomas K. Welty, and Alan T. N. Tita conceived of and designed the study. Jodie Dionne-Odom drafted the initial paper. Rahel Mbah collected the data and provided critical revisions to the paper. Samuel Tancho performed laboratory testing, assisted with data collection, and provided critical revisions to the paper. Nicole J. Rembert performed the data analysis. Rahel Mbah, Gregory E. Halle-Ekane, Comfort Enah, Thomas K. Welty, Pius M. Tih, and Alan T. N. Tita provided critical revisions to the paper. All authors read and approved the final paper.

Acknowledgments

Thanks are due to the trained CBCHS laboratory staff who performed all of the tests on pregnant women and blood donors to reduce the risk of mother to child transmission of these pathogens and to reduce the risk of nosocomial transmission of pathogens in blood transfusions.

References

[1] N. Yeganeh, H. D. Watts, M. Camarca et al., "Syphilis in HIV-infected mothers and infants: results from the NICHD/HPTN 040 study," *The Pediatric Infectious Disease Journal*, vol. 34, no. 3, pp. e52–e57, 2015.

[2] E. Sappenfield, D. J. Jamieson, and A. P. Kourtis, "Pregnancy and susceptibility to infectious diseases," *Infectious Diseases in Obstetrics and Gynecology*, vol. 2013, Article ID 752852, 8 pages, 2013.

[3] S. A. Vishwanathan, A. Burgener, S. E. Bosinger et al., "Cataloguing of potential HIV susceptibility factors during the menstrual cycle of pig-tailed macaques by using a systems biology approach," *Journal of Virology*, vol. 89, no. 18, pp. 9167–9177, 2015.

[4] N. R. Mugo, R. Heffron, D. Donnell et al., "Increased risk of HIV-1 transmission in pregnancy: a prospective study among African HIV-1-serodiscordant couples," *AIDS*, vol. 25, no. 15, pp. 1887–1895, 2011.

[5] A. Swartzendruber, R. J. Steiner, M. R. Adler, M. L. Kamb, and L. M. Newman, "Introduction of rapid syphilis testing in antenatal care: a systematic review of the impact on HIV and syphilis testing uptake and coverage," *International Journal of Gynecology and Obstetrics*, vol. 130, supplement 1, pp. S15–S21, 2015.

[6] S. Bucher, I. Marete, C. Tenge et al., "A prospective observational description of frequency and timing of antenatal care attendance and coverage of selected interventions from sites in Argentina, Guatemala, India, Kenya, Pakistan and Zambia," *Reproductive Health*, vol. 12, supplement 2, article S12, 2015.

[7] M. Ediau, R. K. Wanyenze, S. Machingaidze et al., "Trends in antenatal care attendance and health facility delivery following community and health facility systems strengthening interventions in Northern Uganda," *BMC Pregnancy and Childbirth*, vol. 13, article 189, 2013.

[8] World Health Organization, *Guidelines for the Prevention, Care and Treatment of Persons with Chronic Hepatitis B Infection*, 2015.

[9] WHO, *Practices to Improve Coverage of the Hepatitis B Birth Dose Vaccine*, Department of Immunization, Vaccines and Biologicals, 2013.

[10] Y. Dei-Adomakoh, J. K. Acquaye, I. Ekem, and C. Segbefia, "Second trimester anaemia in pregnant Ghanaians," *West African Journal of Medicine*, vol. 33, no. 4, pp. 229–233, 2014.

[11] T. Pierre-Marie, H.-E. Gregory, D. I. Maxwell, E. M. Robinson, M. Yvette, and F. J. Nelson, "Maternal mortality in Cameroon: a university teaching hospital report," *The Pan African Medical Journal*, vol. 21, article 16, 2015.

[12] E. M. Bloch, M. Vermeulen, and E. Murphy, "Blood transfusion safety in africa: a literature review of infectious disease and organizational challenges," *Transfusion Medicine Reviews*, vol. 26, no. 2, pp. 164–180, 2012.

[13] M. S. Khuroo, N. S. Khuroo, and M. S. Khuroo, "Accuracy of rapid point-of-care diagnostic tests for hepatitis b surface antigen-a systematic review and meta-analysis," *Journal of Clinical and Experimental Hepatology*, vol. 4, no. 3, pp. 226–240, 2014.

[14] R. M. Viani, P. Hubbard, J. Ruiz-Calderon et al., "Performance of rapid HIV testing using Determine® HIV-1/2 for the diagnosis of HIV infection during pregnancy in Tijuana, Baja California, Mexico," *International Journal of STD & AIDS*, vol. 18, no. 2, pp. 101–104, 2007.

[15] P. Chaillet, K. Tayler-Smith, R. Zachariah et al., "Evaluation of four rapid tests for diagnosis and differentiation of HIV-1 and HIV-2 infections in Guinea-Conakry, West Africa," *Transactions of the Royal Society of Tropical Medicine and Hygiene*, vol. 104, no. 9, pp. 571–576, 2010.

[16] H. Syed Iqbal, P. Balakrishnan, K. G. Murugavel, and S. Suniti, "Performance characteristics of a new rapid immunochromatographic test for the detection of antibodies to human immunodeficiency virus (HIV) types 1 and 2," *Journal of Clinical Laboratory Analysis*, vol. 22, no. 3, pp. 178–185, 2008.

[17] K. Malm, S. Andersson, H. Fredlund et al., "Analytical evaluation of nine serological assays for diagnosis of syphilis," *Journal of the European Academy of Dermatology and Venereology*, vol. 29, no. 12, pp. 2369–2376, 2015.

[18] G. Filice, S. Patruno, D. Campisi et al., "Specificity and sensitivity of 3rd generation EIA for detection of HCV antibodies among intravenous drug-users," *The New Microbiologica*, vol. 16, no. 1, pp. 35–42, 1993.

[19] M. Heutmekers, P. Gillet, J. Maltha et al., "Evaluation of the rapid diagnostic test CareStart pLDH Malaria (Pf-pLDH/pan-pLDH) for the diagnosis of malaria in a reference setting," *Malaria Journal*, vol. 11, article 204, 2012.

[20] J. D. Bigoga, L. Manga, V. P. K. Titanji, M. Coetzee, and R. G. F. Leke, "Malaria vectors and transmission dynamics in coastal south-western Cameroon," *Malaria Journal*, vol. 6, article 5, 2007.

[21] P. M. Ndumbe, J. Skalsky, and H. I. Joller-Jemelka, "Seroprevalence of hepatitis and HIV infection among rural pregnant women in Cameroon," *APMIS*, vol. 102, no. 9, pp. 662–666, 1994.

[22] A. Buvé, H. A. Weiss, M. Laga et al., "The epidemiology of gonorrhoea, chlamydial infection and syphilis in four African cities," *AIDS*, vol. 15, supplement 4, pp. S79–S88, 2001.

[23] T. K. Welty, M. Bulterys, E. R. Welty et al., "Integrating prevention of mother-to-child HIV transmission into routine antenatal care: the key to program expansion in Cameroon," *Journal of Acquired Immune Deficiency Syndromes*, vol. 40, no. 4, pp. 486–493, 2005.

[24] C. Fritzsche, F. Becker, C. J. Hemmer et al., "Hepatitis b and c: neglected diseases among health care workers in cameroon," *Transactions of the Royal Society of Tropical Medicine and Hygiene*, vol. 107, no. 3, pp. 158–164, 2013.

[25] J. Pépin, M. Lavoie, O. G. Pybus et al., "Risk factors for hepatitis C virus transmission in colonial Cameroon," *Clinical Infectious Diseases*, vol. 51, no. 7, pp. 768–776, 2010.

[26] E. Nerrienet, R. Pouillot, G. Lachenal et al., "Hepatitis C virus infection in Cameroon: a cohort-effect," *Journal of Medical Virology*, vol. 76, no. 2, pp. 208–214, 2005.

[27] J. Ndjomou, B. Kupfer, B. Kochan, L. Zekeng, L. Kaptue, and B. Matz, "Hepatitis C virus infection and genotypes among human immunodeficiency virus high-risk groups in Cameroon," *Journal of Medical Virology*, vol. 66, no. 2, pp. 179–186, 2002.

[28] Institut National de Statistique, Ministère de Santé Publique, Yaoundé, and Cameroon, "Cameroon 2011 DHS," *Studies in Family Planning*, vol. 44, no. 2, pp. 223–232, 2013.

[29] C. Klingler, A. I. Thoumi, and V. S. Mrithinjayam, "Cost-effectiveness analysis of an additional birth dose of Hepatitis B vaccine to prevent perinatal transmission in a medical setting in Mozambique," *Vaccine*, vol. 31, no. 1, pp. 252–259, 2012.

[30] T. H. Nguyen, M. H. Vu, V. C. Nguyen et al., "A reduction in chronic hepatitis B virus infection prevalence among children

in vietnam demonstrates the importance of vaccination," *Vaccine*, vol. 32, no. 2, pp. 217–222, 2014.

[31] *Cameroon Baptist Convention Health Services Activity Report*, 2014.

[32] *Cameroon Demographic and Health Survey*, 2011.

[33] World Health Organization, *The Global Elimination of Congenital Syphilis: Rationale and Strategy for Action*, WHO, Geneva, Switzerland, 2007.

[34] A. Kuznik, A. G. Habib, Y. C. Manabe, and M. Lamorde, "Estimating the public health burden associated with adverse pregnancy outcomes resulting from syphilis infection across 43 countries in sub-Saharan Africa," *Sexually Transmitted Diseases*, vol. 42, no. 7, pp. 369–375, 2015.

[35] C. E. Eboumbou Moukoko, F. Ngo Sack, E. G. Essangui Same, M. Mbangue, and L. G. Lehman, "HIV, HBV, HCV and *T. pallidum* infections among blood donors and Transfusion-related complications among recipients at the Laquintinie hospital in Douala, Cameroon," *BMC Hematology*, vol. 14, no. 1, article 5, 2014.

[36] C. T. Tagny, A. Diarra, R. Yahaya et al., "Characteristics of blood donors and donated blood in sub-Saharan Francophone Africa," *Transfusion*, vol. 49, no. 8, pp. 1592–1599, 2009.

[37] S. J. Rogerson, L. Hviid, P. E. Duffy, R. F. G. Leke, and D. W. Taylor, "Malaria in pregnancy: pathogenesis and immunity," *The Lancet Infectious Diseases*, vol. 7, no. 2, pp. 105–117, 2007.

[38] A. P. Kourtis, J. S. Read, and D. J. Jamieson, "Pregnancy and infection," *The New England Journal of Medicine*, vol. 370, no. 23, pp. 2211–2218, 2014.

[39] J. J. N. Noubiap, W. Y. A. Joko, J. R. N. Nansseu, U. G. Tene, and C. Siaka, "Sero-epidemiology of human immunodeficiency virus, hepatitis B and C viruses, and syphilis infections among first-time blood donors in Edéa, Cameroon," *International Journal of Infectious Diseases*, vol. 17, no. 10, pp. e832–e837, 2013.

[40] E. Osaro and A. T. Charles, "The challenges of meeting the blood transfusion requirements in Sub-Saharan Africa: the need for the development of alternatives to allogenic blood," *Journal of Blood Medicine*, vol. 2, pp. 7–21, 2011.

5

Mycoplasma genitalium: An Overlooked Sexually Transmitted Pathogen in Women?

Samsiya Ona,[1] **Rose L. Molina,**[2,3] **and Khady Diouf**[1]

[1]*Department of Obstetrics and Gynecology, Brigham and Women's Hospital, 75 Francis Street, Boston, MA 02115, USA*
[2]*Department of Obstetrics and Gynecology, Beth Israel Deaconess Medical Center, 330 Brookline Avenue, Boston, MA 02215, USA*
[3]*Division of Women's Health, Brigham and Women's Hospital, 1620 Tremont Street, OBC-34, Boston, MA 02120, USA*

Correspondence should be addressed to Samsiya Ona; sona@partners.org

Academic Editor: Louise Hafner

Mycoplasma genitalium is a facultative anaerobic organism and a recognized cause of nongonococcal urethritis in men. In women, *M. genitalium* has been associated with cervicitis, endometritis, pelvic inflammatory disease (PID), infertility, susceptibility to human immunodeficiency virus (HIV), and adverse birth outcomes, indicating a consistent relationship with female genital tract pathology. The global prevalence of *M. genitalium* among symptomatic and asymptomatic sexually active women ranges between 1 and 6.4%. *M. genitalium* may play a role in pathogenesis as an independent sexually transmitted pathogen or by facilitating coinfection with another pathogen. The long-term reproductive consequences of *M. genitalium* infection in asymptomatic individuals need to be investigated further. Though screening for this pathogen is not currently recommended, it should be considered in high-risk populations. Recent guidelines from the Centers for Disease Control regarding first-line treatment for PID do not cover *M. genitalium* but recommend considering treatment in patients without improvement on standard PID regimens. Prospective studies on the prevalence, pathophysiology, and long-term reproductive consequences of *M. genitalium* infection in the general population are needed to determine if screening protocols are necessary. New treatment regimens need to be investigated due to increasing drug resistance.

1. Introduction

M. genitalium was first identified in 1980 from the urethral specimens of two men with nongonococcal urethritis (NGU) [1, 2]. Its prevalence in men presenting with urethritis is between 30 and 40% [1, 3]. Further, the presence of *M. genitalium* in men is associated with a 5.5-fold increased risk of NGU [4, 5]. In women, *M. genitalium* has been linked to cervicitis, endometritis, pelvic inflammatory disease (PID), infertility, human immunodeficiency virus (HIV), and adverse birth outcomes [1]. In the United States, the prevalence of *M. genitalium* among women is thought to be around 1%, slightly higher than *Neisseria gonorrhoeae* prevalence (0.4%) and less than *Chlamydia trachomatis* prevalence (3%) based on a nationally representative sample of young adults [3]. Despite initial contradictory findings regarding the association between *M. genitalium* and female

genital tract pathology [6, 7], several studies have since confirmed this association [1, 3, 8], which has recently been reviewed in a meta-analysis [9]. The development of nucleic acid amplification in the 1990s has facilitated several epidemiologic studies that have examined the association of *M. genitalium* with PID [1, 10, 11]. In the 2015 sexually transmitted infection (STI) treatment guidelines, the Centers for Disease Control (CDC) calls attention to *M. genitalium* as an emerging sexually transmitted pathogen in women [12].

PID is a polymicrobial disease commonly diagnosed in women of reproductive age [13]. The prevalence among women aged 15–44 in the United States declined since 1995 from ~8.6% down to ~5.7% in 2002 and leveled off between 2006 and 2010 at 5% [14]. Although a third to half of PID cases have been associated with *N. gonorrhoeae* and/or *C. trachomatis*, many cases have an unknown etiology [12]. It is well known that PID can lead to serious reproductive problems including infertility, chronic pelvic pain, ectopic pregnancy, and recurrent infections. The independent association between *M. genitalium* and PID confirmed by several studies [15] raises concern that *M. genitalium* may play a pathogenic role, particularly in cases where other STIs are not identified. Thus, there is a need for PID treatment regimens to cover *M. genitalium*. Further complicating management, several studies have now identified *M. genitalium* treatment resistance among infected women [15–18].

Most studies on *M. genitalium* are observational studies of variable sample sizes, some very small, with very few randomized trials. Consequently, some of the study findings may not be transferable to most populations. The prevalence of *M. genitalium* from cohort studies done in high-risk populations is considerably higher than the prevalence found in the general population [1, 2]. *M. genitalium* has also been described in sexually abstinent women, putting into question the criteria for screening for this pathogen.

Our objective is to review the evidence in the literature regarding the association of *M. genitalium* with genital tract pathology in women and to identify needed areas of research regarding the pathophysiology, clinical manifestations, screening, and treatment of this pathogen.

2. Materials and Methods

An initial PubMed search was conducted using the terms "*Mycoplasma genitalium*," "*Mycoplasma genitalium* women," and "prevalence of *Mycoplasma genitalium* in asymptomatic women," which identified 1064 articles. Articles were excluded for lack of relevance by reviewing titles, abstracts, and content. English articles presenting relevant data stratified by sex and conducted exclusively in women were included. As a result, 66 articles were included in this review.

3. Results and Discussion

3.1. Clinical Updates on M. genitalium as a Sexually Transmitted Infection in Women

3.1.1. Epidemiology. *M. genitalium* is one of the most common microorganisms associated with genital tract infections and is increasingly recognized as a STI [1, 19–21]. *M. genitalium* infection has several clinical features consistent with sexual transmission, including higher detection among sexually active individuals compared to sexually naïve adolescents, detection in partners of infected individuals, and predominance in younger individuals with multiple sexual partners and men who have sex with men (particularly those infected with HIV) [1, 3, 8, 19, 22, 23]. Several studies that had identified *Mycoplasma* as a STI have showed statistically significant increased rates of infection among sexually active women, with rate/risk of infection increasing with 2 or more sexual partners. One study reported that the prevalence of *M. genitalium* increases by 10% with each additional sexual partner [3]. It has also been shown that women with infected partners are also at increased risk [3] so sexual activity in itself appears to be a major risk factor but is not the only determinant factor for infection. Further, several studies have shown an independent association between *M. genitalium* and genital infection. It however appears that not all carriers are symptomatic as evidenced by general population studies [24].

Several clinical associations with *M. genitalium* infection have been identified. In one prospective study, *M. genitalium* was found most frequently among women aged ≤24 years, those with a history of abortion, and those with first intercourse after 20 years [35]. This last association seems counterintuitive but may be related to a higher chance of clearing the infection when women are first exposed to the organism at a younger age, although there are no studies to date to support this argument. Overall, most evidence suggests a low prevalence of *M. genitalium* among asymptomatic women [25], which may make screening efforts low-yield [21, 25, 28, 35, 36].

Most of the epidemiological studies on *Mycoplasma* infection have been conducted in high-risk populations, such as symptomatic and asymptomatic patients attending STI clinics. This introduces a sampling bias and limits the conclusions regarding *M. genitalium* as an independent STI in the general population [25, 36].

Table 1 summarizes the studies regarding the prevalence of *M. genitalium*. The prevalence in the general population is not known since routine screening is not done but some studies have estimated the global prevalence of *M. genitalium* among women to range between 1 and 6.4% [37–39]. Prevalence studies have usually included women attending STI clinics or those infected with HIV. Clarivet et al. found a low rate of 0.1% in asymptomatic women [25] whereas Gaydos et al. found a rate close to 20% among women attending STI clinic in Baltimore (~70% of these women were symptomatic) [2]. Studies from adolescent clinics, STI clinics, and emergency departments in the United States have identified *M. genitalium* as a genital tract microorganism in 15–20% of young women reporting genitourinary symptoms or at risk for STIs based on clinical history [13].

M. genitalium coinfection with *C. trachomatis* has also been recognized. In a cross-sectional case-control study, 4.5% of asymptomatic patients were found to be positive for *M. genitalium* [27], and ~5% of individuals infected with *C. trachomatis* were coinfected with *M. genitalium* [27]. Asymptomatic study participants, usually recruited from a convenience group of STI clinic attendees reported no genital tract symptoms [21]. The prevalence was higher among younger women 18–24 years of age compared to older women (7.9% for *C. trachomatis* and 2.4% for *M. genitalium*, resp.) [35].

3.1.2. Clinical Manifestations. *M. genitalium* has been associated with typical PID symptoms such as pelvic pain, abnormal vaginal discharge, fever, nausea, and vomiting. Symptomatic women who are positive for *M. genitalium* are more likely to report postcoital bleeding, which could be due to cervicitis, compared to women negative for the organism (AOR 5.8; 95% CI 1.4–23.3, after adjusting for age and coinfections) [36]. Most *M. genitalium* infections are asymptomatic

TABLE 1: Summary of *M. genitalium* prevalence according to various studies in women.

Source	Study design	Study population	Overall *M. genitalium* prevalence (%)
Gaydos et al. [2]	Cross-sectional study	324 women attending STI clinics in Baltimore. Detected by transcription mediated amplification from vaginal, endocervical, and urine swabs	19.2
Oakeshott et al. [8]	Prospective study	2378 sexually active female students (mean age of 21) followed up between 2004 and 2008 in London. Tested vaginal swabs by PCR	3.3
Haggerty et al. [15]	Multicenter randomized controlled prospective study, PEACH study	Stored cervical and endometrial specimens of 682 women treated with cefoxitin and doxycycline for clinically suspected PID tested by PCR	15
Clarivet et al. [25]	Cross-sectional study	743 asymptomatic women attending free and anonymous STI clinics from April to August 2009. Detected by PCR in first void urine (FVU) sample	0.1
Falk et al. [23]	Cross-sectional study	465 female STI clinic attendees (mean age of 24) in Orebro, Sweden. Tested FVU and endocervical samples by PCR	6
Hancock et al. [26]	Cross-sectional study	1090 women attending the Public Health-Seattle & Kig County STI Clinic in Seattle, WA. *M. genitalium* detected by TMA from self-obtained vaginal swabs	7.7
Bjartling et al. [27]	Cross-sectional case-control study	679 women attending a gynecological outpatient clinic from 2003 through 2008. Tested urine and vaginal swabs by PCR	2.1
Uno et al. [28]	Cross-sectional study	200 women visiting the Obstetrics and Gynecology Department in Kizawa Memorial Hospital and Jaysaki Women's Clinic in Japan. Tested cervical swabs using PCR.	6.8
Gomih-Alakija et al. [29]	Cross-sectional study	350 female sex workers aged 18–50 years in Nairobi, Kenya. Tested cervical samples by TMA	12.9
Bradshaw et al. [30]	Prospective study	313 women attending Melbourne Sexual Health Center, Australia, between March 2005 and November 2007 with cervicitis/pelvic inflammatory disease and sexual contacts of proven *M. genitalium*, infected partners. Cervical, vaginal swabs, or FVU samples analyzed by PCR	10
Andersen et al. [31]	Cross-sectional study	921 women aged 21–23 provided self-collected vaginal samples by PCR	2.3

in women [24] and roughly half of women (56.2%) who test positive for the organism are asymptomatic [37]. Like *C. trachomatis, M. genitalium* can lead to "silent" PID infections with mild symptoms relative to *N. gonorrhoeae* associated PID symptoms [13]. Bjartling et al. found comparable rates of abnormal vaginal wet smear, cervical friability or tenderness, fever, and level of serum C-reactive protein (CRP) between *M. genitalium*-positive women and negative controls [27]. However, *M. genitalium*-positive women were more likely to report postcoital bleeding than the negative controls [AOR 2.00 (1.10–3.61)]. Further, women with *M. genitalium* were more likely to have combined cervical tenderness, postcoital bleeding, and abnormal vaginal discharge [AOR 2.71 (1.50–4.90)] compared to women not infected with *M. genitalium* [27].

3.1.3. M. genitalium: An Emerging Cause of Pelvic Inflammatory Disease (PID). PID is an inflammatory disease that can

include one or more of the following conditions: endometritis, salpingitis, tuboovarian abscess, and pelvic peritonitis. PID is described as a polymicrobial syndrome, mainly caused by anaerobic bacterial species [1]. *N. gonorrhoeae* and *C. trachomatis* are the most commonly diagnosed organisms in PID, yet up to 70% of cases are of indeterminate etiology [1, 40]. Organisms of the vaginal flora such as *Mycoplasma, Ureaplasma, Gardnerella vaginalis, Escherichia coli,* and anaerobes have also been associated with PID. With the development of nucleic acid amplification tests (NAATs), the incidence of biopsy-proven endometritis or clinical PID associated with *M. genitalium* has increased [1, 27]. Women positive for *M. genitalium* were found to be twice as likely to have histology-proven endometritis than women testing negative after adjusting for age, race, *N. gonorrhoeae,* and *C. trachomatis* [AOR 2.0 (1.0 to 4.2)] [15, 41]. Despite being less studied, postabortal PID has been shown to be strongly associated with *M. genitalium* [AOR 6.3 (1.6–25.3)] [1, 13]. Several cross-sectional studies have investigated the independent association between *M. genitalium* and PID. For example, one prospective study reported a thirteenfold increased incidence of endometritis in the presence of *M. genitalium* at 30-day follow-up visits among an urban population of women in the United States with clinical PID without concurrent *N. gonorrhoeae* and *C. trachomatis* infection [15]. A recent meta-analysis shows pooled odds ratios of 1.66 [95% CI, 1.35–2.04] for cervicitis and 2.43 for infertility [95% CI, .93–6.34] among *M. genitalium* infected women [9].

3.1.4. Mycoplasma genitalium and Its Association with Other STIs and Malignancies.

M. genitalium has been associated with increased susceptibility to HIV infection [42, 43]. Unlike most other *Mycoplasma* species, *M. genitalium* can attach to the surface of epithelial cells and invade the cells with a specialized tip structure [4]. In an *in vitro* model, Das et al. showed that *M. genitalium* increased the risk of HIV infection by infecting the epithelial layer, reducing its integrity, and activating HIV cell targets beyond the epithelial layer, thereby promoting transmission and reproduction within the host and increasing viral shedding through mucosal surfaces [42]. Vandepitte et al. in their nested case-control study found evidence of a temporal relationship between *M. genitalium* and HIV acquisition [43]. The association was only found among the subgroup that was tested for *M. genitalium* three months prior to first HIV-positive results compared to the group with earlier HIV testing (aOR = 7.19; 95% CI 1.68 to 30.77) [43]. Further studies have shown a positive association between *M. genitalium* and high-risk human papilloma virus (HR-HPV) infection. For example, one study of female sex workers showed that 39.6% were positive for *M. genitalium* and HR-HPV [29]. In addition, Zarei et al. have demonstrated an association between chronic *M. genitalium* infection and ovarian cancer and lymphoma [44]. However, these studies did not control for the sexual behavior of women and their partners, limiting the generalizability of the results.

3.1.5. Mycoplasma in Pregnancy.

All *Mycoplasma* species have been associated with perinatal morbidity and mortality [45]. A US-based cohort study demonstrated a 2.5-fold increase in preterm birth in women with *M. genitalium* infection who presented with contractions between 23 and 32 weeks of gestation compared to noninfected women (AOR 2.5; 95% CI 1.2–6.0) [1]. In a meta-analysis of six studies, *M. genitalium* was associated with preterm birth with a pooled OR of 1.89 (95% CI, 1.25–2.85) and also associated with spontaneous abortion with a pooled OR of 1.82 (95% CI, 1.10–3.03) [9].

Of the *Mycoplasmas*, *M. hominis* and *Ureaplasma* have been most associated with chorioamnionitis and are thought to contribute to these adverse effects [45]. While *M. hominis* has not been associated with PID, it has been associated with upper respiratory infections, nervous system infections, neonatal bacteremia, and meningoencephalitis, unlike *M. genitalium* [46].

3.1.6. Diagnosis and Screening

Mycoplasma Diagnosis. *M. genitalium* is a small bacterium of the Mollicutes class with no cell wall and a genome of only 580 kilobases in size [1, 47]. Consequently, it cannot be detected by gram stain and is extremely difficult to culture requiring up to 6 months for growth [12]. Its genome is most similar to *Mycoplasma pneumonia* [48], which causes atypical bacterial pneumonia. Currently there is no FDA-approved diagnostic test for *M. genitalium* [1]. Given the difficulty with culturing the organism and the lack of standardized serological tests for *M. genitalium*, NAATs in the form of polymerase chain reaction (PCR) assays are almost exclusively carried out for the diagnosis of *M. genitalium* in the research setting. Some PCR assays have demonstrated >95% specificity and sensitivity [49]. A recent study reported loop-mediated isothermal amplification (LAMP) as a novel NAAT, which has similar sensitivity to a PCR assay [50].

To date four types of specimens can be collected for the detection of *M. genitalium*: vaginal swab, first void urine, and endocervical and rectal swabs. Some studies in the United States have shown that NAATs with vaginal swab specimens have the highest relative sensitivity compared to urine and endocervical specimens [10, 51]. Further, self-obtained vaginal swabs have been found to yield similar test sensitivities to clinician-obtained specimens [10]. In an earlier study conducted in Seattle, WA, among symptomatic women attending a STI clinic, the specimen with the highest sensitivities was the vaginal specimen PCR: reported sensitivities were 91%, 53%, and 65% for vaginal, cervical, and urine specimens, respectively [51]. In a subsequent cross-sectional study among women attending a STI clinic in New Orleans, the relative sensitivity of PCR was 85.7% for the vaginal swab specimen, 74.3% for the endocervical swab specimen, 61.4% for the urine specimen, and 24.3% for the rectal swab specimen for the detection of *M. genitalium* in women [10]. Consequently, vaginal swabs are currently the most commonly used specimens for detecting *M. genitalium* through PCR.

To Screen or Not to Screen. The 2015 CDC sexually transmitted disease treatment guidelines recommend that all women diagnosed with PID should also be tested for HIV, gonorrhea, and chlamydia [12]. There are no recommendations regarding *M. genitalium* screening given the lack of data around the utility of screening and the lack of a FDA-approved testing modality for commercial use [12].

Given the higher prevalence of *M. genitalium* in high-risk women [1] and its reported association with PID, infertility, and adverse pregnancy outcomes, it would be reasonable to test symptomatic women for *M. genitalium* if NAAT is available. Further, in patients whose symptoms are refractory to appropriate antibiotic therapy for PID, cervicitis, and endometritis, testing for *M. genitalium* may be clinically beneficial and indicated based on current data.

There is ongoing debate regarding possible cost, benefits, and harm of universal screening for *M. genitalium* among asymptomatic patients given that most carriers are likely asymptomatic. Given limited data, this decision should be based on a discussion between providers and patients in the context of personal risk factors, as official screening recommendations will not be made until better quality data on cost, harm, and benefits are available.

3.2. Treating M. genitalium Infection. Azithromycin and doxycycline are the current first-line treatment for cervicitis and NGU [5]. One of the initial randomized controlled trials on *Mycoplasma genitalium* treatment reported more effective treatment with a single 1 g of azithromycin compared to doxycycline 100 mg BID for 7 days in the USA [52]. Cure rates with azithromycin ranged from 67 to 87% [5]. However, higher treatment failures with single 1 g of azithromycin were reported with a decline in efficacy down to 60% [53, 54] and to 39% in the most recent study [55]. Treatment failure with azithromycin is due to an isolated point mutation on 23 rRNA gene in numerous *M. genitalium* populations [17], with up to 50% of cases reported [12].

Due to these poor efficacy rates, alternative azithromycin regimens have been investigated [5]. Several studies have examined an extended 1.5 g azithromycin (500 mg on day 1, followed by 250 mg daily for 4 days) and a single higher dose of 2 g azithromycin once with the rationale that an extended azithromycin-containing regimen decreases the risk of acquired macrolide resistance when initiated first-line among patients without preexisting macrolide resistance. A similar trend has also been noted with doxycycline [52]. Unfortunately, a recent randomized controlled trial found declining microbiological cure rate for the extended regimen and single 2 g regimen to 25–81% (wide range based on different studies) and 73%, respectively [5].

In light of the rising azithromycin resistance, moxifloxacin had been introduced as a second-line treatment option. Moxifloxacin, a fluoroquinolone, was thought to be a reliable alternative with a reported 100% cure rate initially [30, 56]. According to the 2015 CDC guidelines, women with PID who do not respond to the first-line treatment within 7–10 days should be considered as possibly infected with *M. genitalium* and treated with moxifloxacin 400 mg/day for 14 days [12, 57]. It is not used as first-line due to more significant adverse effects associated with moxifloxacin relative to azithromycin, such as tendon rupture, although these significant adverse effects remain rare. However, as of 2013, increasing treatment failures have also been noted due to bacterial resistance to moxifloxacin with failure rates ranging between 10% and 15% [17, 18, 58]. Given increasing moxifloxacin resistance, monotherapy has the potential to increase the risk of multidrug-resistant strains.

Other fluoroquinolones that have been investigated and proven to remain effective include gatifloxacin and sitafloxacin [59]. Other fluoroquinolones such as gemifloxacin, sparfloxacin, grepafloxacin, trovafloxacin, and garenoxacin have been shown to be effective against *M. genitalium in vitro* but lack human studies [59]. Ciprofloxacin, ofloxacin, and levofloxacin reportedly have poor activity against the microbe relative to moxifloxacin [59]. Pristinamycin is a streptogramin that is used to treat vancomycin-resistant *Enterococcus faecium* bacteremia and complicated skin infections due to MRSA [60]. Treatment

of *M. genitalium* with pristinamycin (1 g 6 hourly for 10 days) led to negative PCR results 28 days after treatment [60]. This regimen appears promising for the treatment of multidrug-resistant *M. genitalium* but has not been well studied to inform optimal dosing and is reportedly expensive with limited availability [60].

Given the organism's propensity for drug resistance, follow-up testing to document treatment response is reasonable. Some authors advocate for a test of cure (TOC) in 3-4 weeks after treatment with resistance profiling in those with persistent infection despite treatment [16]. Most studies on TOC have been conducted in men, with fewer studies done in women. A retrospective cohort study performed TOC at 1 month from the initiation of therapy with azithromycin-containing regimens to identify resistant infections [61]. However, a later prospective cohort study investigated the optimal time for TOC and reported negative TOC within an average of 14 days (12–15 days) for infected patients that were susceptible to a single 1 g of azithromycin, which was used as the first-line treatment [55]. Those that appeared resistant were further treated with moxifloxacin 400 mg daily for 10 days with a negative TOC at 28 days for responders [55]. Furthermore, Falk et al. showed that individuals treated with azithromycin had a negative PCR within 8 days and those treated with moxifloxacin had a negative PCR within 1 week [62]. However, it was further discussed that early negative PCR may be related to low DNA levels for detection soon after treatment initiation with resistance detected at 10 days after treatment initiation with azithromycin and eventually recolonization requiring further treatment [62]. Hence it was concluded that optimal timing for the most reliable TOC should take place 3-4 weeks after treatment [62], which correlates with an earlier Japanese study performed among men [63].

Testing and/or empirical treatment of partners within the preceding 60 days of diagnosis are also strongly recommended for women with confirmed positive *M. genitalium* to prevent reinfection [12]. Partners are recommended to abstain from sexual intercourse until adequate treatment is completed and symptoms resolve if initially present [12]. There is no specific evidence regarding the utility of condom use in these circumstances.

3.3. Long-Term Sequelae of M. genitalium Infection. The long-term reproductive consequences of *M. genitalium* infection have not been clearly determined. However, the association with PID indicates that infertility, chronic pelvic pain, and risk of ectopic pregnancy may be potential sequelae of infection with this pathogen like for *C. trachomatis* and *N. gonorrhoeae* infection [64]. This may be another argument for screening in certain populations. Table 2 summarizes the studies that investigated the association between *M. genitalium* and infertility. *M. genitalium* can persist for months or years in infected individuals [65]. In a recent meta-analysis, it had been reported that women carrying *M. genitalium* infection are usually asymptomatic with reported estimated clearance rate of 15 months based on a large London study [24]. Despite spontaneous clearance, chronic infection may lead to tissue damage prior to clearance causing long-term

TABLE 2: Summary of studies regarding *M. genitalium* and female infertility.

Source	Study design	Study population	Findings
Clausen et al. [32]	Cross-sectional study	308 women undergoing IVF treatment in Aarhus, Denmark	*M. genitalium* was detected in 22% of women with tubal factor infertility (TFI) versus 6.3% in women without TFI
Tosh et al. [19]	Multicenter (North America) randomized controlled prospective study, PEACH study	Stored cervical and endometrial specimens of 682 women treated with cefoxitin and doxycycline for clinically suspected PID	*M. genitalium* was associated with baseline endometritis (AOR 3.0, 95% CI 1.5 to 6.1). Nonsignificant trend towards increased infertility, chronic pelvic pain and recurrent PID, decreased pregnancy, and live birth were found in this study.
Svenstrup et al. [33]	Prospective study	212 couples attending a fertility clinic in Horsens-Brædstrup or the Holstebro fertility clinic in Denmark	*M. genitalium* was found to be independently associated with TFI (AOR 4.5, 95% CI 1.2–15.6)
Grześko et al. [34]	Prospective study	51 patients with primary infertility (24 women with idiopathic infertility) and 23 women with proven fertility	*M. genitalium* was found in 19.6% of all infertile women and 4.4% of fertile women ($P = 0.156$); 29.2% among women with idiopathic infertility versus 4.4% in fertile women ($P = 0.0479$)

health problems. Reinfection due to the partner's carrier state may also lead to reinfection leading to more chronic infection. The PID Evaluation and Clinical Health (PEACH) Study is a multicenter, randomized prospective clinical trial, the largest treatment trial of mild to moderate acute PID in the United States, involving 586 women in several centers in North America who presented with signs and symptoms of PID [41]. This study showed higher rates of infertility (22%), chronic pelvic pain (42%), and recurrent PID (31%) among women in whom *M. genitalium* had been detected on endometrial samples by PCR compared to women testing negative, but these findings were not statistically significant [15, 41]. It is unclear whether the increased risk of other infections such as chlamydia or gonorrhea lead to infertility or if *M. genitalium* itself primarily leads to infertility. Given that untreated PID can lead to long-term adverse reproductive outcomes, *M. genitalium* may contribute to adverse effects on the reproductive tract. One prospective study identified strong *M. genitalium* antibody responses among women with a diagnosis of infertility that were asymptomatic, suggesting an adverse effect of *M. genitalium* on fertility [33]. Another prospective study showed that fertile women were less likely to have PCR-proven *M. genitalium* infection compared to women with idiopathic infertility (4.4% versus 29.2%, $P = 0.0479$) [34]. Consequently, some authors would recommend screening for *M. genitalium* as part of the STI work-up given possible adverse effects such as infertility, chronic pelvic disease, risk of ectopic pregnancy, and preterm labor as well as any other health consequence associated with PID. However, evidence regarding other reproductive sequelae is even more limited, and the few studies that have evaluated reproductive sequelae have not shown any statistically significant difference between women with and without *M. genitalium* infection [41]. A single case-control study on risk of ectopic pregnancy did not find any significant association either (OR 1.0, 95% CI 0.5–2.0) [66]. Well-powered prospective studies

that control for other genital tract infections and compare *M. genitalium* cases to asymptomatic noninfected women are needed to establish the long-term reproductive consequences of chronic *M. genitalium* infection.

4. Conclusions and Areas for Future Research

M. genitalium is now increasingly recognized as a STI and has been associated with PID, endometritis, cervicitis, and HIV in women though clinical manifestations and risk factors overlap with other STIs. The availability of NAAT for PCR detection of this organism will allow further investigation into the effects of *M. genitalium* infection on long-term reproductive health outcomes such as infertility, chronic pelvic pain, ectopic pregnancy, and obstetric outcomes such as preterm deliveries. Due to antibiotic resistance patterns, alternatives to azithromycin and moxifloxacin must be investigated. In the interim, clinicians should consider testing for and treating *M. genitalium* on a case-by-case basis, particularly in women diagnosed with PID or cervicitis without clinical improvement using standard regimens.

Competing Interests

The authors declare that there is no conflict of interests regarding the publication of this paper.

References

[1] L. E. Manhart, "*Mycoplasma genitalium*: an emergent sexually transmitted disease?" *Infectious Disease Clinics of North America*, vol. 27, no. 4, pp. 779–792, 2013.

[2] C. Gaydos, N. E. Maldeis, A. Hardick, J. Hardick, and T. C. Quinn, "*Mycoplasma genitalium* as a contributor to the multiple etiologies of cervicitis in women attending sexually transmitted

disease clinics," *Sexually Transmitted Diseases*, vol. 36, no. 10, pp. 598–606, 2009.

[3] L. E. Manhart, K. K. Holmes, J. P. Hughes, L. S. Houston, and P. A. Totten, "*Mycoplasma genitalium* among young adults in the United States: an emerging sexually transmitted infection," *American Journal of Public Health*, vol. 97, no. 6, pp. 1118–1125, 2007.

[4] D. Taylor-Robinson and J. S. Jensen, "*Mycoplasma genitalium*: from chrysalis to multicolored butterfly," *Clinical Microbiology Reviews*, vol. 24, no. 3, pp. 498–514, 2011.

[5] L. E. Manhart, J. S. Jensen, C. S. Bradshaw, M. R. Golden, and D. H. Martin, "Efficacy of antimicrobial therapy for *Mycoplasma genitalium* infections," *Clinical Infectious Diseases*, vol. 61, supplement 8, pp. S802–S817, 2015.

[6] J. E. Korte, J. B. Baseman, M. P. Cagle et al., "Cervicitis and genitourinary symptoms in women culture positive for *Mycoplasma genitalium*," *American Journal of Reproductive Immunology*, vol. 55, no. 4, pp. 265–275, 2006.

[7] M. J. Schlicht, S. D. Lovrich, J. S. Sartin, P. Karpinsky, S. M. Callister, and W. A. Agger, "High prevalence of genital mycoplasmas among sexually active young adults with urethritis or cervicitis symptoms in La Crosse, Wisconsin," *Journal of Clinical Microbiology*, vol. 42, no. 10, pp. 4636–4640, 2004.

[8] P. Oakeshott, A. Aghaizu, P. Hay et al., "Is Mycoplasma genitalium in women the 'new chlamydia?' A community-based prospective cohort study," *Clinical Infectious Diseases*, vol. 51, no. 10, pp. 1160–1166, 2010.

[9] R. Lis, A. Rowhani-Rahbar, and L. E. Manhart, "*Mycoplasma genitalium* infection and female reproductive tract disease: a meta-analysis," *Clinical Infectious Diseases*, vol. 61, no. 3, pp. 418–426, 2015.

[10] R. A. Lillis, M. J. Nsuami, L. Myers, and D. H. Martin, "Utility of urine, vaginal, cervical, and rectal specimens for detection of *Mycoplasma genitalium* in women," *Journal of Clinical Microbiology*, vol. 49, no. 5, pp. 1990–1992, 2011.

[11] V. L. Mobley, M. M. Hobbs, K. Lau, B. S. Weinbaum, D. K. Getman, and A. C. Seña, "*Mycoplasma genitalium* infection in women attending a sexually transmitted infection clinic: diagnostic specimen type, coinfections, and predictors," *Sexually Transmitted Diseases*, vol. 39, no. 9, pp. 706–709, 2012.

[12] K. A. Workowski and G. A. Bolan, "Sexually transmitted diseases treatment guidelines, 2015," *MMWR Recommendations and Reports*, vol. 64, no. 3, pp. 1–137, 2015.

[13] C. L. Haggerty and B. D. Taylor, "*Mycoplasma genitalium*: an emerging cause of pelvic inflammatory disease," *Infectious Diseases in Obstetrics and Gynecology*, vol. 2011, Article ID 959816, 9 pages, 2011.

[14] STDs in Women and Infants—2014 STD Surveillance. (n.d.), March 2016, http://www.cdc.gov/std/stats14/womenandinf.htm#pid.

[15] C. L. Haggerty, P. A. Totten, S. G. Astete et al., "Failure of cefoxitin and doxycycline to eradicate endometrial *Mycoplasma genitalium* and the consequence for clinical cure of pelvic inflammatory disease," *Sexually Transmitted Infections*, vol. 84, no. 5, pp. 338–342, 2008.

[16] P. Horner, K. Blee, and E. Adams, "Time to manage *Mycoplasma genitalium* as an STI: but not with azithromycin 1 g!," *Current Opinion in Infectious Diseases*, vol. 27, no. 1, pp. 68–74, 2014.

[17] K. A. Tagg, N. J. Jeoffreys, D. L. Couldwell, J. A. Donald, and G. L. Gilbert, "Fluoroquinolone and macrolide resistance-associated mutations in *Mycoplasma genitalium*," *Journal of Clinical Microbiology*, vol. 51, no. 7, pp. 2245–2249, 2013.

[18] D. Chrisment, A. Charron, C. Cazanave, S. Pereyre, and C. Bébéar, "Detection of macrolide resistance in *Mycoplasma genitalium* in France," *The Journal of Antimicrobial Chemotherapy*, vol. 67, no. 11, pp. 2598–2601, 2012.

[19] A. K. Tosh, B. Van Der Pol, J. D. Fortenberry et al., "*Mycoplasma genitalium* among adolescent women and their partners," *Journal of Adolescent Health*, vol. 40, no. 5, pp. 412–417, 2007.

[20] A. R. Thurman, O. Musatovova, S. Perdue, R. N. Shain, J. G. Baseman, and J. B. Baseman, "*Mycoplasma genitalium* symptoms, concordance and treatment in high-risk sexual dyads," *International Journal of STD & AIDS*, vol. 21, no. 3, pp. 177–183, 2010.

[21] J. D. C. Ross, L. Brown, P. Saunders, and S. Alexander, "*Mycoplasma genitalium* in asymptomatic patients: implications for screening," *Sexually Transmitted Infections*, vol. 85, no. 6, pp. 436–437, 2009.

[22] B. Andersen, I. Sokolowski, L. Østergaard, J. K. Møller, F. Olesen, and J. S. Jensen, "*Mycoplasma qenitalium*: prevalence and behavioural risk factors in the general population," *Sexually Transmitted Infections*, vol. 83, no. 3, pp. 237–241, 2007.

[23] L. Falk, H. Fredlund, and J. S. Jensen, "Signs and symptoms of urethritis and cervicitis among women with or without *Mycoplasma genitalium* or *Chlamydia trachomatis* infection," *Sexually Transmitted Infections*, vol. 81, no. 1, pp. 73–78, 2005.

[24] T. Smieszek and P. J. White, "Apparently-different clearance rates from cohort studies of mycoplasma genitalium are consistent after accounting for incidence of infection, recurrent infection, and study design," *PLoS ONE*, vol. 11, no. 2, Article ID 0149087, 2016.

[25] B. Clarivet, E. Picot, H. Marchandin et al., "Prevalence of *Chlamydia trachomatis*, *Neisseria gonorrhoeae* and *Mycoplasma genitalium* in asymptomatic patients under 30 years of age screened in a French sexually transmitted infections clinic," *European Journal of Dermatology*, vol. 24, no. 5, pp. 611–616, 2014.

[26] E. B. Hancock, L. E. Manhart, S. J. Nelson, R. Kerani, J. K. H. Wroblewski, and P. A. Totten, "Comprehensive assessment of sociodemographic and behavioral risk factors for *Mycoplasma genitalium* infection in women," *Sexually Transmitted Diseases*, vol. 37, no. 12, pp. 777–783, 2010.

[27] C. Bjartling, S. Osser, and K. Persson, "*Mycoplasma genitalium* in cervicitis and pelvic inflammatory disease among women at a gynecologic outpatient service," *American Journal of Obstetrics and Gynecology*, vol. 206, no. 6, pp. 476.e1–476.e8, 2012.

[28] M. Uno, T. Deguchi, H. Komeda et al., "*Mycoplasma genitalium* in the cervices of Japanese women," *Sexually Transmitted Diseases*, vol. 24, no. 5, pp. 284–286, 1997.

[29] A. Gomih-Alakija, J. Ting, N. Mugo et al., "Clinical characteristics associated with *Mycoplasma genitalium* among female sex workers in nairobi, Kenya," *Journal of Clinical Microbiology*, vol. 52, no. 10, pp. 3660–3666, 2014.

[30] C. S. Bradshaw, M. Y. Chen, and C. K. Fairley, "Persistence of *Mycoplasma genitalium* following azithromycin therapy," *PLoS ONE*, vol. 3, no. 11, Article ID e3618, 2008.

[31] B. Andersen, I. Sokolowski, L. Østergaard, J. Kjølseth Møller, F. Olesen, and J. S. Jensen, "*Mycoplasma genitalium*: prevalence and behavioural risk factors in the general population," *Sexually Transmitted Infections*, vol. 83, no. 3, pp. 237–241, 2007.

[32] H. F. Clausen, J. Fedder, M. Drasbek et al., "Serological investigation of *Mycoplasma genitalium* in infertile women," *Human Reproduction*, vol. 16, no. 9, pp. 1866–1874, 2001.

[33] H. F. Svenstrup, J. Fedder, S. E. Kristoffersen, B. Trolle, S. Birkelund, and G. Christiansen, "*Mycoplasma genitalium, Chlamydia trachomatis*, and tubal factor infertility-a prospective study," *Fertility and Sterility*, vol. 90, no. 3, pp. 513–520, 2008.

[34] J. Grześko, M. Elias, B. Maczyńska, U. Kasprzykowska, M. Tłaczała, and M. Goluda, "Occurrence of *Mycoplasma genitalium* in fertile and infertile women," *Fertility and Sterility*, vol. 91, no. 6, pp. 2376–2380, 2009.

[35] O. Peuchant, C. Le Roy, C. Desveaux et al., "Screening for *Chlamydia trachomatis, Neisseria gonorrhoeae*, and *Mycoplasma genitalium* should it be integrated into routine pregnancy care in French young pregnant women?" *Diagnostic Microbiology and Infectious Disease*, vol. 82, no. 1, pp. 14–19, 2015.

[36] P. Sonnenberg, C. A. Ison, S. Clifton et al., "Epidemiology of *Mycoplasma genitalium* in British men and women aged 16-44 years: evidence from the third National Survey of Sexual Attitudes and Lifestyles (Natsal-3)," *International Journal of Epidemiology*, vol. 44, no. 6, pp. 1982–1994, 2015.

[37] C. Cazanave, L. E. Manhart, and C. Bébéar, "*Mycoplasma genitalium*, an emerging sexually transmitted pathogen," *Médecine et Maladies Infectieuses*, vol. 42, no. 9, pp. 381–392, 2012.

[38] J. Walker, C. K. Fairley, C. S. Bradshaw et al., "*Mycoplasma genitalium* incidence, organism load, and treatment failure in a cohort of young Australian women," *Clinical Infectious Diseases*, vol. 56, no. 8, pp. 1094–1100, 2013.

[39] H. F. Svenstrup, S. S. Dave, C. Carder et al., "A cross-sectional study of *Mycoplasma genitalium* infection and correlates in women undergoing population-based screening or clinic-based testing for Chlamydia infection in London," *BMJ Open*, vol. 4, no. 2, Article ID e003947, 2014.

[40] R. Quentin and R. Verdon, "Microbiologic basis of diagnosis and treatment of pelvic inflammatory disease," *Journal de Gynecologie Obstetrique et Biologie de la Reproduction*, vol. 41, no. 8, pp. 850–863, 2012.

[41] R. B. Ness, D. E. Soper, J. Peipert et al., "Design of the PID Evaluation and Clinical Health (PEACH) study," *Controlled Clinical Trials*, vol. 19, no. 5, pp. 499–514, 1998.

[42] K. Das, G. De la Garza, E. B. Siwak, V. L. Scofield, and S. Dhandayuthapani, "*Mycoplasma genitalium* promotes epithelial crossing and peripheral blood mononuclear cell infection by HIV-1," *International Journal of Infectious Diseases*, vol. 23, pp. e31–e38, 2014.

[43] J. Vandepitte, H. A. Weiss, J. Bukenya et al., "Association between *Mycoplasma genitalium* infection and HIV acquisition among female sex workers in Uganda: evidence from a nested case-control study," *Sexually Transmitted Infections*, vol. 90, no. 7, pp. 545–549, 2014.

[44] O. Zarei, S. Rezania, and A. Mousavi, "*Mycoplasma genitalium* and cancer: a brief review," *Asian Pacific Journal of Cancer Prevention*, vol. 14, no. 6, pp. 3425–3428, 2013.

[45] D. Taylor-Robinson and R. F. Lamont, "Mycoplasmas in pregnancy," *BJOG: An International Journal of Obstetrics and Gynaecology*, vol. 118, no. 2, pp. 164–174, 2011.

[46] K. B. Waites, R. L. Schelonka, L. Xiao, P. L. Grigsby, and M. J. Novy, "Congenital and opportunistic infections: ureaplasma species and *Mycoplasma hominis*," *Seminars in Fetal and Neonatal Medicine*, vol. 14, no. 4, pp. 190–199, 2009.

[47] J. G. Tully, D. Taylor-Robinson, R. M. Cole, and D. L. Rose, "A newly discovered mycoplasma in the human urogenital tract," *The Lancet*, vol. 317, no. 8233, pp. 1288–1291, 1981.

[48] H. F. Svenstrup, J. S. Jensen, E. Björnelius, P. Lidbrink, S. Birkelund, and G. Christiansen, "Development of quantitative real-time PCR assay for detection of *Mycoplasma genitalium*," *Journal of Clinical Microbiology*, vol. 43, no. 7, pp. 3121–3128, 2005.

[49] S. A. Weinstein and B. G. Stiles, "A review of the epidemiology, diagnosis and evidence-based management of *Mycoplasma genitalium*," *Sexual Health*, vol. 8, no. 2, pp. 143–158, 2011.

[50] T. Edwards, P. Burke, H. B. Smalley et al., "Loop-mediated isothermal amplification (LAMP) for the rapid detection of *Mycoplasma genitalium*," *Diagnostic Microbiology and Infectious Disease*, vol. 83, no. 1, pp. 13–17, 2015.

[51] J. K. H. Wroblewski, L. E. Manhart, K. A. Dickey, M. K. Hudspeth, and P. A. Totten, "Comparison of transcription-mediated amplification and PCR assay results for various genital specimen types for detection of *Mycoplasma genitalium*," *Journal of Clinical Microbiology*, vol. 44, no. 9, pp. 3306–3312, 2006.

[52] L. A. Mena, T. F. Mroczkowski, M. Nsuami, and D. H. Martin, "A randomized comparison of azithromycin and doxycycline for the treatment of *Mycoplasma genitalium*-positive urethritis in men," *Clinical Infectious Diseases*, vol. 48, no. 12, pp. 1649–1654, 2009.

[53] C. S. Bradshaw, J. S. Jensen, S. N. Tabrizi et al., "Azithromycin failure in *Mycoplasma genitalium* urethritis," *Emerging Infectious Diseases*, vol. 12, no. 7, pp. 1149–1152, 2006.

[54] A. Lau, C. S. Bradshaw, D. Lewis et al., "The efficacy of azithromycin for the treatment of genital *Mycoplasma genitalium*: a systematic review and meta-analysis," *Clinical Infectious Diseases*, vol. 61, no. 9, pp. 1389–1399, 2015.

[55] M. Bissessor, S. N. Tabrizi, J. Twin et al., "Macrolide resistance and azithromycin failure in a *Mycoplasma genitalium*-infected cohort and response of azithromycin failures to alternative antibiotic regimens," *Clinical Infectious Diseases*, vol. 60, no. 8, pp. 1228–1236, 2015.

[56] E. Jernberg, A. Moghaddam, and H. Moi, "Azithromycin and moxifloxacin for microbiological cure of *Mycoplasma genitalium* infection: an open study," *International Journal of STD & AIDS*, vol. 19, no. 10, pp. 676–679, 2008.

[57] J. D. C. Ross, H. S. Cronjé, T. Paszkowski et al., "Moxifloxacin versus ofloxacin plus metronidazole in uncomplicated pelvic inflammatory disease: results of a multicentre, double blind, randomised trial," *Sexually Transmitted Infections*, vol. 82, no. 6, pp. 446–451, 2006.

[58] D. L. Couldwell, K. A. Tagg, N. J. Jeoffreys, and G. L. Gilbert, "Failure of moxifloxacin treatment in *Mycoplasma genitalium* infections due to macrolide and fluoroquinolone resistance," *International Journal of STD and AIDS*, vol. 24, no. 10, pp. 822–828, 2013.

[59] T. Deguchi, M. Kikuchi, M. Yasuda, and S. Ito, "Sitafloxacin: antimicrobial activity against ciprofloxacin-selected laboratory mutants of *Mycoplasma genitalium* and inhibitory activity against its DNA gyrase and topoisomerase IV," *Journal of Infection and Chemotherapy*, vol. 21, no. 1, pp. 74–75, 2015.

[60] D. L. Couldwell and D. A. Lewis, "*Mycoplasma genitalium* infection: current treatment options, therapeutic failure, and resistance-associated mutations," *Infection and Drug Resistance*, vol. 8, pp. 147–161, 2016.

[61] Z. Gundevia, R. Foster, M. S. Jamil, and A. McNulty, "Positivity at test of cure following first-line treatment for genital *Mycoplasma genitalium*: follow-up of a clinical cohort," *Sexually Transmitted Infections*, vol. 91, no. 1, pp. 11–13, 2015.

[62] L. Falk, M. Enger, and J. S. Jensen, "Time to eradication of *Mycoplasma genitalium* after antibiotic treatment in men and

women," *The Journal of Antimicrobial Chemotherapy*, vol. 70, no. 11, pp. 3134–3140, 2015.

[63] S. Ito, K. Mizutani, K. Seike et al., "Prediction of the persistence of *Mycoplasma genitalium* after antimicrobial chemotherapy by quantification of leukocytes in firstvoid urine from patients with non-gonococcal urethritis," *Journal of Infection and Chemotherapy*, vol. 20, no. 5, pp. 298–302, 2014.

[64] L. Westrom, R. Joesoef, G. Reynolds, A. Hagdu, and S. E. Thompson, "Pelvic inflammatory disease and fertility: a cohort study of 1,844 women with laparoscopically verified disease and 657 control women with normal laparoscopic results," *Sexually Transmitted Diseases*, vol. 19, no. 4, pp. 185–192, 1992.

[65] J. Vandepitte, H. A. Weiss, N. Kyakuwa et al., "Natural history of *Mycoplasma genitalium* infection in a cohort of female sex workers in Kampala, Uganda," *Sexually Transmitted Diseases*, vol. 40, no. 5, pp. 422–427, 2013.

[66] M. Jurstrand, J. S. Jensen, A. Magnuson, F. Kamwendo, and H. Fredlund, "A serological study of the role of *Mycoplasma genitalium* in pelvic inflammatory disease and ectopic pregnancy," *Sexually Transmitted Infections*, vol. 83, no. 4, pp. 319–323, 2007.

6

Lights and Shadows about the Effectiveness of IVF in HIV Infected Women

Catarina Marques,[1] Cristina Guerreiro,[2] and Sérgio Reis Soares[3]

[1]*Maternidade Dr. Alfredo da Costa, Rua Viriato, 1069-089 Lisboa, Portugal*
[2]*Fetal Maternal Department, Maternidade Dr. Alfredo da Costa, Lisbon, Portugal*
[3]*Instituto Valenciano de Infertilidade (IVI-Lisboa), Lisbon, Portugal*

Correspondence should be addressed to Catarina Marques; catarinaomarques@gmail.com

Academic Editor: Susan Cu-Uvin

Background. HIV infected women have higher rates of infertility. *Objective*. The purpose of this literature review is to evaluate the effectiveness of fresh IVF/ICSI cycles in HIV infected women. *Materials and Methods*. A search of the PubMed database was performed to identify studies assessing fresh nondonor oocyte IVF/ICSI cycle outcomes of serodiscordant couples with an HIV infected female partner. *Results and Discussion*. Ten studies met the inclusion criteria. Whenever a comparison with a control group was available, with the exception of one case, ovarian stimulation cancelation rate was higher and pregnancy rate (PR) was lower in HIV infected women. However, statistically significant differences in both rates were only seen in one and two studies, respectively. A number of noncontrolled sources of bias for IVF outcome were identified. This fact, added to the small size of samples studied and heterogeneity in study design and methodology, still hampers the performance of a meta-analysis on the issue. *Conclusion*. Prospective matched case-control studies are necessary for the understanding of the specific effects of HIV infection on ovarian response and ART outcome.

1. Introduction

The human immunodeficiency virus (HIV) epidemic arose from zoonotic infections with simian immunodeficiency viruses from African primates. Since then, the global epidemiology of HIV infection has changed markedly: the prevalence of HIV has increased from 31 million in 2002 to 36.9 million in 2014, essentially due to prolonged survival caused by antiretroviral therapy, whereas the global incidence has decreased from 3.3 million in 2002 to 2 million in 2014 [1].

Since the introduction of antiretroviral therapies, two major medical achievements have been made, allowing many couples with an HIV positive partner to consider pregnancy planning:

(1) Life expectancy of infected patients as well as their life quality has dramatically improved during the last 10 years [2].

(2) A significant reduction in mother-to-child HIV transmission (MTCT) has been observed, especially in developed countries, with transmission rates lower than 1% to 2%, compared to 14% to 42% without any intervention. This has been achieved with the use of antiretroviral drug combinations during pregnancy and labor/delivery, neonatal prophylaxis, elective caesarean delivery, and avoidance of breast feeding [3].

Over 80% of people infected with HIV are of reproductive age (15 to 44 years old). Reports suggest that there are currently more than 140,000 HIV serodiscordant heterosexual couples in the United States (US), approximately 50% of whom having reproductive plans [4]. According to the National Perinatal HIV Hotline and Clinicians Network, calls pertaining to HIV serodiscordant couples and their options for safer conception have increased significantly between 2006 and 2011 [5].

Managing HIV infected patients with a childbearing wish involves a multidisciplinary approach, ideally including maternal-fetal medicine specialists, HIV/AIDS specialists, neonatologists, pediatricians, psychiatrists, social workers, and reproductive endocrinologists [6]. Preconception counseling is highly recommended among HIV serodiscordant and seroconcordant couples, allowing them to make more informed choices in order to reduce sexual transmission and improving pregnancy outcome [7]. However, a recent survey of HIV infected women who had been or were pregnant at the time of the questionnaire showed that more than half of them did not have preconception counseling [8]. Evaluating the need for antiretroviral therapy should be part of the initial assessment of preconception counseling. Any concurrent sexually transmitted infection should be treated and safe sexual practices should be encouraged [9].

Infertility affects approximately 15% of the general population and HIV infected patients, both men and women, have higher rates of infertility than their HIV negative counterparts [10, 11].

In serodiscordant couples in which the male partner is infected, assisted reproductive technology (ART) is the safest way to prevent sexual transmission. After the sperm-washing (SW) procedure, there are two main options to achieve a pregnancy: intrauterine insemination (IUI) and in vitro fertilization (IVF)/intracytoplasmic sperm injection (ICSI). In couples with a normal fertility evaluation, IUI is an effective approach. If semen analysis is abnormal, then IVF/ICSI is undoubtedly the treatment to be offered [6]. SW eliminates round cells, seminal plasma, and the majority of immotile sperm. Spermatozoa are isolated by sequential density gradient and swim-up techniques and are subsequently tested by PCR assays for the presence of HIV RNA [12]. A systematic review and meta-analysis summarized the experience with serodiscordant couples with an infected male partner until 2013, with 2,393 SW-IUI and 780 SW-IVF treatment cycles documented [13]. The authors concluded that HIV infected men with noninfected partners have pregnancy and live birth rates with ART comparable to seronegative couples.

In serodiscordant couples in which the female partner is infected, pregnancy can be achieved without the risk of sexual transmission by self-insemination around the time of ovulation [6]. If conception does not occur after more than six cycles of self-insemination, or if a preexisting fertility problem was diagnosed, the use of ART should be envisaged [7].

Most of the reports so far published on IUI or IVF treatments performed in serodiscordant couples refer to infected male partners. Very few studies have addressed IVF outcome in serodiscordant couples with an HIV infected female partner. The purpose of this review is to evaluate the effectiveness of fresh nondonor oocyte IVF/ICSI treatments performed in this population. Control over variables that are traditionally known to influence IVF/ICSI outcome, such as female age, ovarian reserve, race/ethnicity, Body Mass Index (BMI), tobacco consumption, the presence of tubal disease, and the number of embryos replaced in the uterus, was ascertained in the studies found.

2. Materials and Methods

A search of the PubMed database was performed in order to identify all studies involving ART including the HIV infected population published until July 2014. The search terms used were "HIV" AND "assisted reproduction," "HIV" AND "assisted reproductive technology," "HIV" AND "in vitro fertilization," and "HIV" AND "infertility". Abbreviations such as "IVF" and "ICSI" were also used. An initial list of 626 studies was obtained. Inclusion criterion was studies assessing fresh nondonor oocyte IVF/ICSI cycle outcomes of serodiscordant couples with an HIV infected female partner. References with abstracts that demonstrated them to be unrelated to the IVF/ICSI cycle outcomes of serodiscordant couples with an HIV infected female partner were excluded without full text assessment, as were reviews and case reports. All original articles with abstracts that indicated them to be within the scope of this study were fully assessed; when this assessment was confirmed, they were included in the review. Articles in languages other than English, Portuguese, Spanish, or French were excluded. Ten studies were finally included. Figure 1 summarizes the steps involved in literature selection based on Preferred Reporting Items for Systematic Reviews and Meta-Analyses (PRISMA) guidelines [24].

3. Results

Studies analyzed reported on ART treatments performed in a total of 342 HIV infected women, with a mean age of 35.4 years, who underwent 516 IVF/ICSI cycles (Table 1). The average CD4 count ranged from ">200" to 712 cells/mm^3, 48% to 100% of patients in each study had undetectable viral loads, and 44% to 95% of them were being treated with combined antiretroviral therapy.

Table 1 shows baseline characteristics of study and control groups and Table 2 shows the outcomes of ovarian stimulation and IVF.

Among the studies included in this review, data concerning ovarian response to stimulation in HIV infected patients can be summarized as follows: some of the initial studies report the need of higher doses of gonadotropin to achieve satisfactory ovarian response (Terriou et al. 2005 [16]; Coll et al. 2006 [17]), while a normal response to stimulation is described in infected women who are in good general health conditions and reach egg pick-up (Martinet et al. 2006 [18]). Data from most recent studies suggest that a normal ovarian response is seen in these patients (Manigart et al. 2006 [19], Douglas et al. 2009 [20], Prisant et al. 2010 [21], Santulli et al. 2011 [22], and Nurudeen et al. 2013 [23]) (Table 2). However, in the nine studies that assessed the cancellation rate of ovarian stimulation in HIV infected patients, although significance was observed in only one of them (15.2% versus 4.9% in the control group), in all the instances in which a comparison could be made cancellation rate was higher in the study group than in controls (Table 2).

In study groups, the clinical PR per stimulation cycle initiated varied from 6.7% to 24.1% and the clinical PR per embryo transfer varied from 9.1% to 63% (Table 2). Unfortunately, not all studies mentioned the rate per cycle initiated. A summary of the conclusions of the six studies that compared the PRs in HIV infected women with those from noninfected controls is (Table 2) as follows:

TABLE 1: Summary of the published studies on fresh nondonor oocyte IVF/ICSI cycles in serodiscordant couples with an HIV infected female partner and baseline characteristics of study and control groups.

Study	Type of study	Treatment cycles/couples (n)	Control group	Mean female age	Body Mass Index		Tubal disease (%)		Markers of ovarian reserve	
					Study	Control	Study	Control	Study	Control
Ohl et al. 2003 [14]	Clinical prospective	12/9	49 cycles HIV noninfected women with HIV infected male partners	35.9	NM	NM	NM	NM	Day 3 FSH = 9 IU/L	Day 3 FSH = 7 IU/L*
Ohl et al. 2005 [15]	Clinical prospective	62/50	NA	35	NM	NA	32%	NA	Day 3 FSH = 7.1 IU/L	NA
Terriou et al. 2005 [16]	Age-matched cohort	66/29	66 age-matched cycles HIV noninfected women undergoing ICSI during the same period	35.8	NM	NM	30%	18%	Day 3 FSH = 7.4 IU/L	Day 3 FSH = 7.3 IU/L
Coll et al. 2006 [17]	Age-matched cohort	50/35	100 age-matched cycles HIV noninfected women with HIV noninfected male	NM	NM	NM	NM	NM	NM	NM
Martinet et al. 2006 [18]	Retrospective case-matched control	27/27	77 cycles HIV noninfected women matched for age, etiology and duration of infertility, history of pelvic surgery, and type of pituitary inhibition	35.5	NM	NM	70.8%	68.83%	NM	NM
Manigart et al. 2006 [19]	Prospective cohort	56/33	62 cycles Non-HIV infected women with HIV infected male partners	35.6	NM	NM	NM	NM	NM	NM
Douglas et al. 2009 [20]	Retrospective age-matched cohort	29/14	42 age-matched cycles HIV noninfected women undergoing ICSI for male factor infertility	36.5	NM	NM	35%	NM	Day 2 FSH = 7.7 IU/L	Day 2 FSH = 6.9 IU/L
Prisant et al. 2010 [21]	Retrospective case-matched control	94/52	94 cycles HIV noninfected women matched for age, etiology of infertility, rank of oocyte retrieval, and type of ART	34.7	NM	NM	NM	NM	NM	NM
Santulli et al. 2011 [22]	Prospective age-matched cohort	57/57	171 age-matched cycles HIV noninfected women with HIV noninfected male partners	34.2	24.2	22.9*	Unilateral defect 8% Bilateral defect 54%	4.6% 25.2%*	Day 3 FSH 6.5 IU/L AFC: 12.9	Day 3 FSH 7.1 IU/L AFC 13.9
Nurudeen et al. 2013 [23]	Retrospective age-matched cohort	<35 y: 8 ≥35 y: 52/36	8 age-matched cycles 52 age-matched cycles HIV noninfected controls undergoing treatment for male factor infertility	37.7	<35 y: 21 ≥35 y: 28	24.4 24.7	<35 y: 43% ≥35 y: 32%	20% 0%*	<35 y: FSH = 6.8 IU/L AMH: NM ≥35 y: FSH = 8.5 IU/L AMH: 0.92 ng/mL	<35 y: FSH = 5.3 IU/L AMH: NM ≥35 y: FSH = 7.7 IU/L AMH: 0.6 ng/mL

* p value < 0.05. NA: not available. NM: not mentioned.

TABLE 2: Summary of ovarian stimulation and IVF outcomes of study and control groups.

Study	Cancellation rate (%)		Mean gonadotrophin dose/stimulation (IU)		Mean number of oocytes/retrieval		Mean number of embryos replaced		Implantation rate		PR/cycle (%)	PR/ET (%)	
	Study	Control	Study	Control	Study	Control	Study	Control	Study	Control	Study	Study	Control
Ohl et al. 2003 [14]	NM	NM	2893	1972	8.6	9	1.9 ± 0.6	1.7 ± 0.5	NM	NM	6.7	9.1	48.8*
Ohl et al. 2005 [15]	9,7	NA	2793	NA	8.4	NA	1.8 ± 0.6	NA	11.8	NA	15.8	23.9	NM
Terriou et al. 2005 [16]	15.2	4.9*	2898	2429*	10.6	8.3	2	2.4	NM	NM	16.1	NM	NM
Coll et al. 2006 [17]	26	20	3721	3743	NM	NM	NM	NM	NM	NM	12	16.2	37,5*
Martinet et al. 2006 [18]	18.5	14.29	4200	3348	6.55	8.27	1.3	1.94*	NM	NM	11	14	24
Manigart et al. 2006 [19]	42.9	24.2	NM	NM	6	8	NM	NM	NM	NM	16.1	NM	NM
Douglas et al. 2009 [20]	17.2	NM	NM	NM	11.2	12.4	2.7 ± 0.3	3 ± 0.2	15	19	24.1	33	NM
Prisant et al. 2010 [21]	5.7	4.9	NM	NM	6.4	7.3	1.96 ± 0.5	1.94 ± 0.3	10.8	7.1	15.96**	17.65	11,5
Santulli et al. 2011 [22]	16.2	9.5	2408	2283	8.3	9.6	1.5 ± 0.7	1.9 ± 0.7*	21.9	27.4	NM	26.3**	36.3
Nurudeen et al. 2013 [23]	20	NM	<35 y: 2105 ≥35 y: 3677	3103 4318	<35 y: 13.7 ≥35 y: 10.7	20.3 11.1	<35 y: 2.6 ± 0.8 ≥35 y: 2.7 ± 1.5	2.1 ± 0.6 2.9 ± 1.7	NM	NM	NM	<35 y: 63 ≥35 y: 17	57 25

* p value < 0.05. ** PR per oocyte retrieval. NA: not available. NM: not mentioned.

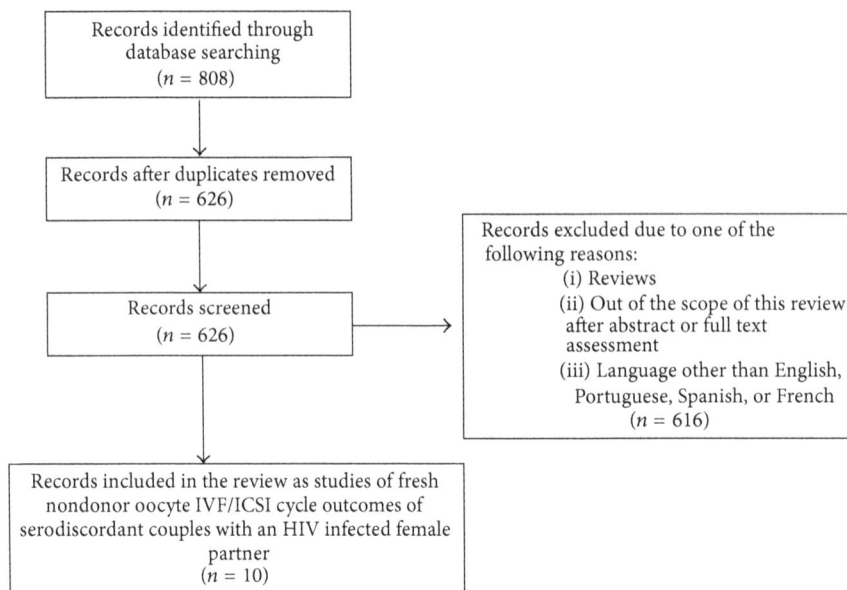

FIGURE 1: Flow chart for the search methodology.

(i) In two studies, HIV infected women had a statistically significantly lower PR (Ohl et al. 2003 [14], Coll et al. 2006 [17]).

(ii) In three studies, the PR of HIV infected women was not statistically significantly different from that of control subjects, but lower values were observed (Martinet et al. 2006 [18], Santulli 2011 et al. [22], and Nurudeen et al. 2013 [23]).

(iii) In one study, the PR of HIV infected women was not statistically significantly different from that of control subjects, but a higher value was observed (Prisant et al. 2010 [21]).

In all studies, PR was reported per embryo transfer, with the exception of two cases of PR per cycle initiated [16, 19] and one of PRs per oocyte retrieval [22]. Noteworthy, vertical transmission of HIV infection was zero.

Concerning variables that are traditionally known to influence IVF/ICSI outcome, data from studies can be summarized as follows.

3.1. Female Age. Seven studies included in this review were age-matched. In only one study, ART results were stratified by age: in both age groups (<35 and ≥35 years), infected and control patients had similar IVF/ICSI clinical outcomes with similar clinical PRs per embryo transfer [23].

3.2. Ovarian Reserve. Six studies included in this review evaluated the ovarian reserve, but only five of them had a control group (Table 1):

(i) In one of them, the comparison between early follicular phase serum FSH of HIV infected women and controls showed a statistically significant difference (9.0 ± 2.4 versus 7.0 ± 2.9 IU/L, resp., $p < 0.001$) (Ohl et al. 2003 [14]).

(ii) In the other four studies, HIV infected women and controls had similar values for markers of ovarian reserve. FSH and HAM levels and antral follicle count (AFC) were evaluated (Terriou et al. 2005 [16]; Douglas et al. 2005 [20]; Santulli et al. 2011 [22]; Nurudeen et al. 2013 [23]).

3.3. Race/Ethnicity. In our review, only two studies documented patients' race/ethnicity [18, 23]. In both of them, the proportion of black women was significantly higher in the study group and this was mentioned as a possible source of bias.

3.4. Body Mass Index (BMI). Only two of the studies analyzed evaluated BMI (Table 1):

(i) In one of them, HIV infected women had higher BMI than control subjects (24.2 versus 22.9, $p = 0.032$) (Santulli et al. 2011 [22]).

(ii) In the other one, HIV infected women and controls had similar BMI (Nurudeen et al. 2013 [23]).

3.5. Tobacco. Of the studies analyzed in this review, only two controlled for tobacco consumption:

(i) In the first of them, no differences were found between HIV infected women and controls (Santulli et al. 2011 [22]).

(ii) In the other one, in the group of women ≥35 years of age, infected patients smoked significantly more often than controls (16% versus 0%; $p < 0.05$). Although parameters of ovarian reserve, the number of mature oocytes retrieved, and fertilization and clinical PRs per embryo transfer were similar in HIV infected women and controls, live birth rates per embryo transfer were significantly lower for HIV infected women (6% versus 24%, $p = 0.04$) (Nurudeen et al. 2013 [23]). Unfortunately, cancelation rates were not compared between groups.

3.6. Tubal Disease. In four of the studies reviewed, the incidence of tubal disease could be compared between the study and control groups and in all of them a higher proportion of tubal disease in HIV infected women was documented, confirming previous reports on the literature [25] (Table 1). In two of them, a statistically significant difference was observed (Santulli et al. 2011 [22] and Nurudeen et al. 2013 [23]).

3.7. Number of Embryos Replaced per Transfer. In the studies analyzed, different criteria were adopted regarding embryo transfer (Table 2). In three of them, the authors reported they were more likely to replace a lower number of embryos in infected women (Terriou et al. 2005 [16]; Martinet et al. 2006 [18]; Santulli et al. 2011 [22]). However, documentation of a significant reduction in the mean number of embryos transferred was seen in only two of these (Martinet et al. 2006 [18]; Santulli et al. 2011 [22]).

4. Discussion

The variability of results observed in the studies analyzed can be mostly related to the small size of the samples studied, heterogeneity in study design, and methodology and incomplete control over potential confounding data. These limitations do not allow for the implementation of a statistical approach that might lead to solid conclusions, such as a meta-analysis.

Variables that are traditionally known to influence IVF/ICSI outcome and should therefore be controlled for are the following:

(1) Female age.

(2) Ovarian reserve.

(3) Race/ethnicity.

(4) Body Mass Index (BMI).

(5) Tobacco consumption.

(6) Tubal disease.

(7) Number of embryos replaced.

A summary of the variables controlled per study is available in Table 3 and aspects to be considered regarding each of them are as follows.

4.1. Female Age. Population studies from areas where no consistent methods of birth control are applied show that natural fertility starts to decline after the age of 30, has its decline accelerated in the mid-30s, and ends at a mean age of 41 years [26]. The age-related effect on female fertility has also been shown in numerous reports on the results of IVF treatments due to a progressive decline on oocyte quality and quantity. The implantation rate per embryo clearly decreases after the age of 35 and the same has been shown for the probability of a live birth in IVF [27].

Due to this knowledge, control over female age is of paramount importance in any study on IVF treatment outcome. Such was not seen in three of the ten studies included in this review.

4.2. Ovarian Reserve. ART requires controlled ovarian stimulation for the achievement of improved efficacy. Currently, it is not consensual that HIV infection affects ovarian reserve. Seifer et al. evaluated the markers of ovarian follicular reserve and reproductive ageing in 187 HIV infected women not diagnosed as infertile [28]. Early follicular phase FSH, estradiol, inhibin B, and anti-Mullerian hormone (AMH) levels were measured. No evidence was found that HIV infection affects ovarian ageing. On the other hand, Ohl et al. measured serum FSH, inhibin B, AMH, and the antral follicle count (AFC) in 78 HIV infected women [29]. Mean FSH was 36% higher than that seen in the control group, whereas mean inhibin B and AMH were 57% and 23% lower, respectively. AFC was also significantly lower in the study group.

The possible influence of combined antiretroviral therapy on ovarian reserve and ovarian response to stimulation is not clear either. Side effects of the use of antiretroviral drugs such as mitochondrial dysfunction or modification in the lipid metabolism and insulin resistance could have consequences on folliculogenesis and ovulation regulatory processes [2, 30]. Oocytes from infertile HIV infected women on combined antiretroviral therapy were reported to have 32% depletion in mtDNA in comparison to infertile uninfected controls ($p < 0.05$) and depletion was even stronger in patients who failed to become pregnant in IVF treatments [31].

4.3. Race/Ethnicity. A growing number of studies have investigated the association between race/ethnicity and ART outcomes. Most of the studies have focused on comparisons between white Caucasian and black women and some have identified that the last group is more likely to have a diagnosis of tubal factor infertility, leiomyoma/uterine factor infertility, a longer duration of infertility before ART, and higher miscarriage/stillbirth rates [32–36]. Race/ethnicity as a risk factor for poor ART outcomes has been consistently acknowledged in recent large studies, even after adjusting for many confounding factors [37]. This may certainly be a source of bias for data collected in this review.

4.4. Body Mass Index (BMI). Overweight and obesity are well-described risk factors for infertility, particularly as they relate to ovulation disorders. In spite of conflicting results of studies regarding the effect of high BMI on ART outcome, a systematic review and meta-analysis published in 2011 showed that overweight or obese women (BMI ≥ 25) had significantly lower clinical pregnancy (RR = 0.90, 95% CI 0.85–0.94) and live birth rates (RR = 0.84, 95% CI 0.77–0.92) and a significantly higher miscarriage rate (RR = 1.31, 95% CI 1.18–1.45) [38]. The analysis of overweight women alone (BMI ≥ 25–29.9) also showed lower clinical pregnancy (RR = 0.91, 95% CI 0.86–0.96) and live birth rates (RR = 0.91, 95% CI 0.85–0.98) and higher miscarriage rate (RR = 1.24, 95% CI 1.13–1.35), compared to women with BMI < 25. In conclusion, increased BMI is associated with adverse outcomes in women

TABLE 3: Summary of the variables that influence IVF/ICSI outcome which were controlled in each study.

Study	Female age	Ovarian reserve	Race/ethnicity	Body Mass Index	Tobacco consumption	Tubal disease	Number of embryos replaced per transfer
Ohl et al. 2003 [14]	—	Yes	—	—	—	—	Yes
Ohl et al. 2005 [15]	—	Yes	—	—	—	Yes	Yes
Terriou et al. 2005 [16]	Yes	Yes	—	—	—	Yes	Yes
Coll et al. 2006 [17]	Yes	—	Yes	—	—	—	—
Martinet et al. 2006 [18]	Yes	—	—	—	—	Yes	Yes
Manigart et al. 2006 [19]	—	—	—	—	—	—	—
Douglas et al. 2009 [20]	Yes	Yes	—	—	—	Yes	Yes
Prisant et al. 2010 [21]	Yes	—	—	—	—	—	Yes
Santulli et al. 2011 [22]	Yes	Yes	—	Yes	Yes	Yes	Yes
Nurudeen et al. 2013 [23]	Yes	Yes	Yes	Yes	Yes	Yes	Yes

undergoing IVF/ICSI treatment, including lower live birth rates.

Increasing overweight and obesity in the HIV infected population were not seen until two decades ago. This relatively new reality has been attributed to several factors, such as better health due to combined antiretroviral therapy and improved life expectancy, which leads to obesity trends similar to those seen in the general population [39]. This parameter was not properly controlled for in the majority of studies analyzed here.

4.5. Tobacco. Over the last few decades, the prevalence of cigarette smoking among women of reproductive age has increased, reaching, in 2006, 33% in Europe and 28% in the USA [40], and is highly prevalent among persons infected with HIV [41]. Studies on IVF showed that cigarette smoking has deleterious effects on many aspects of treatment: ovarian responsiveness to gonadotropins, number of oocytes retrieved, fertilization, implantation, and early placentation [42].

4.6. Tubal Disease. In the studies reviewed, a higher proportion of tubal disease in HIV infected women was documented, confirming previous reports on the literature [25]. It is important to notice that many studies collected data at times during which it was still not a standard procedure to remove hydrosalpinx before IVF, which may have reduced live birth rates and constituted a source of bias [43].

Another factor associated with tubal disease that should be considered is the personal history of pelvic inflammatory disease. This condition has been shown to reduce ovarian response to stimulation due to direct damage to the ovaries and follicle loss or due to mechanical alterations of follicular development [18].

4.7. Number of Embryos Replaced per Transfer. The rate of preterm delivery and multiple gestations after ART is of particular concern for HIV infected women. Preterm labor or premature rupture of membranes may increase the risk of HIV vertical transmission [44]. Elective single embryo transfer for HIV infected women shall be considered in order to reduce the risk of multiple gestations [15]. A lower number of embryos replaced in HIV positive women may obviously contribute to lower pregnancy and live birth rates per transfer.

5. Conclusions

Data on PR in IVF/ICSI treatments performed in couples with HIV infected women are conflicting and it is still not clear if these patients display worse clinical outcomes per cycle initiated when compared to the general population. The same can be said specifically about ovarian response to stimulation, though a tendency for higher cancellation rates seems to be observed.

The small size of the samples studied and heterogeneity in study design and methodology make it difficult to draw clear conclusions about the impact of HIV infection in women on IVF outcome. Incomplete control over confounding variables (such as age, race/ethnicity, BMI, tobacco consumption, tubal disease, history of pelvic inflammatory disease, duration of infertility, and the number of embryos replaced) is of special concern. Altogether, such limitations hamper the performance of a proper meta-analysis.

In the future, prospective matched case-control studies are needed to understand the specific effects of HIV infection on ovarian response and ART outcome. Available data suggest some impact of HIV infection on ovarian function and IVF outcome, but noncontrolled sources of bias in published studies do not allow for definitive conclusions.

Conflict of Interests

The authors declare that there is no conflict of interests regarding the publication of this paper.

References

[1] UNAIDS, *How AIDS Changed Everything*, UNAIDS, Geneva, Switzerland, 2015.

[2] Y. Englert, B. Lesage, J.-P. Van Vooren et al., "Medically assisted reproduction in the presence of chronic viral diseases," *Human Reproduction Update*, vol. 10, no. 2, pp. 149–162, 2004.

[3] A. P. Kourtis and M. Bulterys, "Mother-to-child transmission of HIV: pathogenesis, mechanisms and pathways," *Clinics in Perinatology*, vol. 37, no. 4, pp. 721–737, 2010.

[4] M. A. Lampe, D. K. Smith, G. J. E. Anderson, A. E. Edwards, and S. R. Nesheim, "Achieving safe conception in HIV-discordant couples: the potential role of oral preexposure prophylaxis (PrEP) in the United States," *American Journal of Obstetrics and Gynecology*, vol. 204, no. 6, pp. 488.e1–488.e8, 2011.

[5] S. Weber, J. F. Waldura, and D. Cohan, "Safer conception options for HIV serodifferent couples in the United States: the experience of the National Perinatal HIV Hotline and Clinicians' Network," *Journal of Acquired Immune Deficiency Syndromes*, vol. 63, no. 4, pp. e140–e141, 2013.

[6] S. J. Estes and E. S. Ginsburg, "Use of assisted reproduction in HIV and hepatitis infected couples," *UpToDate*, 2014.

[7] V. Savasi, L. Mandia, A. Laoreti, and I. Cetin, "Reproductive assistance in HIV serodiscordant couples," *Human Reproduction Update*, vol. 19, no. 2, pp. 136–150, 2013.

[8] K. E. Squires, S. L. Hodder, J. Feinberg et al., "Health needs of HIV-infected women in the United States: insights from the women living positive survey," *AIDS Patient Care and STDs*, vol. 25, no. 5, pp. 279–285, 2011.

[9] V. A. Kushnir and W. Lewis, "Human immunodeficiency virus/acquired immunodeficiency syndrome and infertility: emerging problems in the era of highly active antiretrovirals," *Fertility and Sterility*, vol. 96, no. 3, pp. 546–553, 2011.

[10] G. F. Homan, M. Davies, and R. Norman, "The impact of lifestyle factors on reproductive performance in the general population and those undergoing infertility treatment: a review," *Human Reproduction Update*, vol. 13, no. 3, pp. 209–223, 2007.

[11] V. A. Moragianni, "Why are we still, 20 years later, depriving human immunodeficiency virus-serodiscordant couples of equal access to fertility care?" *Fertility and Sterility*, vol. 102, no. 2, pp. 352–353, 2014.

[12] A. C. Eke and C. Oragwu, "Sperm washing to prevent HIV transmission from HIV-infected men but allowing conception in sero-discordant couples," *Cochrane Database of Systematic Reviews*, no. 1, Article ID CD008498, 2011.

[13] A. Barnes, D. Riche, L. Mena et al., "Efficacy and safety of intrauterine insemination and assisted reproductive technology in populations serodiscordant for human immunodeficiency virus: a systematic review and meta-analysis," *Fertility and Sterility*, vol. 102, no. 2, pp. 424–434, 2014.

[14] J. Ohl, M. Partisani, C. Wittemer et al., "Assisted reproduction techniques for HIV serodiscordant couples: 18 months of experience," *Human Reproduction*, vol. 18, no. 6, pp. 1244–1249, 2003.

[15] J. Ohl, M. Partisani, C. Wittemer, J.-M. Lang, S. Viville, and R. Favre, "Encouraging results despite complexity of multidisciplinary care of HIV-infected women using assisted reproduction techniques," *Human Reproduction*, vol. 20, no. 11, pp. 3136–3140, 2005.

[16] P. Terriou, P. Auquier, V. Chabert-Orsini et al., "Outcome of ICSI in HIV-1-infected women," *Human Reproduction*, vol. 20, no. 10, pp. 2838–2843, 2005.

[17] O. Coll, A. Suy, F. Figueras et al., "Decreased pregnancy rate after in-vitro fertilization in HIV-infected women receiving HAART," *AIDS*, vol. 20, no. 1, pp. 121–123, 2006.

[18] V. Martinet, Y. Manigart, S. Rozenberg, B. Becker, M. Gerard, and A. Delvigne, "Ovarian response to stimulation of HIV-positive patients during IVF treatment: a matched, controlled study," *Human Reproduction*, vol. 21, no. 5, pp. 1212–1217, 2006.

[19] Y. Manigart, S. Rozenberg, P. Barlow, M. Gerard, E. Bertrand, and A. Delvigne, "ART outcome in HIV-infected patients," *Human Reproduction*, vol. 21, no. 11, pp. 2935–2940, 2006.

[20] N. C. Douglas, J. G. Wang, B. Yu, S. Gaddipati, M. M. Guarnaccia, and M. V. Sauer, "A systematic, multidisciplinary approach to address the reproductive needs of HIV-seropositive women," *Reproductive BioMedicine Online*, vol. 19, no. 2, pp. 257–263, 2009.

[21] N. Prisant, R. Tubiana, G. Lefebvre et al., "HIV-1 or hepatitis C chronic infection in serodiscordant infertile couples has no impact on infertility treatment outcome," *Fertility and Sterility*, vol. 93, no. 3, pp. 1020–1023, 2010.

[22] P. Santulli, V. Gayet, P. Fauque et al., "HIV-positive patients undertaking ART have longer infertility histories than age-matched control subjects," *Fertility and Sterility*, vol. 95, no. 2, pp. 507–512, 2011.

[23] S. K. Nurudeen, L. C. Grossman, L. Bourne, M. M. Guarnaccia, M. V. Sauer, and N. C. Douglas, "Reproductive outcomes of HIV seropositive women treated by assisted reproduction," *Journal of Women's Health*, vol. 22, no. 3, pp. 243–249, 2013.

[24] D. Moher, A. Liberati, J. Tetzlaff, and D. G. Altman, "Preferred reporting items for systematic reviews and meta-analyses: the PRISMA statement," *Annals of Internal Medicine*, vol. 151, no. 4, pp. 264–269, 2009.

[25] J. D. Sobel, "Gynecologic infections in human immunodeficiency virus-infected women," *Clinical Infectious Diseases*, vol. 31, no. 5, pp. 1225–1233, 2000.

[26] E. R. te Velde and P. L. Pearson, "The variability of female reproductive ageing," *Human Reproduction Update*, vol. 8, no. 2, pp. 141–154, 2002.

[27] F. J. Broekmans, J. Kwee, D. J. Hendriks, B. W. Mol, and C. B. Lambalk, "A systematic review of tests predicting ovarian reserve and IVF outcome," *Human Reproduction Update*, vol. 12, no. 6, pp. 685–718, 2006.

[28] D. B. Seifer, E. T. Golub, G. Lambert-Messerlian et al., "Biologic markers of ovarian reserve and reproductive aging: application in a cohort study of HIV infection in women," *Fertility and Sterility*, vol. 88, no. 6, pp. 1645–1652, 2007.

[29] J. Ohl, M. Partisani, C. Demangeat, F. Binder-Foucard, I. Nisand, and J.-M. Lang, "Alterations of ovarian reserve tests in Human Immunodeficiency Virus (HIV)-infected women," *Gynecologie Obstetrique Fertilite*, vol. 38, no. 5, pp. 313–317, 2010.

[30] C. de Mendoza, M. Sanchez-Conde, E. Ribera, P. Domingo, and V. Soriano, "Could mitochondrial DNA quantitation be a surrogate marker for drug mitochondrial toxicity?" *AIDS Reviews*, vol. 6, no. 3, pp. 169–180, 2004.

[31] S. López, O. Coll, M. Durban et al., "Mitochondrial DNA depletion in oocytes of HIV-infected antiretroviral-treated infertile women," *Antiviral Therapy*, vol. 13, no. 6, pp. 833–838, 2008.

[32] F. I. Sharara and H. D. McClamrock, "Differences in in vitro fertilization (IVF) outcome between white and black women in an inner-city, university-based IVF program," *Fertility and Sterility*, vol. 73, no. 6, pp. 1170–1173, 2000.

[33] E. C. Feinberg, F. W. Larsen, W. H. Catherino, J. Zhang, and A. Y. Armstrong, "Comparison of assisted reproductive technology utilization and outcomes between Caucasian and African American patients in an equal-access-to-care setting," *Fertility and Sterility*, vol. 85, no. 4, pp. 888–894, 2006.

[34] D. B. Seifer, R. Zackula, D. A. Grainger, and Society for Assisted Reproductive Technology Writing Group Report, "Trends of racial disparities in assisted reproductive technology outcomes in black women compared with white women: Society for Assisted Reproductive Technology 1999 and 2000 vs. 2004–2006," *Fertility and Sterility*, vol. 93, no. 2, pp. 626–635, 2010.

[35] D. B. Seifer, L. M. Frazier, and D. A. Grainger, "Disparity in assisted reproductive technologies outcomes in black women compared with white women," *Fertility and Sterility*, vol. 90, no. 5, pp. 1701–1710, 2008.

[36] V. Y. Fujimoto, B. Luke, M. B. Brown et al., "Racial and ethnic disparities in assisted reproductive technology outcomes in the United States," *Fertility and Sterility*, vol. 93, no. 2, pp. 382–390, 2010.

[37] S. F. Butts and D. B. Seifer, "Racial and ethnic differences in reproductive potential across the life cycle," *Fertility and Sterility*, vol. 93, no. 3, pp. 681–690, 2010.

[38] V. Rittenberg, S. Seshadri, S. K. Sunkara, S. Sobaleva, E. Oteng-Ntim, and T. El-Toukhy, "Effect of body mass index on IVF treatment outcome: an updated systematic review and meta-analysis," *Reproductive BioMedicine Online*, vol. 23, no. 4, pp. 421–439, 2011.

[39] N. Crum-Cianflone, R. Tejidor, S. Medina, I. Barahona, and A. Ganesan, "Obesity among patients with HIV: the latest epidemic," *AIDS Patient Care and STDs*, vol. 22, no. 12, pp. 925–930, 2008.

[40] C. Dechanet, T. Anahory, J. C. Mathieu Daude et al., "Effects of cigarette smoking on reproduction," *Human Reproduction Update*, vol. 17, no. 1, pp. 76–95, 2011.

[41] N. R. Reynolds, "Cigarette smoking and HIV: more evidence for action," *AIDS Education and Prevention*, vol. 21, no. 3, pp. 106–121, 2009.

[42] The Practice Committee of the American Society for Reproductive Medicine, "Smoking and infertility: a committee opinion," *Fertility and Sterility*, vol. 98, no. 6, pp. 1400–1406, 2012.

[43] P. Devroey, B. C. J. M. Fauser, and K. Diedrich, "Approaches to improve the diagnosis and management of infertility," *Human Reproduction Update*, vol. 15, no. 4, pp. 391–408, 2009.

[44] L. Mandelbrot, M. J. Mayaux, A. Bongain et al., "Obstetric factors and mother-to-child transmission of human immunodeficiency virus type 1: the French perinatal cohorts. SEROGEST French Pediatric HIV Infection Study Group," *American Journal of Obstetrics & Gynecology*, vol. 175, no. 3, part 1, pp. 661–667, 1996.

7

Development of a Novel Test for Simultaneous Bacterial Identification and Antibiotic Susceptibility

Jonathan Faro,[1] Malika Mitchell,[2] Yuh-Jue Chen,[2] Sarah Kamal,[2] Gerald Riddle,[1] and Sebastian Faro[1]

[1]*The Woman's Hospital of Texas, 7400 Fannin Suite 930, Houston, TX 77054, USA*
[2]*The University of Texas Health Science Center at Houston, Medical College, Houston, TX 77054, USA*

Correspondence should be addressed to Jonathan Faro; jonfaro@yahoo.com

Academic Editor: Bryan Larsen

Background. Elucidation of a pathogen's antimicrobial susceptibility requires subculture after the organism is first isolated. This takes several days, requiring patients to be treated with broad-spectrum antibiotics. This approach contributes to the development of bacterial resistance. *Methods.* Microtiter wells were coated with a polyclonal antibody targeting the pathogen of interest. Bacterial suspensions were added in the presence/absence of selected antibiotics. After washing, captured bacteria were detected. *Findings.* Group B streptococcus (GBS), *Enterococcus faecalis*, and *Neisseria gonorrhoeae* were each detected at 10^5 bacteria/mL following a 20-minute incubation period. Susceptibility to select antibiotics was discernable following a 6-hour incubation period (GBS and *Enterococcus*). Sensitivity was increased to 10^{-2} bacteria/mL for GBS, 10^{-1} bacteria/mL for *E. faecalis*, and 10^1 bacteria/mL for *N. gonorrhoeae* following 18–24-hour culture. *Conclusion.* This novel assay allows for the highly sensitive and specific identification of a pathogen and simultaneous determination of its antimicrobial susceptibility in a reduced time.

1. Introduction

When confronted with a patient battling an infectious disease, elucidation of the offending pathogen requires great effort. Time is critical: broad-spectrum antibiotics are initiated after cultures are collected, as identification of the offending microbe requires 24–48 hours. To increase the sensitivity of culture, an enrichment step may be added [1]. The workup is not completed once a pathogen is identified: antimicrobial susceptibility must next be ascertained following additional subculture in the presence of select antibiotics for another 24–48 hours [2].

Several techniques have been developed to aid in reducing the time required to identify a pathogen. These techniques include the use of chromogenic agar/broth and nucleic acid amplification technology (NAAT) [3, 4]. While both of these techniques have been employed in screening for antenatal GBS colonization, the Centers for Disease Control and Prevention still recommend that culture be performed [5]. This is an absolute requirement for patients allergic to penicillin, as NAAT is not capable of providing antimicrobial susceptibility profiles. Additionally, the resources and highly specialized training required to perform NAAT are not universally available [6].

Recently, the Infectious Diseases Society of America released a paper detailing the current approach towards identifying clinical pathogens. Described is a process characterized as having inadequate sensitivity and significant time delays, thereby contributing to the development of greater and greater antimicrobial resistance [7]. These concerns are all too-well illustrated in our approach towards treatment for GBS prophylaxis, in which increasing resistance to penicillin has been observed, and resistance to clindamycin is on the rise [8, 9]. Additionally, there is concern that this practice will contribute to *E. coli* resistance observed in premature neonates [10]. Already, we have seen the implications of antimicrobial resistance with *Enterococcus*, and hospital acquired infections with this pathogen are estimated to add $27,000.00 per infection [11, 12]. *N. gonorrhoeae* resistance has been increasing steadily, and multidrug resistance has recently been confirmed [13]. These three disparate organisms demonstrate a range in the microbial response to our directed approach to both prophylaxis and treatment.

Through a modification of a recently reported test, we have developed a method for the simultaneous identification of a pathogen and determination of its antibiotic susceptibility [14]. We have modified this test so that GBS, *E. faecalis*, and *N. gonorrhoeae* may be detected at dilute concentrations after 6-hour incubation. Additionally, we show that inducible resistance of GBS against clindamycin may be determined. Finally, we show that following an overnight incubation, test organisms may be detected at concentrations rivaling those published for PCR. As this test allows one to simultaneously identify a pathogen and determine its antimicrobial susceptibility, this novel technique provides a change in the clinician's approach to managing infectious diseases.

2. Methods

2.1. Bacterial Strains and Antibodies. Group B streptococcus clinical isolates 12386 and 01.12.76 were shown by disk diffusion to be susceptible or resistant to clindamycin, respectively. *Enterococcus faecalis* ATCC 29212 was confirmed to be susceptible to vancomycin by disk diffusion, and ATCC strain 51299 was confirmed to be resistant. *Neisseria gonorrhoeae* ATCC strain 31426 was shown to be resistant to penicillin. Strain 1279, a clinical isolate, was shown to be susceptible to penicillin. *E. coli, S. aureus, Candida albicans,* and Beta streptococcus groups A, C, F, and G were all clinical isolates.

Rabbit polyclonal anti-GBS antibody (1521), HRP-conjugated rabbit polyclonal anti-GBS antibody (1524), rabbit polyclonal anti-*Enterococcus* antibody (3711), and HRP-conjugated rabbit polyclonal anti-*Enterococcus* antibody (3714) were all obtained from Virostat (Portland, Maine). Rabbit polyclonal anti-*N. gonorrhoeae* antibody (PA1-7233) and HRP-conjugated rabbit polyclonal anti-*N. gonorrhoeae* antibody (PA1-73144) were purchased from ThermoFisher (Waltham, MA).

2.2. Bacterial Detection and Competition Experiments. 96-well Immulon microtiter plates (ThermoFisher, Waltham, MA) were coated with specified antibody. For the GBS assay, anti-GBS antibody was first diluted 1 : 30 in bicarbonate buffer (Sigma, St. Louis MO). For the *N. gonorrhoeae* or *Enterococcus* assays, antibodies were diluted 1 : 200 or 1 : 100, respectively. 100 μL of the antibody dilutions was placed in respective wells, and the plates were incubated at 4°C overnight. Wells were then washed three times with phosphate-buffered saline (PBS, Sigma Aldrich, St. Louis, MO) supplemented with 0.05% Tween-20 (Fisher Scientific, Pittsburg, PA). The plates were blocked for 30 minutes at room temperature with 200 μL of StartingBlock™ (ThermoScientific, Rockford, IL) followed by washing three times with PBS-Tw at room temperature.

Bacterial isolates were individually prepared at a concentration of approximately 10^8 bacteria/mL based on 0.5 McFarland and confirmed by OD$_{600}$ nm. Aliquots were plated on appropriate agar (Columbia colistin nalidixic acid blood agar, for GBS and *Enterococcus*, and Chocolate agar, for

N. gonorrhoeae, Fisher Scientific, Pittsburg, PA), and colony forming units (CFUs) were determined following a 24–48-hour culture. Inoculates were prepared further in tenfold dilutions down to 10^{-3} bacteria/mL. For the Time Zero Test, isolates were diluted in PBS and incubated at room temperature for 20 minutes. For growth experiments, Fastidious Broth (Remel, Lenexa, KS) was substituted for PBS, and inoculates were diluted out in test tubes and incubated prior to being transferred to wells. Competing organisms were prepared at a concentration of 10^8 bacteria/mL. Varying concentrations of inoculates were added to tubes containing an amount of competing organisms held steady at 10^8 bacteria/mL in Fastidious Broth. After a prespecified incubation timepoint (6 hours for antimicrobial susceptibility testing with GBS and *Enterococcus*, 9 hours for inducible resistance of GBS to clindamycin, or overnight for determining the limit of detection of all three organisms or determination of antimicrobial susceptibility with *N. gonorrhoeae*) organisms were transferred to microtiter wells and plates were then incubated for 20 minutes at room temperature. For the Time Zero assay, this transfer step was omitted, as inoculates were prepared directly in the wells. For growth experiments, 10 μL of the incubated bacterial suspensions was added to 90 μL of PBS in each well. Following 20-minute incubation, wells were washed three times with PBS. Horseradish peroxidase (HRP) conjugated antibody was next added in 100 μL aliquots and plates were incubated for 10 minutes at room temperature. HRP-conjugated antibodies for all tests were diluted 1 : 100 in PBS.

After washing three times with PBS-Tw, TMB peroxidase substrate (KPL, Gaithersburg, MD) was added to the wells in 100 μL aliquots. Plates were incubated for 3 minutes at room temperature. Reactions were terminated using Stop Solution (Thermo Scientific, Rockford, IL). Plates were read in an ELX 808 BioTek (Winooski, Vermont) plate reader at 450 nm.

3. Results

3.1. Time Zero Test. Serial dilutions of each bacterium were prepared starting with a 0.5 McFarland and diluted down to 10^1 bacteria/mL in PBS. When processed on the pathogen-specific ELISAs, Group B streptococcus, *E. faecalis*, and *N. gonorrhoeae* each individually showed detection in the range of 10^2–10^8 bacteria/mL after 20-minute incubation (Figures 1(a)–1(c)). GBS was detected down to 10^2 bacteria/mL, *E. faecalis* down to 10^5 bacteria/mL, and *N. gonorrhoeae* down to 10^3 bacteria/mL. In order to determine the specificity of the test, suspensions were tested in which the bacterium to be identified was diluted out, but the level of a competing bacterium was held constant at 10^8 bacteria/mL in PBS. Testing of several commonly found vaginal cocolonizers mixed with the bacterium of interest revealed little to no interference with the assays (Supplemental Figures 1(A)–1(L) in Supplementary Material available online at http://dx.doi.org/10.1155/2016/5293034).

3.2. Limit of Detection. Bacteria were next diluted in Fastidious Broth after first preparing a 0.5 McFarland. The ability

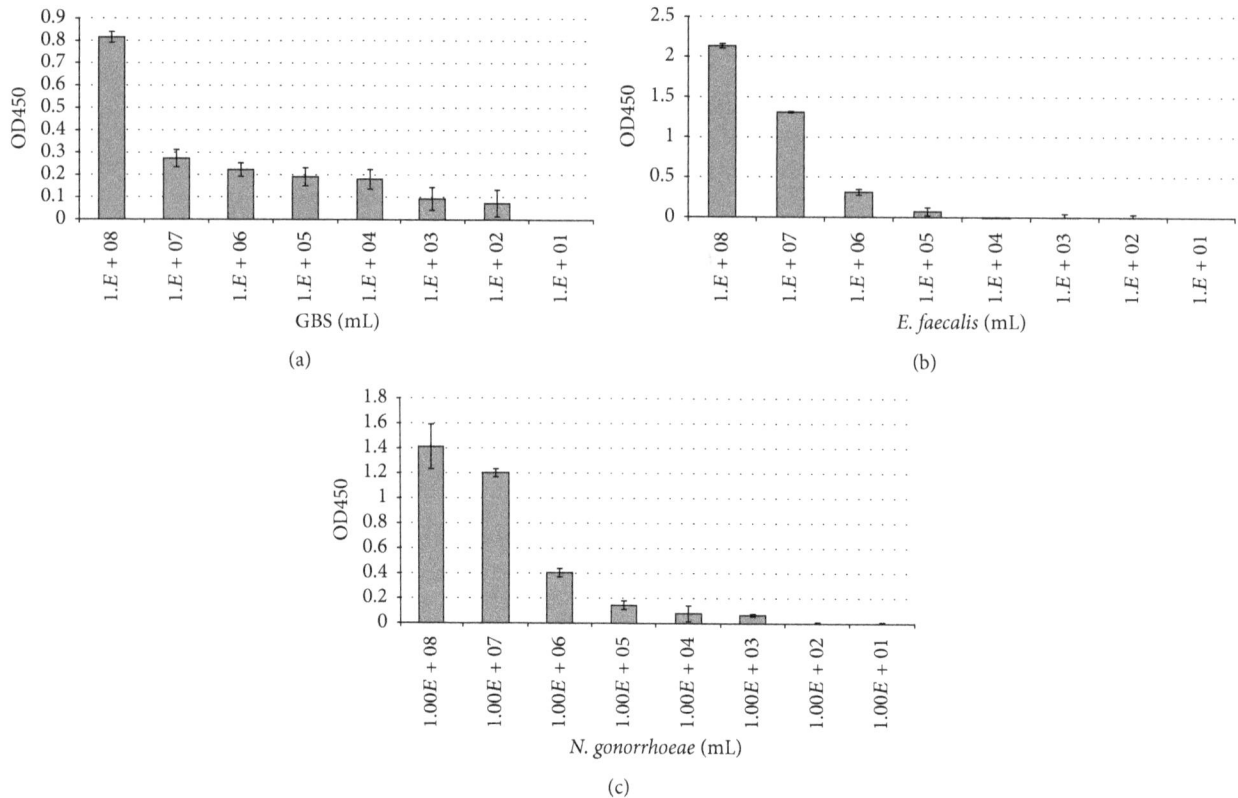

FIGURE 1: Determination of the limit of detection for the Time Zero Test. GBS (a), *Enterococcus* (b), and *N. gonorrhoeae* (c) were prepared at 0.5 McFarland in PBS and diluted out serially. Following 20-minute incubation at room temperature, wells were washed and then HRP-conjugated antibody directed against the bacterium of interest was used to detect any bound organism. Three distinct strains of GBS were tested, two strains of *Enterococcus*, and *N. gonorrhoeae* each. Results shown are of GBS clinical isolate 01.12.76 (a), *Enterococcus* ATCC strain 29212 (b), and *N. gonorrhoeae* strain 19424 (c); each study was performed in triplicate and representative of three individual experiments. Bacterial concentrations were confirmed by CFUs following plating on agar for 24–48 hours.

to detect the test organism at greater dilutions increased when the incubation times were lengthened. GBS was detected down to 10^2 bacteria/mL after 2-hour incubation, 10^1 bacteria/mL after 6 hours, and 10^{-2} bacteria/mL after incubating overnight (Figure 2(a)).

A series of dilutions of *E. faecalis* starting at 0.5 McFarland was prepared similarly to that of GBS, and after incubating overnight (18 hrs) in Fastidious Broth, the tubes surrounding the turbidity point were assayed. Turbidity was observed down to 10^{-1} bacteria/mL. This tube was assayed directly, as well as was a series of dilutions of this sample. This same procedure was performed on the subsequent nonturbid dilutions, so that 10^{-2} and 10^{-3} bacteria/mL tubes were both assayed directly and then when diluted out further. *E. faecalis* was detected at 10^{-1} bacteria/mL, and when this sample was diluted out further, bacteria were capable of being detected following both 10-fold and 100-fold dilution (Figure 2(b)). In the nonturbid overnight culture tubes, no *E. faecalis* was detected (10^{-2} and 10^{-3} bacteria/mL).

N. gonorrhoeae was diluted out serially in Fastidious Broth, first starting with a 0.5 McFarland. After overnight incubation, the assay was run. *N. gonorrhoeae* was detected

strongly at high concentrations, as well as at very low concentrations, 10^2 and 10^1 bacteria/mL (Figure 2(c)). The test was not capable of detecting bacteria less than 10^1 bacteria/mL following 24-hour incubation.

3.3. *Determination of Antimicrobial Susceptibility.* Isolates were individually prepared in the presence or absence of selected antibiotics. After culturing for 6 hours, the assay was performed and susceptibility profiles were obtained. A strain of GBS sensitive to penicillin was cultured in the presence of increasing concentrations of the following antibiotics: penicillin, cefazolin, erythromycin, and clindamycin. At all concentrations of penicillin tested, growth of this strain of GBS was inhibited and no GBS was detected at 10^5 bacteria/mL (Figure 3(a)). Incubation of GBS with increasing concentrations of cefazolin showed a dose effect, in which growth was observed at a more dilute concentration of antibiotic, 0.005 μg/mL, but not when increasing amounts were used (Supplemental Figure 2(A)). Similar results were observed when the same strain was tested in the presence of either clindamycin or erythromycin (Supplemental Figures 2(B) and 3(C)).

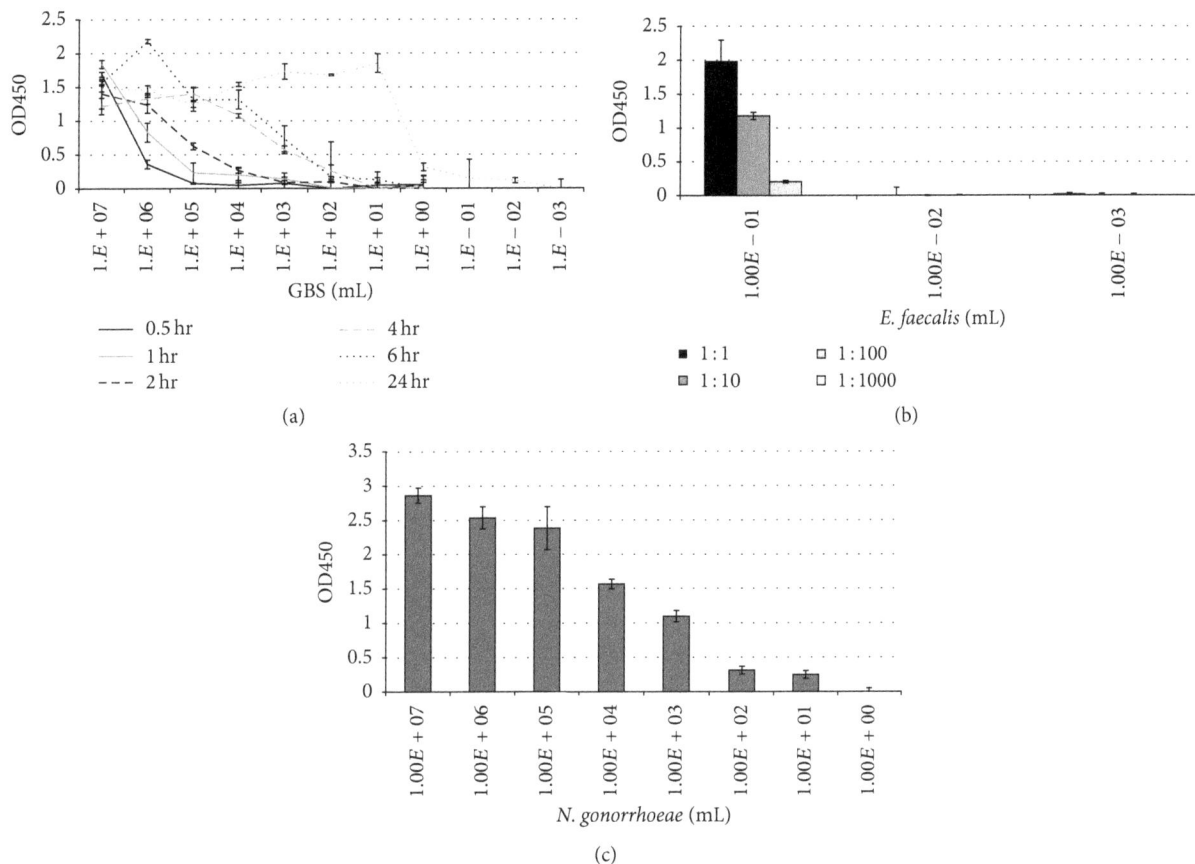

FIGURE 2: Determination of the limit of detection following incubation at 37° Celsius. GBS (a), *Enterococcus* (b), and *N. gonorrhoeae* (c) were prepared at 0.5 McFarland in Fastidious Broth and diluted out serially. For GBS, samples were incubated for either 0.5, 1, 2, 4, 6 or 24 hours at 37° Celsius (a). For *E. faecalis*, samples were incubated overnight at 37° Celsius. Tubes were noted to be turbid down to 10^0 bacteria per mL, and this sample and the following two dilutions, 10^{-1} and 10^{-2} bacteria per mL, were prepared further by diluting in PBS out to 1:1,000. For *N. gonorrhoeae*, samples were prepared at a 0.5 McFarland in Fastidious Broth and then incubated overnight at 37° Celsius (c). Following these incubation time-points for each study, 10 μL of each sample was transferred to microtiter wells containing 90 μL PBS and allowed to stand for 20 minutes at room temperature. Any bound organism was detected by HRP-conjugated antibody against the specific pathogen. As with Figure 1, three distinct strains of GBS were tested, as were two strains of *Enterococcus* and *N. gonorrhoeae* each. Results shown are of GBS clinical isolate 01.12.76 (a), *Enterococcus* ATCC strain 29212 (b), and *N. gonorrhoeae* strain 19424 (c), each performed in triplicate and representative of three individual experiments. Again, bacterial concentrations were confirmed by CFUs following plating on agar for 24–48 hours.

Next, a GBS strain resistant to clindamycin but sensitive to erythromycin was prepared, as above. Supplemental Figure 2(D) shows that, at 0.25 μg erythromycin, growth of the GBS strain was inhibited at 10^5 bacteria/mL. Antibiotic concentrations were selected based on CLSI breakpoints. Conversely, at all concentrations of clindamycin tested, GBS was detected at levels similar to that of the no antibiotic control for this strain of GBS (Supplemental Figure 2(E), strain 165).

Enterococcus faecalis was tested by methods similar to that of GBS. When vancomycin sensitive *E. faecalis* was diluted out in the presence of vancomycin, no growth was detected at 10^5 bacteria/mL (Figure 3(b)). When a vancomycin resistant strain was substituted under test conditions, however, this organism was detected at 10^5 bacteria/mL after 6-hour incubation (Supplemental Figure 2(F)).

Strains of *N. gonorrhoeae* were prepared and diluted out as above, in the presence of either penicillin or ceftriaxone.

Following 24-hour incubation, a strain of *N. gonorrhoeae* shown to be sensitive to penicillin was assayed. This strain was detected at 10^5 bacteria/mL when tested in the absence of penicillin, but no bacteria were detected at this inoculum in wells which received penicillin (Figure 3(c)). When a penicillin-resistant strain of *N. gonorrhoeae* was tested, bacteria were strongly detected at 10^5 bacteria/mL following 24-hour incubation in wells receiving less than 2 μg/mL, with slight detection at 2 μg/mL (Supplemental Figure 2(G)). A strain of *N. gonorrhoeae* sensitive to ceftriaxone was next tested and showed similar results: bacteria cultured in the absence of ceftriaxone were detected at 10^5 bacteria/mL, but not when cultured in the presence of either 0.0625 μg/mL or 0.125 μg/mL ceftriaxone at this inoculum (Supplemental Figure 2(H)). Both antibiotic concentrations used were less than the recommended level of 0.25 μg/mL in determining resistance to ceftriaxone [15].

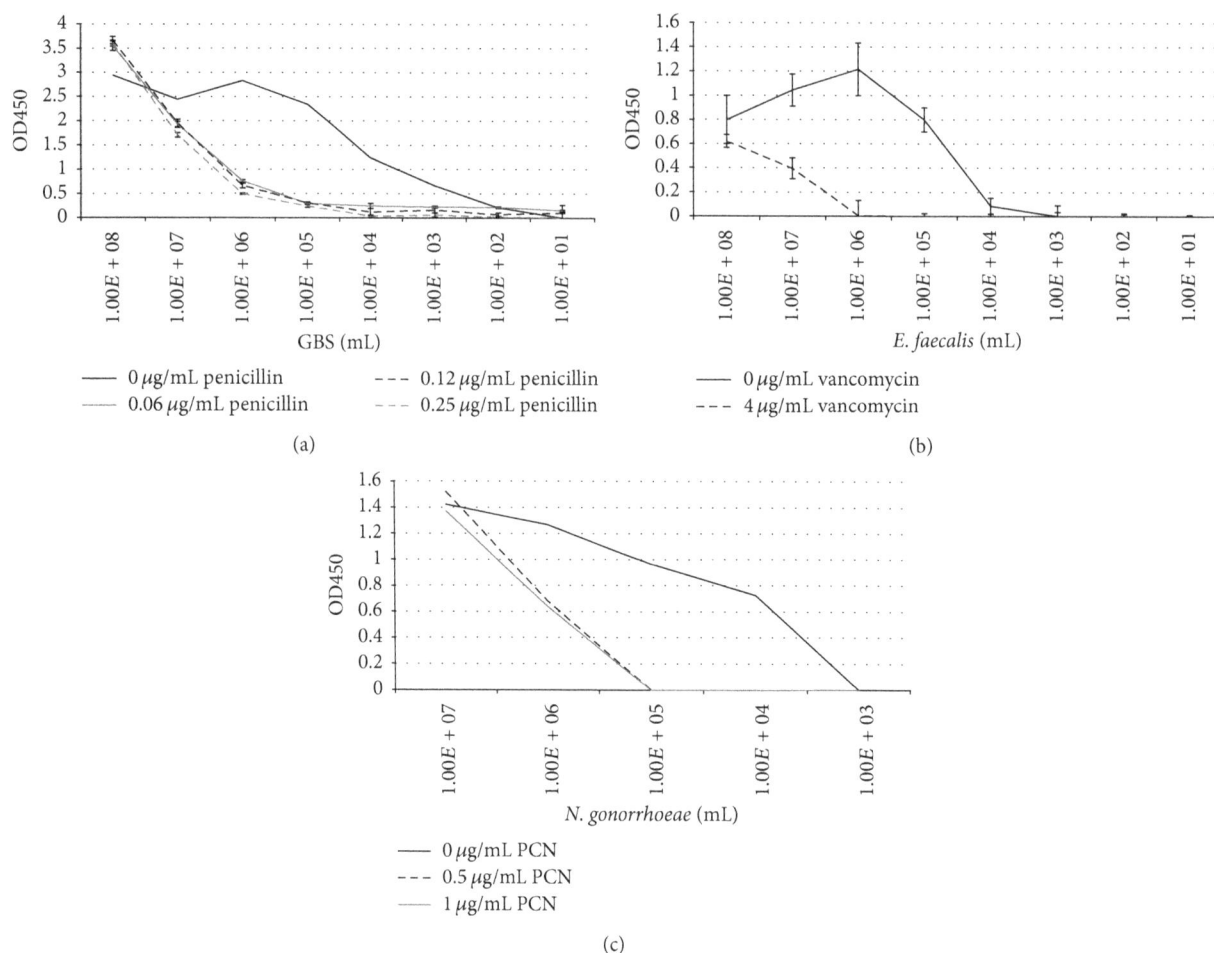

FIGURE 3: Bacterial identification and demonstration of susceptibility to selected antibiotics following a 6-hour culture. After first preparing a 0.5 McFarland in Fastidious Broth and then diluting bacterial isolates out, antibiotics were added to the wells giving the final concentrations indicated. (a) Dilutions of GBS strain 12386 (confirmed to be susceptible to penicillin by disk diffusion), in the presence of 0, 0.06, 0.12, or 0.25 μg/mL penicillin. (b) E. faecalis was diluted out in Fastidious Broth in the presence (4 μg/mL) or absence of vancomycin. *Enterococcus faecalis* ATCC strain 29212 was confirmed to be susceptible to vancomycin by disk diffusion. (c) N. gonorrhoeae was prepared and diluted out, as above, in 0, 0.5, or 1 μg/mL penicillin. Strain 1279, a clinical isolate of N. gonorrhoeae, was shown to be susceptible to penicillin by disk diffusion. Each test was performed in triplicate and data shown are representative of three individual experiments. Again, bacterial concentrations were confirmed by CFUs following plating on agar for 24–48 hours.

3.4. Inducible Resistance of GBS against Clindamycin. GBS strains previously determined to show either noninducible (Isolate A) or inducible (Isolate B) resistance to clindamycin in the presence of erythromycin were tested following 9-hour incubation. In the noninducible resistance strain (Isolate A), GBS was detected only in wells which did not receive clindamycin (Table 1). When a strain capable of showing inducible resistance was tested, GBS was detected down to a 10^3 bacteria/mL dilution, with very strong detection at 10^6 bacteria/mL, moderate detection at 10^5 bacteria/mL, and light detection at 10^4 bacteria/mL.

4. Discussion

The development of microbial resistance to antibiotics has plagued contemporary clinicians. Following the introduction of each new antibiotic, resistant isolates have been detected,

with resistance of *Staphylococcus* to Methicillin noted 2 yrs after the first use of this antibiotic in 1960, resistance of *Enterococcus* to vancomycin was noted 16 yrs after its introduction in 1972, and resistance of *Staphylococcus* to Linezolid was noted just 1 yr after its first use in 1996 [16]. The development of microbial resistance to an antibiotic has become the norm, and anticipated resistance has been confirmed again as recently as 2011 with the multidrug resistant N. gonorrhoeae strain reported in Japan [17].

That antimicrobial resistance has developed and continues to do so is not surprising. What is concerning is that the approach to managing patients with suspected infection/colonization has remained static, and in fact this approach continues to be reestablished, with the recent example of intrapartum GBS prophylaxis as recommended by the CDC in 2010 [5]. It is agreed that intrapartum GBS prophylaxis has led to a reduction in early-onset GBS sepsis:

TABLE 1: Detection of GBS following 9-hour incubation in the presence of erythromycin and dilutions of clindamycin. Isolate A (noninducible resistance to clindamycin) compared with isolate B (inducible resistance capable). ++++ OD > 3.0. +++ OD 2.0–2.9. ++ OD 1.0–1.9. + OD 0.1–0.9. − OD 0–0.099.

	10^7 bacteria/mL		10^6 bacteria/mL		10^5 bacteria/mL		10^4 bacteria/mL	
	Isolate A	Isolate B	Isolate A	Isolate B	Isolate A	Isolate B	Isolate A	Isolate B
Clindamycin 0 μg/mL Erythromycin 1.0 μg/mL	++++	++++	++++	++++	++++	++++	++++	+++
Clindamycin 0.5 μg/mL Erythromycin 1.0 μg/mL	−	++++	−	++	−	+	−	+
Clindamycin 0.05 μg/mL Erythromycin 1.0 μg/mL	−	++++	−	+++	−	+	−	+
Clindamycin 0.005 μg/mL Erythromycin 1.0 μg/mL	−	++++	−	+++	−	+	−	+

However, there is concern that this practice may promote resistant strains of E. coli [13]. The increased prevalence of vancomycin resistant Enterococcus in hospitalized patients is yet another example. As Enterococci are to a large degree resistant to cephalosporins, use of this class of antibiotic for surgical prophylaxis allows for overgrowth of Enterococcus at sites previously colonized by cephalosporin-sensitive organisms and may contribute to the increased number of hospital associated surgical site infections [18]. Perhaps nowhere is this battle between pathogen and microbicide more apparent than with N. gonorrhoeae. From the first use of sulfonamides in the 1940s, this bacterium has countered the development of resistant strains [19]. After showing that this pathogen is capable of developing resistance to any antibiotic directed against it, including sulfonamides, penicillin, tetracycline, spectinomycin, quinolones, macrolides, and now cephalosporins, it is apparent that novel approaches are needed beyond the two-drug counterattack recommended just last year [20].

We recently developed an immunoassay in which membranes coated with antibody against GBS are exposed to bacterial suspensions, and after incubating for a series of time-points, bound GBS is detected [14]. This assay was tested on patients' vaginal-rectal specimens and was found to have a high degree of sensitivity and specificity, with the added benefit of being capable of detecting nonbeta hemolytic streptococcal strains of GBS [21]. In order to decrease the interobserver variation seen with dot-blot assays, we converted the test to an ELISA format. In this study, we have substituted the anti-GBS antibodies for those directed against either N. gonorrhoeae or Enterococcus. We show that these polyclonal antibodies provide a great deal of sensitivity in a nonselective broth, with little interference from other commonly isolated cocolonizers Figure 1 and Supplemental Figure 1.

Following a six-hour incubation period, the limit of detection increased to 10^1 bacteria per mL for GBS (Figure 2). Furthermore, we show that antibiotic susceptibility may be determined (Supplemental Figure 2). From this, one may envision a panel in which a series of wells are set up in which multiple clinically relevant antibiotics are tested, providing the clinician with a targeted approach to treatment in a greatly reduced timeframe (Figure 3).

A central facet of this assay involves cellular viability: the concentration of bacteria present in the well is related specifically to the incubation times utilized. By incubating overnight, the sensitivity of the test was increased significantly as live bacteria continued to grow and divide, with GBS being detected at 10^{-2} bacteria per mL, Enterococcus detected at 10^{-1} bacteria per mL, and N. gonorrhoeae detected at 10^1 bacteria per mL (Figure 2). This allows for a sensitivity greater than published results for several PCR-based methods of detection following an enrichment step, with the unique advantage being that this test is capable of detecting viable cells [22–25].

This assay provides the unique approach of targeting the growth of a specific clinically relevant pathogen through the use of a capture antibody. An immediate binding assay demonstrates whether a pathogen is present or not. By then culturing the organism in the presence or absence of selected antibiotics, one may show that cells are viable and susceptible to specific antimicrobials, thereby allowing the clinician to then make an informed decision more rapidly.

Competing Interests

The authors report no financial interest in Nanologix, Inc. Dr. Jonathan Faro is named as a coinventor of the ELISA method utilized in this study, Patent 9034583, granted May 19, 2015. All authors report no conflict of interests.

References

[1] W. F. Vincent, W. E. Gibbons, and H. A. Gaafar, "Selective medium for the isolation of streptococci from clinical specimens," Applied Microbiology, vol. 22, no. 5, pp. 942–943, 1971.

[2] S. S. Altaie and D. Dryja, "Detection of group B Streptococcus comparison of solid and liquid culture media with and without selective antibiotics," Diagnostic Microbiology and Infectious Disease, vol. 18, no. 3, pp. 141–144, 1994.

[3] T. Block, E. Munson, A. Culver, K. Vaughan, and J. E. Hryciuk, "Comparison of carrot broth- and selective Todd-Hewitt broth-enhanced PCR protocols for real-time detection of Streptococcus agalactiae in prenatal vaginal/anorectal specimens," Journal of Clinical Microbiology, vol. 46, no. 11, pp. 3615–3620, 2008.

[4] W. P. Dela Cruz, J. Y. Richardson, J. M. Broestler, J. A. Thornton, and P. J. Danaher, "Rapid determination of macrolide and lincosamide resistance in group B streptococcus isolated from

vaginal-rectal swabs," *Infectious Diseases in Obstetrics and Gynecology*, vol. 2007, Article ID 46581, 6 pages, 2007.

[5] J. R. Verani, L. McGee, and S. J. Schrag, "Prevention of perinatal group B streptococcal disease, revised guidelines from CDC," *Morbidity and Mortality Weekly Report*, vol. 59, no. 10, pp. 1–36, 2010.

[6] J. Daniels, J. Gray, H. Pattison et al., "Rapid testing for group B streptococcus during labour: a test accuracy study with evaluation of acceptability and cost-effectiveness," *Health Technology Assessment*, vol. 13, no. 42, pp. 1–154, 2009.

[7] A. M. Caliendo, D. N. Gilbert, C. C. Ginocchio et al., "Better tests, better care: improved diagnostics for infectious diseases," *Clinical Infectious Diseases*, vol. 57, supplement 3, pp. S139–S170, 2013.

[8] Y. W. Chu, C. Tse, G. K.-L. Tsang, D. K.-S. So, J. T.-L. Fung, and J. Y.-C. Lo, "Invasive group B *Streptococcus* isolates showing reduced susceptibility to penicillin in Hong Kong," *Journal of Antimicrobial Chemotherapy*, vol. 60, no. 6, pp. 1407–1409, 2007.

[9] S. Dahesh, M. E. Hensler, N. M. Van Sorge et al., "Point mutation in the group B streptococcal pbp2x gene conferring decreased susceptibility to β-lactam antibiotics," *Antimicrobial Agents and Chemotherapy*, vol. 52, no. 8, pp. 2915–2918, 2008.

[10] K. A. Simonsen, A. L. Anderson-Berry, S. F. Delair, and H. D. Davies, "Early-onset neonatal sepsis," *Clinical Microbiology Reviews*, vol. 27, no. 1, pp. 21–47, 2014.

[11] C. D. Salgado, "The risk of developing a vancomycin-resistant *Enterococcus* bloodstream infection for colonized patients," *American Journal of Infection Control*, vol. 36, no. 10, pp. S175.e5–S175.e8, 2008.

[12] Centers for Disease Control and Prevention, "Recommendations for preventing the spread of vancomycin resistance recommendations of the Hospital Infection Control Practices Advisory Committee (HICPAC)," *Morbidity and Mortality Weekly Report*, vol. 44, no. 12, pp. 1–13, 1995.

[13] M. Unemo, D. Golparian, M. Potočnik, and S. Jeverica, "Treatment failure of pharyngeal gonorrhoea with internationally recommended first-line ceftriaxone verified in Slovenia, September 2011," *Eurosurveillance*, vol. 17, no. 25, pp. 1–4, 2012.

[14] J. Faro, A. Katz, K. Bishop, G. Riddle, and S. Faro, "Rapid diagnostic test for identifying group B *Streptococcus*," *American Journal of Perinatology*, vol. 28, no. 10, pp. 811–814, 2011.

[15] CLSI, "Performance standards for antimicrobial susceptibility testing; twenty-second informational supplement," CLSI Document M100-S22, Clinical and Laboratory Standards Institute, Wayne, Pa, USA, 2012.

[16] L. Ventola, "The antibiotic resistance crisis," *Pharmacy and Therapeutics*, vol. 40, no. 4, pp. 277–283, 2015.

[17] M. Ohnishi, T. Saika, S. Hoshina et al., "Ceftriaxone- resistant Neisseria gonorrhoeae, Japan," *Emerging Infectious Diseases*, vol. 17, no. 1, pp. 148–149, 2011.

[18] S. J. Dancer, "The problem with cephalosporins," *Journal of Antimicrobial Chemotherapy*, vol. 48, no. 4, pp. 463–478, 2001.

[19] M. Unemo and W. M. Shafer, "Antimicrobial resistance in *Neisseria gonorrhoeae* in the 21st Century: past, evolution, and future," *Clinical Microbiology Reviews*, vol. 27, no. 3, pp. 587–613, 2014.

[20] Centers for Disease Control and Prevention, "Sexually transmitted diseases treatment guidelines," *MMWR Recommendations and Reports*, vol. 64, no. 3, pp. 1–137, 2015.

[21] J. Faro, K. Bishop, G. Riddle et al., "Accuracy of an accelerated, culture-based assay for detection of group B *Streptococcus*," *Infectious Diseases in Obstetrics and Gynecology*, vol. 2013, Article ID 367935, 4 pages, 2013.

[22] S. A. Miller, E. Deak, and R. Humphries, "Comparison of the AmpliVue, BD max system, and *illumigene* molecular assays for detection of group B Streptococcus in antenatal screening specimens," *Journal of Clinical Microbiology*, vol. 53, no. 6, pp. 1938–1941, 2015.

[23] http://www.bd.com/ds/technicalCenter/inserts/max_gbs_pkgin-sert.pdf.

[24] L. Chui, T. Chiu, J. Kakulphimp, and G. J. Tyrrell, "A comparison of three real-time PCR assays for the confirmation of Neisseria gonorrhoeae following detection of N. gonorrhoeae using Roche COBAS AMPLICOR," *Clinical Microbiology and Infection*, vol. 14, no. 5, pp. 473–479, 2008.

[25] C. M. Sedgley, A. C. Nagel, C. E. Shelburne, D. B. Clewell, O. Appelbe, and A. Molander, "Quantitative real-time PCR detection of oral *Enterococcus faecalis* in humans," *Archives of Oral Biology*, vol. 50, no. 6, pp. 575–583, 2005.

8

A Systematic Review of Point of Care Testing for *Chlamydia trachomatis*, *Neisseria gonorrhoeae*, and *Trichomonas vaginalis*

Sasha Herbst de Cortina,[1] Claire C. Bristow,[2]
Dvora Joseph Davey,[3] and Jeffrey D. Klausner[1,3]

[1]*Division of Infectious Diseases, Department of Medicine, University of California Los Angeles, 10833 Le Conte Avenue,*
 Los Angeles, CA 90095, USA
[2]*Division of Global Public Health, Department of Medicine, University of California San Diego, 9500 Gilman Drive 0507,*
 La Jolla, CA 92093, USA
[3]*Department of Epidemiology, Fielding School of Public Health, University of California Los Angeles,*
 640 Charles E. Young Drive S., Los Angeles, CA 90024, USA

Correspondence should be addressed to Sasha Herbst de Cortina; sherbstdecortina@mednet.ucla.edu

Academic Editor: Louise Hafner

Objectives. Systematic review of point of care (POC) diagnostic tests for sexually transmitted infections: *Chlamydia trachomatis* (CT), *Neisseria gonorrhoeae* (NG), and *Trichomonas vaginalis* (TV). *Methods*. Literature search on PubMed for articles from January 2010 to August 2015, including original research in English on POC diagnostics for sexually transmitted CT, NG, and/or TV. *Results*. We identified 33 publications with original research on POC diagnostics for CT, NG, and/or TV. Thirteen articles evaluated test performance, yielding at least one test for each infection with sensitivity and specificity ≥90%. Each infection also had currently available tests with sensitivities <60%. Three articles analyzed cost effectiveness, and five publications discussed acceptability and feasibility. POC testing was acceptable to both providers and patients and was also demonstrated to be cost effective. Fourteen proof of concept articles introduced new tests. *Conclusions*. Highly sensitive and specific POC tests are available for CT, NG, and TV, but improvement is possible. Future research should focus on acceptability, feasibility, and cost of POC testing. While pregnant women specifically have not been studied, the results available in nonpregnant populations are encouraging for the ability to test and treat women in antenatal care to prevent adverse pregnancy and neonatal outcomes.

1. Introduction

Globally, *Chlamydia trachomatis* (CT), *Neisseria gonorrhoeae* (NG), and *Trichomonas vaginalis* (TV) are responsible for over 351.7 million infections per year [1]. Though curable, those infections can lead to long-term sequelae in both men and women, especially among pregnant women and their children. CT, NG, and TV can cause preterm birth, fetal growth retardation, low birth weight, pelvic inflammatory disease (PID) which can lead to ectopic pregnancy or infertility, perinatal diseases such as conjunctivitis and pneumonia, and infant death [2–5]. It has been demonstrated that up to 40% of women with STIs will develop PID, and

these women are up to 10 times more likely to have an ectopic pregnancy [5], resulting in loss of pregnancy and even death. Maternal to child transmission of HIV has also been demonstrated to occur at higher rates among mothers who are coinfected with CT or NG [6]. Additionally, an estimated 4,000 infants globally are born blind each year due to maternal to child transmission of CT and NG [7]. Despite those sobering outcomes, the global response to controlling STIs has been inadequate. The World Health Organization (WHO) estimates that the global incidences of CT, NG, and TV have been steadily rising since 1995 and increased from 2005 to 2008 by 11.7% [1]. Antenatal care provides an excellent opportunity for screening for STIs, and this strategy has largely been successful in preventing mother to child transmission of HIV. An estimated 180,000 HIV infections in infants were averted globally between 2005 and 2008 due to screening and treatment of HIV-infected pregnant women [8]. International studies have shown antenatal screening for CT, NG, and TV to be feasible and acceptable as well as effective at reducing rates of infection and adverse outcomes [9–12]. Therefore, antenatal screening and treatment not only is important in preventing sequelae of CT, NG, and TV in women and neonates but also is a feasible intervention for infection control at the population level. More needs to be done to ensure pregnant women receive treatment for STIs starting with improving access to rapid, accurate, and inexpensive screening.

Globally, the standard of care increasingly focuses on point of care (POC) diagnostic tools for STIs. In 2002, the WHO Special Program for Research and Training in Tropical Disease identified POC testing as a key priority for controlling curable STIs [13]. POC tests can potentially be defined in multiple ways, and the WHO Special Program outlined the ASSURED criteria: affordable, sensitive, specific, user-friendly, rapid and robust, equipment-free, and deliverable. However, others also define a POC test as any diagnostic tool that can provide accurate results and facilitate treatment within the same clinical visit as testing [14]. That definition includes some nucleic acid amplification tests (NAATs), although they do not fit classic ASSURED criteria.

The purposes of POC testing are to reduce the frequency of patients who do not receive results and improve the ability to treat cases in the same clinical visit as testing. In resource-poor environments, patients may not be able to return quickly or at all for treatment, leading to morbidity in the infected individual as well as potential transmission from mother to child or to sex partners. Mathematical models demonstrate that even a POC test with 63% sensitivity ensures greater rates of treatment than a test with high sensitivity and a poor patient return rate [15]. Furthermore, while syndromic management may allow treatment without a follow-up visit, syndromic management misses most infections with CT, NG, and TV, as most are asymptomatic [2–4, 16]. Therefore, although syndromic management may identify individual cases, it is unlikely to be an effective public health tool in reducing the burden of disease on population levels. One study of an emergency department in North Carolina, USA, found that while syndromic management led to the treatment for presumed CT or NG of 28% patients studied, only 7.6% of all patients were actually infected, and 63.6% of those infected went untreated [17]. Syndromic management and presumptive treatment have the additional drawback of causing inappropriate treatment or treatment of uninfected individuals, contributing to the growing global problem of antibiotic resistance. Therefore, accurate testing facilitating same-visit treatment is crucial to reducing the burden of disease, especially among pregnant women and their children.

This systematic review aims to evaluate the current status of POC diagnostics for CT, NG, and TV and makes recommendations for the future of POC testing in low resource settings.

2. Methods

We used PRISMA guidelines [18] to focus our systematic review of recent literature published between January 2010 and August 2015 that reported on POC diagnostics for NG, CT, and TV. A comprehensive search term using a compilation of medical subject headings, text words, and subheadings was used to search PubMed (Figure 1). Abstracts of all search results and the full text of all potentially eligible articles were reviewed. This search yielded sixty-one articles whose abstracts we evaluated to determine whether they fit inclusion criteria. The inclusion criteria were (1) publications including CT, NG, or TV as STIs; (2) publications that date from January 2010 through August 2015; (3) publications relating to diagnostics; (4) publications published in English; and (5) original research. The exclusion criteria were (1) publications not covering CT, NG, or TV; (2) publications including those infections but not in the sexually transmissible form; (3) publications published before 2010; and (4) publications not evaluating POC diagnostics. Articles were sorted into the following subject categories and stratified based on disease: (1) performance evaluations, (2) cost analyses, (3) acceptability and feasibility trials, and (4) proof of concept studies.

3. Results

We analyzed results from 61 publications on POC testing for CT, NG, and/or TV from 2010 to 2015. Twenty-eight articles were excluded from analysis, yielding 33 articles for the review (Figure 1).

3.1. Performance Evaluations. Our search yielded thirteen articles that evaluated the performance of POC tests [19–31]. Eight reports evaluated ten CT tests [19–26], four reports evaluated four NG tests [21, 25, 27, 28], and three reports evaluated six TV tests [29–31]. Two reports evaluated tests for both CT and NG [21, 25]. We further stratified the results when available for different populations (i.e., male versus female and/or high versus low risk) and different collection sources (i.e., urine versus vaginal swab versus cervical swab). Results are summarized in Tables 1–3. For each disease, the sensitivities and specificities of various tests varied widely. However, for each STI there was at least one test which consistently had sensitivity and specificity of ≥90%.

3.1.1. Chlamydia trachomatis. For CT, the ten diagnostics evaluated were the Gram stained urethral smear [19, 20], GeneXpert® Xpert CT/NG (Xpert CT/NG) (Cepheid, Sunnyvale, CA, USA) [21], aQcare Chlamydia TRF kit (Medisensor, Inc., Daegu, Korea) [22], Chlamydia Rapid Test (CRT) (Diagnostics for the Real World (Europe), Cambridge, UK) [23, 24], ACON Plate CT Rapid Test (ACON CT) (ACON Laboratories, San Diego, CA, USA) [23, 25], ACON NG and CT Duo test combo (ACON Duo) (ACON Laboratories, San Diego, CA, USA) [25], QuickVue Chlamydia Rapid Test (QuickVue) (Quidel Corporation, San Diego, CA, USA) [25, 26], Automated Urine Flow Cytometry (AUFC) of first void

TABLE 1: Performance evaluations of point of care tests for *Chlamydia trachomatis* from 2010 to 2015.

Study authors and year	Location	Test used	Sample type	Reference test	Sample size and population	Sensitivity (95% CI)	Specificity (95% CI)	Positive predictive value (95% CI) or LR+	Negative predictive value (95% CI) or LR−
Bartelsman et al. 2015 [19]	Amsterdam, Netherlands	Gram stained urethral smear (2008-2009: including asymptomatic)	Urethral swab	APTIMA CT assay (Hologic, USA)	7,185 "high risk" men at STI clinic, both symptomatic and asymptomatic	83.8% (81.2–86.1%)	74.1% (73.0–75.2%)	31.7% (29.8–33.6%)	97.0% (96.4%–97.4%)
Bartelsman et al. 2015 [19]	Amsterdam, Netherlands	Gram stained urethral smear (2010-2011: only symptomatic)	Urethral swab	APTIMA CT assay (Hologic, USA)	18,852 "high risk," symptomatic men at STI clinic	91.0% (89.5–92.3%)	53.1% (51.8–54.4%)	35.6% (34.1–37.1%)	95.4% (94.6–96.1%)
Pond et al. 2015 [20]	London, UK	Gram stained urethral smear	Urethral swab	BD Viper Qx System (BD, USA)	208 symptomatic male patients (mean age 31 years) without NG at genitourinary medicine clinic	93.7% (67.7–99.6%)	N/A	16.1% (9.6–25.5%)	99.1% (94.5–99.9%)
Gaydos et al. 2013 [21]	USA	Cepheid GeneXpert CT/NG (nucleic acid amplification test (NAAT))	Vaginal swab (self-collected)	Aptima Combo 2 assay (Hologic, USA) & ProbeTec ET System (BD, USA)	1,722 sexually active females, symptomatic and asymptomatic, at OB-GYN, STD, teen, public health, or family planning clinics	98.7% (93.1–100%)	99.4% (98.9–99.7%)	88.6%	99.9%
Gaydos et al. 2013 [21]	USA	Cepheid GeneXpert CT/NG (NAAT)	Endocervical swab	Aptima Combo 2 assay (Hologic, USA) & ProbeTec ET System (BD, USA)	1,722 sexually active females, symptomatic and asymptomatic, at OB-GYN, STD, teen, public health, or family planning clinics	97.4% (91.0–99.7)	99.6% (99.1–99.8%)	91.6%	99.9%
Gaydos et al. 2013 [21]	USA	Cepheid GeneXpert CT/NG (NAAT)	Urine	Aptima Combo 2 assay (Hologic, USA) & ProbeTec ET System (BD, USA)	1,722 sexually active females, symptomatic and asymptomatic, at OB-GYN, STD, teen, public health, or family planning clinics	97.6% (91.5–99.7%)	99.8% (99.5–100%)	96.4%	99.9%
Gaydos et al. 2013 [21]	USA	Cepheid GeneXpert CT/NG (NAAT)	Urine	Aptima Combo 2 assay (Hologic, USA) & ProbeTec ET System (BD, USA)	1,387 sexually active males, symptomatic and asymptomatic, at OB-GYN, STD, teen, public health, or family planning clinics	97.5% (91.4–99.7%)	99.9% (99.6–100%)	98.7%	99.8%

TABLE 1: Continued.

Study authors and year	Location	Test used	Sample type	Reference test	Sample size and population	Sensitivity (95% CI)	Specificity (95% CI)	Positive predictive value (95% CI) or LR+	Negative predictive value (95% CI) or LR−
Ham et al. 2015 [22]	South Korea	aQcare Chlamydia TRF kit (lateral flow immunoassay (LFIA))	Endocervical and urethral swabs, urine overall results	AccuPower CT & NG Real-Time PCR Kit (Bioneer, Korea)	340 women and 101 men, age 20–80, who visited a hospital for the evaluation of STD symptoms	93.0% (88.0–96.3%)	96.3% (94.6–97.5%)	89.8% (85.0–93.0%)	97.5% (95.8–98.7%)
Ham et al. 2015 [22]	South Korea	aQcare Chlamydia TRF kit (LFIA)	Endocervical and urethral swabs	AccuPower CT & NG Real-Time PCR Kit (Bioneer, Korea)	8 urethral swabs and 340 endocervical swabs from women and men, age 20–80, who visited a hospital for the evaluation of STD symptoms	93.8% (88.6–97.0%)	96.8% (94.8–98.1%)	91.9% Calculated by review authors	97.6% Calculated by review authors
Ham et al. 2015 [22]	South Korea	aQcare Chlamydia TRF kit (LFIA)	Urine	AccuPower CT & NG Real-Time PCR Kit (Bioneer, Korea)	93 men and women, age 20–80, who visited a hospital for the evaluation of STD symptoms	88.2% (67.4–97.7%)	94.7% (90.1–96.9%)	79.0% Calculated by review authors	97.3% Calculated by review authors
Hurly et al. 2014 [23]	Port Vila, Vanuatu	Chlamydia Rapid Test, Diagnostics for the Real World (Signal Amplification System (SAS))	Urine	COBAS TaqMan Analyzer CT assay (Roche, USA)	156 men, age 18+, at reproductive health clinic	41.4% (23.5–61.1%)	89.0% (82.2–93.8%)	46.2% Calculated by review authors	86.9% Calculated by review authors
Hurly et al. 2014 [23]	Port Vila, Vanuatu	Chlamydia Rapid Test, Diagnostics for the Real World (SAS)	Vaginal swab (self-collected)	COBAS TaqMan Analyzer CT assay (Roche, USA)	223 women, age 18+, at reproductive health clinic, pregnant women not excluded	74.2% (61.5–84.5%)	95.7% (91.3–98.2%)	86.8% Calculated by review authors	90.6% Calculated by review authors
van der Helm et al. 2012 [24]	Paramaribo, Suriname	Chlamydia Rapid Test, Diagnostics for the Real World (SAS)	Vaginal swab (nurse-collected)	Aptima CT assay (Hologic, USA)	912 women (median age 30 years) at either STI clinic or sexual health clinic	41.2% (31.9–50.9%)	96.4% (95.0–97.5%)	59.2% (47.5–70.1%)	92.9% (91.0–94.5%)
van der Helm et al. 2012 [24]	Paramaribo, Suriname	Chlamydia Rapid Test, Diagnostics for the Real World (SAS)	Vaginal swab (nurse-collected)	Aptima CT assay (Hologic, USA)	159 women seeking STI care at STI clinic, "high risk"	39.4% (24.0–56.6%)	94.4% (89.3–97.5%)	65.0% (42.7–83.2%)	85.6% (79.0–90.7%)
van der Helm et al. 2012 [24]	Paramaribo, Suriname	Chlamydia Rapid Test, Diagnostics for the Real World (SAS)	Vaginal swab (nurse-collected)	Aptima CT assay (Hologic, USA)	753 women at sexual health/family planning clinic, "low risk"	42.0% (30.8–53.9%)	96.8% (95.3–97.9%)	56.9% (43.1–69.9%)	94.3% (92.4–95.8%)
Hurly et al. 2014 [23]	Port Vila, Vanuatu	ACON Chlamydia Rapid Test Device (immunoassay)	Urine	COBAS TaqMan Analyzer CT assay (Roche, USA)	133 men, age 18+, at reproductive health clinic	43.8% (19.8–70.1%)	98.3% (93.9–99.8%)	77.8% Calculated by review authors	92.7% Calculated by review authors

TABLE 1: Continued.

Study authors and year	Location	Test used	Sample type	Reference test	Sample size & population	Sensitivity (95% CI)	Specificity (95% CI)	Positive predictive value (95% CI) or LR+	Negative predictive value (95% CI) or LR−
Hurly et al. 2014 [23]	Port Vila, Vanuatu	ACON Chlamydia Rapid Test Device (immunoassay)	Vaginal swab (self-collected)	COBAS TaqMan Analyzer CT assay (Roche, USA)	75 women, age 18+, at reproductive health clinic, pregnant women not excluded	66.7% (22.3–95.7%)	91.3% (82.0–96.7%)	40.0% Calculated by review authors	96.9% Calculated by review authors
Nuñez-Forero et al. 2016 [25]	Bogota, Colombia	ACON Chlamydia Rapid Test Device (immunoassay)	Endocervical swab	COBAS AMPLICOR Analyzer CT/NG assay (Roche, USA)	229 sexually active females, age 14–49, w/lower UTI symptoms (pregnant women excluded)	22.7% (2.9–42.5%)	100% (99.7–100%)	Not quantifiable (LR+)	0.8 (LR−)
Nuñez-Forero et al. 2016 [25]	Bogota, Colombia	ACON CT/NG Duo test (immunoassay)	Endocervical swab	COBAS AMPLICOR Analyzer CT/NG assay (Roche, USA)	491 sexually active females, age 14–49, w/lower UTI symptoms (pregnant women excluded)	30.5% (17.9–43.1%)	99.8% (99.2–100%)	131.8 (LR+)	0.7 (LR−)
Nuñez-Forero et al. 2016 [25]	Bogota, Colombia	QuickVue Chlamydia Rapid Test (immunoassay)	Endocervical swab	COBAS AMPLICOR Analyzer CT/NG assay (Roche, USA)	664 sexually active females, age 14–49, w/lower UTI symptoms (pregnant women excluded)	37.7% (23.7–51.7%)	99.4% (98.6–100%)	57.6 (LR+)	0.6 (LR−)
Van Dommelen et al. 2010 [26]	Maastricht, Netherlands	QuickVue Chlamydia Rapid Test (immunoassay)	Vaginal swab (self-collected)	COBAS AMPLICOR Analyzer CT/NG assay (Roche, USA)	763 females, age 16+, at STI clinic	25.0% (15.7–34.3%)	99.7% (99.3–100%)	91.3%	91.5%
Pond et al. 2015 [20]	London, UK	Automated Urine Flow Cytometry of first void urine	Urine	BD Viper Qx System (BD, USA)	208 symptomatic male patients (mean age 31 years) without NG at genitourinary medicine clinic	93.7% (67.7–99.6%)	N/A	28.3% (17.1–42.5%)	99.3% (95.8–99.9%)
Van Dommelen et al. 2010 [26]	Maastricht, Netherlands	Handilab-C (enzyme detection)	Vaginal swab (self-collected)	COBAS AMPLICOR Analyzer CT/NG assay (Roche, USA)	735 females, age 16+, at STI clinic	22.5% (13.0–31.7%)	88.9% (86.4–91.3%)	90.4%	4.8%
Van Dommelen et al. 2010 [26]	Maastricht, Netherlands	Biorapid Chlamydia Ag test (antigen detection)	Vaginal swab (self-collected)	COBAS AMPLICOR Analyzer CT/NG assay (Roche, USA)	763 females, age 16+, at STI clinic	17.1% (8.9–25.2%)	93.7% (91.9–95.5%)	24.6%	90.4%

TABLE 2: Performance evaluations of point of care tests for *Neisseria gonorrhoeae* from 2010 to 2015.

Study authors and year	Location	Test used	Sample type	Reference test	Sample size and population	Sensitivity (95% CI)	Specificity (95% CI)	Positive predictive value (95% CI) or LR+	Negative predictive value (95% CI) or LR−
Bartelsman et al. 2014 [27]	Amsterdam, Netherlands	Gram stained urethral or cervical smear (2008-2009)	Urethral and cervical swabs	Culture	10,952 "high risk" men and women attending STI clinic, symptomatic and asymptomatic	87.2% (83.3–90.4%)	99.9% (99.8–100%)	97.0% (94.5–98.5%)	99.6% (99.4–99.7%)
Bartelsman et al. 2014 [27]	Amsterdam, Netherlands	Gram stained urethral or cervical smear (2010-2011)	Urethral and cervical swabs	Culture	11,755 "high risk" men and women attending STI clinic, only symptomatic	84.8% (82.3–87.1%)	99.8% (99.7–99.9%)	97.7% (96.3–98.6%)	98.8% (98.5–99.0%)
Bartelsman et al. 2014 [27]	Amsterdam, Netherlands	Gram stained cervical smear (2008-2009)	Cervical swab	Culture	3767 "high risk" women attending STI clinic, symptomatic and asymptomatic	32.0% (19.5–46.7%)	100% (99.9–100%)	100% (82.9–100%)	99.1% (98.7–99.4%)
Bartelsman et al. 2014 [27]	Amsterdam, Netherlands	Gram stained cervical smear (2010-2011)	Cervical swab	Culture	4530 "high risk" women attending STI clinic, only symptomatic	23.1% (16.1–31.3%)	99.9% (99.8–100%)	90.9% (75.7–98.1%)	98.7% (97.3–98.2%)
Bartelsman et al. 2014 [27]	Amsterdam, Netherlands	Gram stained urethral smear (2008-2009)	Urethral swab	Culture	7185 "high risk" men attending STI clinic, symptomatic and asymptomatic	95.9% (93.1–97.8%)	99.9% (99.7–99.9%)	96.8% (94.2–98.5%)	99.8% (99.7–99.9%)
Bartelsman et al. 2014 [27]	Amsterdam, Netherlands	Gram stained urethral smear (2010-2011)	Urethral swab	Culture	7225 "high risk" men attending STI clinic, only symptomatic	95.4% (93.7–96.8%)	99.8% (99.6–99.9%)	98.0% (96.7–98.9%)	99.5% (99.3–99.6%)
Gaydos et al. 2013 [21]	USA	Cepheid GeneXpert CT/NG (NAAT)	Vaginal swab (self-collected)	Aptima Combo 2 assay (Hologic, USA) & ProbeTec ET System (BD, USA)	1,722 sexually active females, symptomatic and asymptomatic, at OB-GYN, STD, teen, public health, or family planning clinics	100% (87.3–100%)	99.9% (99.6–100%)	91.7%	100%
Gaydos et al. 2013 [21]	USA	Cepheid GeneXpert CT/NG (NAAT)	Endocervical swab	Aptima Combo 2 assay (Hologic, USA) & ProbeTec ET System (BD, USA)	1,722 sexually active females, symptomatic and asymptomatic, at OB-GYN, STD, teen, public health, or family planning clinics	100% (87.3–100%)	100% (99.8–100%)	100%	100%

TABLE 2: Continued.

Study authors and year	Location	Test used	Sample type	Reference test	Sample size and population	Sensitivity (95% CI)	Specificity (95% CI)	Positive predictive value (95% CI) or LR+	Negative predictive value (95% CI) or LR−
Gaydos et al. 2013 [21]	USA	Cepheid GeneXpert CT/NG (NAAT)	Urine	Aptima Combo 2 assay (Hologic, USA) & ProbeTec ET System (BD, USA)	1,722 sexually active females, symptomatic and asymptomatic, at OB-GYN, STD, teen, public health, or family planning clinics	95.6% (78.1–99.9%)	99.9% (99.7–100%)	95.6%	99.9%
Gaydos et al. 2013 [21]	USA	Cepheid GeneXpert CT/NG (NAAT)	Urine	Aptima Combo 2 assay (Hologic, USA) & ProbeTec ET System (BD, USA)	1,387 sexually active males, symptomatic and asymptomatic, at OB-GYN, STD, teen, public health, or family planning clinics	98.0% (89.4–99.9%)	99.9% (99.6–100%)	98.0%	99.9%
Nuñez-Forero et al. 2016 [25]	Bogota, Colombia	ACON CT/NG Duo test (immunoassay)	Endocervical swab	COBAS AMPLICOR Analyzer CT/NG assay (Roche, USA)	491 sexually active females, age 14–49, symptomatic (pregnant women excluded)	12.5% (0–41.7%)	99.8% (99.3–100%)	60.4 (LR+)	0.4 (LR−)
Nuñez-Forero et al. 2016 [25]	Bogota, Colombia	ACON NG individual test (immunoassay)	Endocervical swab	COBAS AMPLICOR Analyzer CT/NG assay (Roche, USA)	773 sexually active females, age 14–49, asymptomatic (pregnant women excluded)	Not quantifiable (no true positives)	97.2% (96–98.5%)	Not quantifiable (LR+)	Not quantifiable (LR−)
Samarawickrama et al. 2014 [28]	London, UK	BioStar Optical ImmunoAssay	Urine	Aptima Combo 2 assay (Hologic, USA)	52 men, age 18+, attending sexual health clinic	100% (57–100%)	98% (98–100%)	83% (44–97%)	100% (92–100%)
Samarawickrama et al. 2014 [28]	London, UK	BioStar Optical ImmunoAssay	Urine	Microscopy	33 men, age 18+, attending sexual health clinic	100% (51–100%)	93% (78–98%)	67% (30–90%)	100% (88–100%)
Samarawickrama et al. 2014 [28]	London, UK	BioStar Optical ImmunoAssay	Urine	Culture	32 men, age 18+, attending sexual health clinic	100% (51–100%)	93% (77–98%)	67% (30–90%)	100% (87–100%)

TABLE 3: Performance evaluations of point of care tests for *Trichomonas vaginalis* from 2010 to 2015.

Study authors and year	Location	Test used	Sample type	Reference test	Sample size and population	Sensitivity (95% CI)	Specificity (95% CI)	Positive predictive value (95% CI)	Negative predictive value (95% CI)
Hegazy et al. 2012 [29]	Mansoura, Dakahlia Governorate, Egypt	OSOM Trichomonas Rapid Test (antigen detection)	Vaginal swab (care provider-collected)	Positive on either wet mount microscopy or culture	258 women, age 18–50, attending gynecology and fertility clinic	98.0%	99.4%	99.0%	98.8%
Khatoon et al. 2015 [30]	North India	OSOM Trichomonas Rapid Test (antigen detection)	Vaginal swab (collector not specified)	Culture	835 females, age 15–45, at gynecological clinic, symptomatic, excluded pregnant women	88.2%	99.6%	95.2%	98.9%
Nathan et al. 2015 [31]	UK	OSOM Trichomonas Rapid Test (antigen detection)	Vaginal swab (care provider-collected)	Positive on 2+ of 5 tests: microscopy, culture, OSOM Trichomonas Rapid Test (Sekisui, USA), in-house real time PCR, and Aptima TV assay (Hologic, USA)	246 women, age 18+, at sexual/reproductive health clinic, symptomatic	92% (73–99%)	100% (98.3–100%)	100% (84–100%)	99.1% (96.8–99.9%)
Khatoon et al. 2015 [30]	North India	Acridine orange staining	Vaginal swab (collector not specified)	Culture	835 females, age 15–45, at gynecological clinic, symptomatic, excluded pregnant women	73.5%	99.6%	94.3%	97.7%
Khatoon et al. 2015 [30]	North India	Wet mount microscopy	Vaginal swab (collector not specified)	Culture	835 females, age 15–45, at gynecological clinic, symptomatic, excluded pregnant women	58.8%	99.3%	88.9%	96.5%
Nathan et al. 2015 [31]	UK	Wet mount microscopy	Vaginal swab (care provider-collected)	Positive on 2+ of 5 tests: microscopy, culture, OSOM Trichomonas Rapid Test (Sekisui, USA), in-house real time PCR, and Aptima TV assay (Hologic, USA)	246 women, age 18+, at sexual/reproductive health clinic, symptomatic	38% (19–59%)	100% (98.3–100%)	100% (66–100%)	93.7% (89.8–96.4%)
Nathan et al. 2015 [31]	UK	Real-time in-house PCR	Vaginal swab (care provider-collected)	Positive on 2+ of 5 tests: microscopy, culture, OSOM Trichomonas Rapid Test (Sekisui, USA), in-house real time PCR, and Aptima TV assay (Hologic, USA)	246 women, age 18+, at sexual/reproductive health clinic, symptomatic	88% (68–97%)	99.6 (97.5–99.99%)	96% (77–99.2%)	98.7% (96.1–99.7%)
Nathan et al. 2015 [31]	UK	Culture	Vaginal swab (care provider-collected)	Positive on 2+ of 5 tests: microscopy, culture, OSOM Trichomonas Rapid Test (Sekisui, USA), in-house real time PCR, and Aptima TV assay (Hologic, USA)	246 women, age 18+, at sexual/reproductive health clinic, symptomatic	88% (68–97%)	100% (98.3–100%)	100% (84–100%)	98.7% (96.2–99.7%)

Search criteria:

(Sexually transmitted diseases or sexually transmitted infection* and (chlamydia or gonorrh* or trichom*)) and (point-of-care and (rapid test or diagnostic or screening or test)) in last 5 years

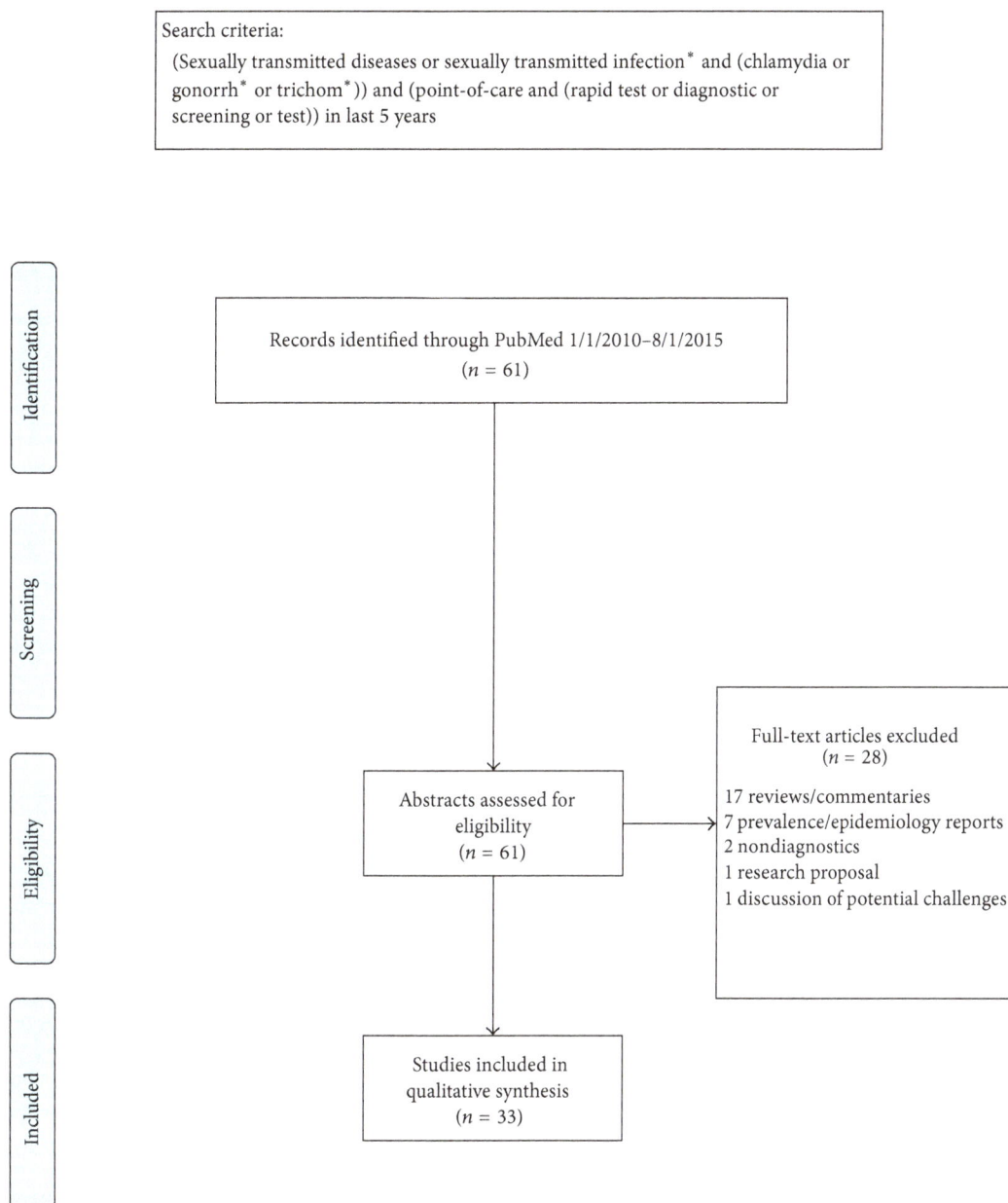

FIGURE 1: PRISMA flow diagram of publications searched. * refers to the search function of including all words which have the same beginning as the starred word and can have any ending after the star. For example: "gonorrh*" will search for "gonorrhea," "gonorrhoea," and "gonorrhoeae."

urine [20], Handilab-C (Zonda, Dallas, TX, USA) [26], and Biorapid Chlamydia Ag test (Biokit, S.A., Barcelona, Spain) [26]. The performance results are summarized in Table 1. All evaluations used NAAT as a reference test. The best performing test was the Xpert CT/NG, an FDA cleared real-time PCR platform, which consistently had sensitivities and specificities >97% across sample types [21]. The aQcare Chlamydia TRF kit and AUFC also performed well, with sensitivities and specificities above 90%, although they were each evaluated in one study [20, 22]. The remainder of the diagnostics did not perform adequately, with either sensitivities or specificities <75% and often <50% [19, 20, 23–26]. The highly sensitive

Xpert CT/NG and aQcare Chlamydia TRF kit, a rapid NAAT and lateral flow immunoassay, respectively, were the only tests of their test type evaluated [20, 21]. The other test types did not perform as accurately.

For both the Xpert CT/NG and aQcare Chlamydia TRF kit, the authors did not report significant differences in accuracy depending on sample type [21, 22]. For the Xpert CT/NG, there were not any significant differences between detecting infections in men using urine and women using urine, vaginal swabs, or endocervical swabs [21]. However, when Hurly et al. compared men and women for the CRT and ACON CT test, they found lower sensitivities for men than women, for both tests [23]. The authors attribute this difference in accuracy to the difference in sample type—urine versus vaginal swabs—and the organism load in each type of sample [23].

3.1.2. Neisseria gonorrhoeae. For NG, the five diagnostics evaluated were the Xpert CT/NG [21], ACON Duo [25], NG ACON Plate (ACON NG) (ACON Laboratories, San Diego, CA, USA) [25], Gram stain urethral or cervical smear [27], and BioStar Optical ImmunoAssay-Gonorrhea (BioStar) (BioStar, Inc., Boulder, CO, USA) [28]. The performance results are summarized in Table 2. The Gram stain was compared to culture [27]; the BioStar assay to NAAT, culture, and microscopy [28]; and the remainder to NAAT as the reference standard. All five tests were each only evaluated in one study. The Xpert CT/NG had the highest sensitivities and specificities, consistently >95% between sample types for both men and women [21]. The BioStar assay had similar sensitivities and specificities [28], although with a much smaller sample size. Although the BioStar assay and the ACON NG and ACON Duo tests are all immunoassays, the BioStar assay was far more sensitive than the ACON tests [25, 28]. As with the CT studies, the ACON Duo and ACON NG tests had sensitivities <35% [25]. Gram staining had dramatically and significantly different sensitivities between urethral smears for men and cervical smears for women. Among men, the Gram stain urethral smear had sensitivities >95%, but for women, the sensitivities of Gram stain cervical smear were <35% [27].

3.1.3. Trichomonas vaginalis. For TV, the six diagnostics evaluated were the OSOM Trichomonas Rapid Test (Sekisui Diagnostics, Lexington, MA, USA) [29–31], acridine orange staining [30], wet mount microscopy [30, 31], real-time in-house PCR [31], and culture [31]. The performance results are summarized in Table 3. All diagnostics were compared to culture [30] or a composite of multiple tests as the reference standard [29, 31]. Across three different studies, the OSOM Test performed well, with sensitivities and specificities >88% [29–31]. This was in contrast to the traditionally used POC diagnostic, wet mount microscopy, which had sensitivities <60% in two studies [30, 31]. All the studies were conducted on women using vaginal swabs, so no differences between samples types were reported, although one article mentioned that the higher organism load required for detection by culture and microscopy may have reduced the accuracy of those two tests as compared to other tests using the same sample type [31].

3.2. Cost and Cost Effectiveness. Our search found three publications which analyzed the cost effectiveness of POC diagnostics for CT and/or NG [27, 32, 33]. One study was a retrospective analysis of results from actual patients [27], while the other two used mathematical models [32, 33]. All three found that POC tests were a cost effective strategy for diagnosing those STIs, supporting the conclusion of Gift et al. in 1999 that a reasonably accurate POC test can be a cost effective diagnostic by minimizing loss to follow-up [15].

In 2014, Bartelsman et al. performed a study on women attending an STI clinic in Amsterdam between 2008 and 2011 [27]. In 2008-2009, all "high risk" (as determined by physicians) patients at the clinic were offered Gram stains for NG, but in 2010-2011 this was limited to only women who had urogenital symptoms. That change saved €2.34 (US$2.54 using 2015 conversion rate) per correctly managed consultation without significantly changing loss to follow-up and while maintaining an equivalent diagnostic accuracy as the standard of care, culture.

In 2014, Turner et al. created a simulation of 1.2 million attendees at a sexual health clinic in England to compare the use of a POC NAAT with the standard protocol for CT and NG [32]. Using the NAAT instead of standard protocol saved £11.7 million (US$17.7 million using 2015 conversion rate) and an additional 47 Quality-Adjusted Life Years over all patients. They therefore found the POC NAAT to be a cost effective diagnostic, improving both cost and health outcomes. In a 2013 model, Huang et al. created a decision tree for a scenario of 10,000 women visiting an STI clinic with a hypothetical CT POC test [33]. With a test sensitivity of 92.9%, test cost of $33.48, and 47.5% of women willing to wait the 40 minutes for a test result, the POC test saved $5,050 for each case of PID averted compared with a non-POC NAAT. They found the POC test would save money compared to a non-POC NAAT as long as the POC tests had a sensitivity of 87.1% or greater or if it cost less than $41.52.

3.3. Feasibility and Acceptability. Our search yielded five articles which discussed feasibility and acceptability of using POC diagnostics in clinical settings [24, 34–37]. Three studies, by van der Helm et al. and Huppert et al. in 2010 and 2011, surveyed female patients about their preferences [24, 34, 35]. The other two, by Hsieh et al. in 2010 and 2011, instead surveyed health care providers for their opinions on averting potential challenges of POC testing [36, 37]. All of the referenced reports agreed that POC testing would be feasible and acceptable to perform in a clinical setting.

van der Helm et al. and Hsieh et al. in 2010 and 2011 focused on wait time as a potential challenge for POC testing. In 2012, van der Helm et al. interviewed women at an STI clinic in Maastricht, the Netherlands, regarding the acceptability of waiting for the results of a rapid CT test, in this case CRT [24]. They found that 98.7% of women agreed to wait for half an hour for results, and 26.7% of this group would be willing to wait for an hour. These results correspond with qualitative studies performed by Hsieh et al. in 2010 and 2011. In 2010, focus groups of clinicians and other professionals working in STIs highlighted long wait times as a major barrier to use of current POC tests, in addition to complex protocols and difficulty of interpreting results [36]. As a follow-up to these surveys, Hsieh et al. performed an online survey in 2011 for STI clinicians who also identified time as a barrier for current POC diagnostic use [37]. In the focus groups, themes for the ideal POC test prioritized fast turnaround time, ease of use, accuracy, and user-friendliness. The online surveys confirmed this result with accuracy as the highest priority for an ideal test, followed by low cost. Both groups selected CT as their priority organism to target with a new POC test.

In 2010 and 2011, Huppert et al. studied the feasibility and acceptability of self-testing for TV among urban teens in Cincinnati, OH, USA. In 2010, sexually active women aged 14–22 years old recruited at a teen health center or emergency department collected vaginal swabs and used the sample for the OSOM Test [34]. All participants correctly performed the test, and 99% interpreted the results correctly. The results agreed with the physician-collected and physician-performed tests in 95.7% of cases. As a follow-up to the earlier study with a similar group of participants in 2011, Huppert et al. surveyed women to evaluate their trust and comfort of self-collected versus clinician-collected samples before and after testing [35]. They found that women's trust in their ability to perform a self-test increased after having done so. Their comfort was higher for self-testing than clinician-testing both before and after performing the test. These results were in agreement with women's attitudes toward self-testing: both at baseline and after testing, 93% of women were definitely or probably willing to test themselves at home. As in the 2010 study, 99% of women were able to correctly perform the test and interpret the results.

3.4. Proof of Concept. Our search yielded fourteen proof of concept articles for new POC diagnostics [38–51]. Eleven reports introduced CT diagnostics [38–48], five introduced NG diagnostics [39, 47–50], and two introduced TV diagnostics [47, 51]. The diagnostic methods and performance, if provided, for those novel tests are summarized in Tables 4–6. Those diagnostics varied widely in method and in performance. Some, such as the BioStar assay, have been the subject of later articles with encouraging results [28]. Whereas some, such as the Xpert CT/NG, are already commercially available, others do not appear to have been followed up with later published research or development.

4. Discussion

We reviewed 33 articles on POC testing for CT, NG, and/or TV from 2010 to 2015. We analyzed the publications to report results on (1) performance evaluations, (2) feasibility and acceptability analyses, (3) cost effectiveness, and (4) proof of concept reports.

For performance evaluations, we found that six publications had tests with >80% sensitivity and specificity, at least one test for each CT, NG, and TV [21, 22, 28–31]. However, many commercially available or commonly used diagnostics, while their specificities were >90%, had sensitivities <50%, such as the QuickVue Chlamydia Rapid Test (with sensitivities of 25.0 [26]–37.7% [25], specificities of 99.4 [25]–99.7% [26]), ACON NG test (with sensitivities of 0–12.5% [25], specificities of 97.2–99.8% [25]), and wet mount microscopy for TV (with sensitivities of 38.0 [31]–58.8% [30], specificities of 99.3 [30]–100% [31]). Furthermore, these tests were usually analyzed in high risk or symptomatic populations, potentially giving them an inflated accuracy compared to the general population, which has lower rates of

infection. However, articles such as Gaydos et al. in 2013 [21], Hurly et al. in 2014 [23], and Hegazy et al. in 2012 [29], which evaluated both symptomatic and asymptomatic women at reproductive health clinics, showed very good accuracy for the Xpert CT/NG, CRT, and OSOM Test, respectively. Indeed, in 2012, van der Helm et al. did not find a significant difference in the performance of CRT between women attending an STI clinic (with sensitivity of 39.4%, specificity of 94.4%) and those at a sexual health and family planning clinic (with sensitivity of 42.0%, specificity of 95.8%) [24]. While that study only evaluated one relatively poorly sensitive test, it shows that a diagnostic test will not necessarily perform worse in a lower risk patient population.

Among the tests available for women that had sensitivities ≥90%, the Xpert CT/NG and aQcare Chlamydia TRF kit were the only two tested with multiple sample types and neither had significantly different performances between sample types [21, 22]. AUFC [20], the BioStar assay [28], and the OSOM Test [29–31] were each only evaluated using one sample type. Gram stain urethral smear also had a sensitivity >90% for CT [19, 20] and NG [27], but this test is only available to men. Gram stained cervical smears were not as accurate for NG [27] and were never studied for CT. Other tests which were studied across sample types, such as CRT, ACON CT test, and QuickVue Chlamydia Rapid Test, had some variability in sensitivities based on sample type, but no sample type ever reached specificity >75%. [23–26].

Those tests available for women with sensitivities ≥90% varied in their style of detection: a rapid NAAT (the Xpert CT/NG) [21], immunoassays (the aQcare Chlamydia TRF kit and BioStar assay) [22, 28], an antigen detection test (the OSOM Test) [29–31], and AUFC [20]. Those data are encouraging for the continued pursuit of multiple types of test. However, other tests of the same types did not perform with adequate sensitivities for use: the ACON CT, ACON NG, ACON Duo, and QuickVue immunoassays and the Biorapid Chlamydia Ag antigen detection test all performed with sensitivities <70% [23, 25, 26]. Overall, the highly sensitive performance of some immunoassays, antigen detection tests, and rapid NAATs in comparison with the low sensitivities of traditional diagnostics such as Gram stains, culture, and microscopy [19, 20, 27, 30, 31] underline the importance of continuing development and improvement of POC tests.

The cost and cost effectiveness articles about POC testing for STIs were similarly encouraging. However, as with the acceptability and feasibility articles, the small number of total studies as well as the emphasis on modeling rather than observational data leaves room for additional research. Models are important to pave the way for a potential new strategy, but now that POC diagnostics are in use around the world, more work should be done on evaluating the actual costs of implementing POC tests. While Bartelsman et al.'s study in the Netherlands [27] is a good first example of that, more studies should be done in varied economic settings and with different tests.

The articles on acceptability and feasibility showed that POC testing is a priority for health care professionals and is feasible to implement for patients. However, the low number of total reports and focus on surveys about potential POC

TABLE 4: Summary of proof of concept articles on point of care tests for *Chlamydia trachomatis* from 2010 to 2015.

Study authors and year	Summary of results (summaries are based on descriptions in abstracts and articles)	Performance
Dean et al. 2012 [38]	Microfluidic Multiplex PCR Assay: microfluidic assay that simultaneously identifies nine CT genetic markers. The assay is based on microfluidic modules that purify DNA from clinical samples, performs highly multiplexed amplification, and separates the amplicons electrophoretically with laser-induced fluorescence detection	Comparison with Roche-AMPLICOR NAAT: Multiplex sensitivity and specificity, PPV and NPV: 91.5% and 100%, 100% and 91% AMPLICOR sensitivity and specificity, PPV and NPV: 62.4% and 95.9%, 94.1% and 68.6%
Doseeva et al. 2011 [39]	Thermophilic helicase dependent amplification (tHDA) assay: helicase unwinds double-stranded DNA at constant temperature. This is treated with a sequence-specific sample preparation on magnetic beads and homogeneous endpoint fluorescence detection using dual-labeled probes.	Not measured
Hesse et al. 2011 [40]	BioVei, Inc., vaginal swab prototype: self-contained, two-step enzyme-based detection system that contains a chromogenic substrate for the specific enzyme coupled to a fluorescent tag in an aqueous solution. When exposed to Chlamydia, the substrate undergoes an enzymatic reaction. Evaluators utilized rapid communication with the manufacturers to maximize performance	Of final prototype: Sensitivity: 80% (CI 28%–99%) Specificity of cervical swabs: 37% (CI 22–53%) Specificity of vaginal swabs: 25% (CI 13–40%)
Jung et al. 2010 [41]	Simplified colorimetric detection method to identify PCR-amplified nucleic acids: after PCR amplification reaction, unmodified gold nanoparticles (AuNPs) are added to the reaction tube followed by the addition of NaCl to induce the aggregation of AuNPs. The PCR products strongly bind to the surface of AuNPs, preventing the salt-induced aggregation. The unaggregated AuNPs are red while aggregated change to blue. This color change is visible to naked eye and shown to be effective in human urine sample	Not measured
Krõlov et al. 2014 [42]	Recombinase polymerase amplification: a recombinase complex from T4 bacteriophage introduces primers to specific DNA sites to initiate an amplification reaction by the strand, displacing DNA polymerase. Results in 20 minutes using unpurified urine	Specificity of 100% (95% CI, 92%–100%) and a sensitivity of 83% (95% CI, 51%–97%) Detection limit of 5 to 12 pathogens per test
Lehmusvuori et al. 2010 [43]	Rapid homogenous PCR assay with GenomEra technology: bacteria are first concentrated by a centrifugation-based urine pretreatment method, followed by a rapid closed-tube PCR performed by automated GenomEra technology and including time-resolved fluorometric detection of the target using lanthanide chelate labeled probes. Results in 1 hour	Sensitivity and specificity of 98.7% and 97.3%, respectively
Linnes et al. 2014 [44]	Paper-based molecular diagnostic: incorporates cell lysis, isothermal nucleic acid amplification, and lateral flow visual detection using only a pressure source and heat block on a paper-based test. Results in less than an hour	Limit of detection of 1000 cells, more sensitive than current rapid immunoassays used for chlamydia diagnosis

TABLE 4: Continued.

Study authors and year	Summary of results (summaries are based on descriptions in abstracts and articles)	Performance
Melendez et al. 2013 [45]	Microwave-accelerated metal-enhanced fluorescence (MAMEF) assays: Microwave exposure accelerates the transport of DNA targets. Two assays were developed: the first targets the *C. trachomatis* 16S rRNA gene, and the second targets the *C. trachomatis* cryptic plasmid	Sensitivity 73.3%; specificity 92.9% if both assays are required to determine a positive Sensitivity 82.2% for only cryptic plasmid assay Sensitivity 75.5% for only 12S rRNA assay (all tested with vaginal swabs)
Pearce et al. 2011 [46]	Velox™ electrochemical assay: a fully integrated fluidic card with a novel electrochemical label technique. Steps include extraction of DNA from a clinical sample, specific amplification of a small segment of the DNA sequence by PCR, and detection of the amplified DNA using an electrochemically labeled ferrocene-based DNA probe. Results in less than 25 minutes	Benchtop (non-POC) version of assay: Sensitivity of 98.1% and specificity of 98.0% on genital swabs
Spizz et al. 2012 [47]	Rheonix CARD® STI CARD® assay: a patented lamination process incorporates all pumps, valves, microchannels, and reaction compartments into an inexpensive disposable plastic device that automatically performs all assay steps. Amplicons detected with Reverse Dot Blot assay	Able to detect a minimum of 10 copies of each of the four pathogens (*N. gonorrhoeae*, *C. trachomatis*, *T. pallidum*,and *T. vaginalis*)
Tabrizi et al. 2013 [48]	Cepheid GeneXpert CT/NG assay: amplifies one chromosomal target (CT1) for the detection of *C. trachomatis*, two chromosomal targets (NG2 and NG4) for detection of *N. gonorrhoeae*, a single-copy human gene which should be present in each specimen to act as a sample adequacy control (SAC), and *Bacillus globigii* DNA added to each cartridge to serve as a sample-processing/internal control (SPC)	All 15 serovars of *C. trachomatis* were detectable to 10 genome copies per reaction. The GeneXpert CT/NG assay was also able to detect the Swedish new variant of *C. trachomatis* (nvCT) and the L2b strain

testing demonstrate a need for additional research studying the actual use of POC diagnostics and how patients and providers respond to them. The articles by Huppert et al., which evaluated the actual use of the OSOM Test, showed promising feasibility and acceptability of the self-test and yielded an important insight into women's comfort with self-testing versus clinician-testing [34, 35]. Additional studies to evaluate the best way to optimize the use of POC diagnostics among different populations with varying prevalences are needed.

The proof of concept articles show a promising number of novel tests and methods from the past five years, some of which have already gone on to become commercially available tests. However, the small number of TV and NG tests compared to CT demonstrates that there is still room for more innovation. As more tests become available, the cost to produce, distribute, and use these tests will also decline, increasing availability in low resource settings, where STI prevalence is highest and the burden of adverse outcomes is greatest.

Previous literature reviews of POC diagnostics for STIs, including CT, NG, and/or TV, demonstrate the growth of the field in the last five years. As with our findings, reviews in 2011 showed the consensus that traditional diagnostics or strategies such as microscopy, syndromic management, and culture are not sufficient tools for diagnosing STIs [4, 52]. However, in 2011, the accuracy of alternative rapid assays was still not as high as desired, and the authors called for continued research into more accurate immunoassays. In recent years, more assays have been developed and rapid NAATs such as the GeneXpert have entered the market. In 2013, Gaydos and Hardick found the Xpert CT/NG for CT and NG and the OSOM Test for TV to be promising new developments in an otherwise unsatisfactorily inaccurate POC testing scene [53]. The optimism for the OSOM Test was shared by McGowin et al. in their 2014 review of TV diagnostics [54], and we, too, have found that these tests perform well. With additional data from articles published in 2014-2015, our review has confirmed those results and found new tests that have been demonstrated to have high accuracies [21, 22, 28, 30, 31]. One previous review also commented on the patient populations studied in performance evaluations [55]. Watchirs Smith et al. found that, unsurprisingly, tests demonstrated more accuracy when studied in symptomatic populations [55]. However,

TABLE 5: Summary of proof of concept articles on point of care tests for *Neisseria gonorrhoeae* from 2010 to 2015.

Study authors and year	Summary of results (summaries are based on descriptions in abstracts and articles)	Performance
Cho et al. 2015 [49]	Smartphone based microfluidic paper analytical device (μPAD): anti-*N. gonorrhoeae* antibodies are conjugated to submicron particles then preloaded and dried in the center of each paper microfluidic channel. The device simultaneously filters urine and performs the assay, so no pretreatment is necessary. The smartphone optically detects immunoagglutination to perform the assay. The total μPAD assay time is less than 30 seconds	Spiked urine samples: Detection limit of 10 CFU/mL
Doseeva et al. 2011 [39]	Thermophilic helicase dependent amplification (tHDA) assay: Helicase unwinds double-stranded DNA at constant temperature. This is treated with a sequence-specific sample preparation on magnetic beads and homogeneous endpoint fluorescence detection using dual-labeled probes	Not measured
Samarawickrama et al. 2011 [50]	The BioStar Optical ImmunoAssay: immunochromatographic strip test that detects a specific epitope on the L7/L12 ribosomal protein, reducing cross-reactivity with other neisseriae for a highly specific test. Visual results within 30 minutes	A laboratory-based evaluation: Sensitivity 99.4%, specificity 88.7% 7 false positives (six strains of *N. meningitidis* and one nonspeciated *Neisseria* sp.) 1 false negative
Spizz et al. 2012 [47]	Rheonix CARD STI CARD assay: a patented lamination process incorporates all pumps, valves, microchannels, and reaction compartments into an inexpensive disposable plastic device that automatically performs all assay steps. Amplicons detected with Reverse Dot Blot assay	Able to detect a minimum of 10 copies of each of the four pathogens (*N. gonorrhoeae*, *C. trachomatis*, *T. pallidum*, and *T. vaginalis*)
Tabrizi et al. 2013 [48]	Cepheid GeneXpert CT/NG assay: amplifies one chromosomal target (CT1) for the detection of *C. trachomatis*, two chromosomal targets (NG2 and NG4) for detection of *N. gonorrhoeae*, a single-copy human gene which should be present in each specimen to act as a sample adequacy control (SAC), and *Bacillus globigii* DNA added to each cartridge to serve as a sample-processing/internal control (SPC)	Limit of detection was 10 genome copies per reaction. No false positives resulted, but four out of 11 *Neisseria mucosa* isolates and two of 42 *Neisseria subflava* isolates were positive in one (NG4) of two NG targets, which led to correct interpretation as negative

TABLE 6: Summary of proof of concept articles on point of care tests for *Trichomonas vaginalis* from 2010 to 2015.

Study authors and year	Summary of results (summaries are based on descriptions in abstracts and articles)	Performance
Pearce et al. 2013 [51]	Electrochemical endpoint assay prototype: a single card performs target DNA extraction, amplification, and electrochemical detection via electrochemical endpoint detection. This prototype is designed to work with the Atlas io platform	Sensitivity and specificity of 95.5% (42/44) and 95.7% (44/46), respectively Limit of detection: 5 TV cells No cross-reactivity with the nucleic acids from organisms commonly associated with the genitourinary tract
Spizz et al. 2012 [47]	Rheonix CARD STI CARD assay: a patented lamination process incorporates all pumps, valves, microchannels, and reaction compartments into an inexpensive disposable plastic device that automatically performs all assay steps. Amplicons detected with Reverse Dot Blot assay	Able to detect a minimum of 10 copies of each of the four pathogens (*N. gonorrhoeae*, *C. trachomatis*, *T. pallidum*, and *T. vaginalis*)

they did not comment on the accuracy of results for low versus high risk patients in contexts such as STI clinics versus family planning clinics.

Just as we found few articles on acceptability, feasibility, and cost effectiveness of implementing POC diagnostics, other reviews have also called for more research on these subjects [56, 57]. Previous reviews also noted the disproportionate number of studies on and diagnostics available for CT compared to NG [57]. This is in agreement with our review, in which twice as many articles evaluated the performance of CT as NG or TV, and for which we found no articles on the cost or cost effectiveness of TV testing.

5. Limitations

Our review had several limitations. Firstly, we only used PubMed to find relevant articles. Secondly, there are some existing commercial tests, such as the GeneXpert TV test, which are approved for use but were not evaluated in any publications between January 2010 and August 2015, preventing their inclusion in our study. Due to the small number of articles on cost effectiveness, feasibility, and acceptability of implementing POC testing, it is difficult to draw strong conclusions. Similarly, the lack of studies on NG and TV demonstrates a need for more research and development in order to control these diseases. There were some diagnostics, such as the Xpert CT/NG, aQcare Chlamydia TRF, and BioStar assay which had good sensitivity and specificity but were each only evaluated in one trial among one group [21, 22, 28]. Continued evaluation should be done with those diagnostics to confirm their accuracy across settings and populations. For TV particularly, it has not been clearly demonstrated that screening pregnant women is beneficial, so additional research on this topic with highly sensitive and specific POC tests should be performed. Of the publications on TV we reviewed, all used culture or a composite of imperfect tests as the reference standard rather than NAAT, the usual comparator for all CT and most NG studies. Additional trials should more rigorously compare TV diagnostics to a more sensitive reference standard, NAAT. The use of different reference tests in various studies undermined our ability to compare accuracy across articles, as some reference tests such as culture and microscopy have been demonstrated to have low sensitivities. Finally, especially given the vulnerability among pregnant women and neonates, more research is needed on diagnostics in pregnant women. We did not identify any research which specifically studied pregnant women, and most studies excluded pregnant women.

6. Conclusion

Overall, this review demonstrates that recent progress has occurred for developing diagnostics for CT, NG, and TV that have high accuracy. However, we still need more studies of those tests for acceptability, feasibility, cost (especially for low and middle income countries), and sensitivity and specificity among populations not considered to be at risk (especially for NG and TV). While pregnant women specifically have not been studied, the results available in nonpregnant populations are encouraging for the ability to screen and treat women in antenatal care to prevent adverse pregnancy and neonatal outcomes.

Competing Interests

The authors declare that they have no competing interests.

Acknowledgments

Claire C. Bristow acknowledges funding from NIDA T32 DA023356 and NIDA R01 DA037773-01A1. Additional funding was received from UCLA Center for AIDS Research (CFAR) NIH/NIAID AI028697 and UCLA Center for HIV Identification, Prevention, and Treatment Services (CHIPTS) NIH P30MH058107.

References

[1] L. Newman, J. Rowley, S. Vander Hoorn et al., "Global estimates of the prevalence and incidence of four curable sexually transmitted infections in 2012 based on systematic review and global reporting," *PLOS ONE*, vol. 10, no. 12, Article ID e0143304, 2015.

[2] M. Romoren, F. Hussein, T. W. Steen et al., "Costs and health consequences of chlamydia management strategies among pregnant women in sub-Saharan Africa," *Sexually Transmitted Infections*, vol. 83, no. 7, pp. 558–566, 2007.

[3] V. J. Johnston and D. C. Mabey, "Global epidemiology and control of *Trichomonas vaginalis*," *Current Opinion in Infectious Diseases*, vol. 21, no. 1, pp. 56–64, 2008.

[4] W. H. Su, T. S. Tsou, and C. S. Chen, "Are we satisfied with the tools for the diagnosis of gonococcal infection in females?" *Journal of the Chinese Medical Association*, vol. 74, no. 10, pp. 430–434, 2011.

[5] K. Adachi, J. D. Klausner, J. Xu et al., "*Chlamydia trachomatis* and *Neisseria gonorrhea* in HIV-infected pregnant women and adverse infant outcomes," *Pediatric Infectious Disease Journal*, In press.

[6] K. Adachi, J. D. Klausner, C. C. Bristow et al., "Chlamydia and gonorrhea in HIV-infected pregnant women and infant HIV transmission," *Sexually Transmitted Diseases*, vol. 42, no. 10, pp. 554–565, 2015.

[7] N. Ortayli, K. Ringheim, L. Collins, and T. Sladden, "Sexually transmitted infections: progress and challenges since the 1994 International Conference on Population and Development (ICPD)," *Contraception*, vol. 90, supplement 6, pp. S22–S31, 2014.

[8] UNAIDS and World Health Organization, *AIDS Epidemic Update: December 2009*, UNAIDS/09.36E/JC1700E, 2009.

[9] K. S. H. Kwan, C. M. Giele, B. Combs, and D. B. Mak, "Improvement in antenatal testing for sexually transmissible infections and blood-borne viruses in Western Australian hospitals, 2007 to 2010," *Sexual Health*, vol. 9, no. 4, pp. 349–354, 2012.

[10] U. S. Sangkomkamhang, P. Lumbiganon, W. Prasertcharoensuk, and M. Laopaiboon, "Antenatal lower genital tract infection screening and treatment programs for preventing preterm delivery," *Cochrane Database of Systematic Reviews*, vol. 2, Article ID CD006178, 2015.

[11] J. Cabeza, P. J. García, E. Segura et al., "Feasibility of *Chlamydia trachomatis* screening and treatment in pregnant women in Lima, Peru: a prospective study in two large urban hospitals," *Sexually Transmitted Infections*, vol. 91, no. 1, pp. 7–10, 2015.

[12] A. Wynn, D. Ramogola-Masire, P. Gaolebale et al., "Acceptability and feasibility of sexually transmitted infection testing and treatment among pregnant women in Gaborone, Botswana, 2015," *BioMed Research International*, vol. 2016, Article ID 1251238, 6 pages, 2016.

[13] World Health Organization, *Mapping the Landscape of Diagnostics for Sexually Transmitted Infections: Key Findings and Recommendations*, World Health Organization, Geneva, Switzerland, 2004.

[14] M. Pai, M. Ghiasi, and N. P. Pai, "Point-of-care diagnostic testing in global health: what is the point?" *Microbe*, vol. 10, no. 3, pp. 103–107, 2015.

[15] T. L. Gift, M. S. Pate, E. W. Hook III, and W. J. Kassler, "The rapid test paradox: when fewer cases detected lead to more cases treated: a decision analysis of tests for *Chlamydia trachomatis*," *Sexually Transmitted Diseases*, vol. 26, no. 4, pp. 232–240, 1999.

[16] S. C. Francis, T. T. Ao, F. M. Vanobberghen et al., "Epidemiology of curable sexually transmitted infections among women at increased risk for HIV in Northwestern Tanzania: inadequacy of syndromic management," *PLoS ONE*, vol. 9, no. 7, Article ID e101221, 2014.

[17] J. B. Hack and C. Hecht, "Emergency physicians' patterns of treatment for presumed gonorrhea and chlamydia in women: one center's practice," *Journal of Emergency Medicine*, vol. 37, no. 3, pp. 257–263, 2009.

[18] D. Moher, A. Liberati, J. Tetzlaff et al., "Preferred reporting items for systematic reviews and meta-analyses: the PRISMA statement," *PLoS Medicine*, vol. 6, no. 7, Article ID e1000097, 2009.

[19] M. Bartelsman, M. S. Van Rooijen, S. Alba et al., "Point-of-care management of urogenital *Chlamydia trachomatis* via Gram-stained smear analysis in male high-risk patients. Diagnostic accuracy and costeffectiveness before and after changing the screening indication at the STI Clinic in Amsterdam," *Sexually Transmitted Infections*, vol. 91, no. 7, pp. 479–484, 2015.

[20] M. J. Pond, A. V. Nori, S. Patel et al., "Performance evaluation of automated urine microscopy as a rapid, non-invasive approach for the diagnosis of non-gonococcal urethritis," *Sexually Transmitted Infections*, vol. 91, no. 3, pp. 165–170, 2015.

[21] C. A. Gaydos, B. Van Der Pol, M. Jett-Goheen et al., "Performance of the cepheid CT/NG Xpert rapid PCR test for detection of *Chlamydia trachomatis* and *Neisseria gonorrhoeae*," *Journal of Clinical Microbiology*, vol. 51, no. 6, pp. 1666–1672, 2013.

[22] J. Y. Ham, J. Jung, B.-G. Hwang et al., "Highly sensitive and novel point-of-care system, aQcare Chlamydia TRF kit for detecting *Chlamydia trachomatis* by using europium (Eu) (III) chelated nanoparticles," *Annals of Laboratory Medicine*, vol. 35, no. 1, pp. 50–56, 2015.

[23] D. S. Hurly, M. Buhrer-Skinner, S. G. Badman et al., "Field evaluation of the CRT and ACON chlamydia point-of-care tests in a tropical, low-resource setting," *Sexually Transmitted Infections*, vol. 90, no. 3, pp. 179–184, 2014.

[24] J. J. van der Helm, L. O. A. Sabajo, A. W. Grunberg, S. A. Morré, A. G. C. L. Speksnijder, and H. J. C. de Vries, "Point-of-care test for detection of urogenital chlamydia in women shows low sensitivity. A performance evaluation study in two clinics in suriname," *PLoS ONE*, vol. 7, no. 2, Article ID e32122, 2012.

[25] L. Nuñez-Forero, L. Moyano-Ariza, H. Gaitán-Duarte et al., "Diagnostic accuracy of rapid tests for sexually transmitted infections in symptomatic women," *Sexually Transmitted Infections*, vol. 92, no. 1, pp. 24–28, 2016.

[26] L. Van Dommelen, F. H. Van Tiel, S. Ouburg et al., "Alarmingly poor performance in *Chlamydia trachomatis* point-of-care testing," *Sexually Transmitted Infections*, vol. 86, no. 5, pp. 355–359, 2010.

[27] M. Bartelsman, M. Straetemans, K. Vaughan et al., "Comparison of two Gram stain point-of-care systems for urogenital gonorrhoea among high-risk patients: Diagnostic accuracy and cost-effectiveness before and after changing the screening algorithm at an STI clinic in Amsterdam," *Sexually Transmitted Infections*, vol. 90, no. 5, pp. 358–362, 2014.

[28] A. Samarawickrama, E. Cheserem, M. Graver, J. Wade, S. Alexander, and C. Ison, "Pilot study of use of the BioStar Optical ImmunoAssay GC point-of-care test for diagnosing gonorrhoea in men attending a genitourinary medicine clinic," *Journal of Medical Microbiology*, vol. 63, no. 8, pp. 1111–1112, 2014.

[29] M. M. Hegazy, N. L. El-Tantawy, M. M. Soliman, E. S. El-Sadeek, and H. S. El-Nagar, "Performance of rapid immunochromatographic assay in the diagnosis of *Trichomoniasis vaginalis*," *Diagnostic Microbiology and Infectious Disease*, vol. 74, no. 1, pp. 49–53, 2012.

[30] R. Khatoon, N. Jahan, S. Ahmad, H. Khan, and T. Rabbani, "Comparison of four diagnostic techniques for detection of *Trichomonas vaginalis* infection in females attending tertiary care hospital of North India," *Indian Journal of Pathology and Microbiology*, vol. 58, no. 1, pp. 36–39, 2015.

[31] B. Nathan, J. Appiah, P. Saunders et al., "Microscopy outperformed in a comparison of five methods for detecting *Trichomonas vaginalis* in symptomatic women," *International Journal of STD and AIDS*, vol. 26, no. 4, pp. 251–256, 2015.

[32] K. M. Turner, J. Round, P. Horner et al., "An early evaluation of clinical and economic costs and benefits of implementing point of care NAAT tests for *Chlamydia trachomatis* and *Neisseria gonorrhoea* in genitourinary medicine clinics in England," *Sexually Transmitted Infections*, vol. 90, no. 2, pp. 104–111, 2014.

[33] W. Huang, C. A. Gaydos, M. R. Barnes, M. Jett-Goheen, and D. R. Blake, "Comparative effectiveness of a rapid point-of-care test for detection of *Chlamydia trachomatis* among women in a clinical setting," *Sexually Transmitted Infections*, vol. 89, no. 2, pp. 108–114, 2013.

[34] J. S. Huppert, E. Hesse, G. Kim et al., "Adolescent women can perform a point-of-care test for trichomoniasis as accurately as clinicians," *Sexually Transmitted Infections*, vol. 86, no. 7, pp. 514–519, 2010.

[35] J. S. Huppert, E. A. Hesse, M. A. Bernard et al., "Acceptability of self-testing for trichomoniasis increases with experience," *Sexually Transmitted Infections*, vol. 87, no. 6, pp. 494–500, 2011.

[36] Y.-H. Hsieh, M. T. Hogan, M. Barnes et al., "Perceptions of an ideal point-of-care test for sexually transmitted infections—a qualitative study of focus group discussions with medical providers," *PLoS ONE*, vol. 5, no. 11, Article ID e14144, 2010.

[37] Y.-H. Hsieh, C. A. Gaydos, M. T. Hogan et al., "What qualities are most important to making a point of care test desirable for clinicians and others offering sexually transmitted infection testing?" *PLoS ONE*, vol. 6, no. 4, Article ID e19263, 2011.

[38] D. Dean, R. S. Turingan, H.-U. Thomann et al., "A multiplexed microfluidic PCR assay for sensitive and specific point-of-care detection of *Chlamydia trachomatis*," *PLoS ONE*, vol. 7, no. 12, Article ID e51685, 2012.

[39] V. Doseeva, T. Forbes, J. Wolff et al., "Multiplex isothermal helicase-dependent amplification assay for detection of Chlamydia trachomatis and Neisseria gonorrhoeae," Diagnostic Microbiology and Infectious Disease, vol. 71, no. 4, pp. 354–365, 2011.

[40] E. A. Hesse, S. A. Patton, J. S. Huppert, and C. A. Gaydos, "Using a rapid communication approach to improve a POC Chlamydia test," IEEE Transactions on Biomedical Engineering, vol. 58, no. 3, pp. 837–840, 2011.

[41] Y. L. Jung, C. Jung, H. Parab, T. Li, and H. G. Park, "Direct colorimetric diagnosis of pathogen infections by utilizing thiol-labeled PCR primers and unmodified gold nanoparticles," Biosensors and Bioelectronics, vol. 25, no. 8, pp. 1941–1946, 2010.

[42] K. Krõlov, J. Frolova, O. Tudoran et al., "Sensitive and rapid detection of Chlamydia trachomatis by recombinase polymerase amplification directly from urine samples," Journal of Molecular Diagnostics, vol. 16, no. 1, pp. 127–135, 2014.

[43] A. Lehmusvuori, E. Juntunen, A.-H. Tapio, K. Rantakokko-Jalava, T. Soukka, and T. Lövgren, "Rapid homogeneous PCR assay for the detection of Chlamydia trachomatis in urine samples," Journal of Microbiological Methods, vol. 83, no. 3, pp. 302–306, 2010.

[44] J. C. Linnes, A. Fan, N. M. Rodriguez, B. Lemieux, H. Kong, and C. M. Klapperich, "Paper-based molecular diagnostic for Chlamydia trachomatis," RSC Advances, vol. 4, no. 80, pp. 42245–42251, 2014.

[45] J. H. Melendez, J. S. Huppert, M. Jett-Goheen et al., "Blind evaluation of the microwave-accelerated metal-enhanced fluorescence ultrarapid and sensitive Chlamydia trachomatis test by use of clinical samples," Journal of Clinical Microbiology, vol. 51, no. 9, pp. 2913–2920, 2013.

[46] D. M. Pearce, D. P. Shenton, J. Holden, and C. A. Gaydos, "Evaluation of a novel electrochemical detection method for Chlamydia trachomatis: application for point-of-care diagnostics," IEEE Transactions on Biomedical Engineering, vol. 58, no. 3, pp. 755–758, 2011.

[47] G. Spizz, L. Young, R. Yasmin et al., "Rheonix CARD® technology: an innovative and fully automated molecular diagnostic device," Point Care, vol. 11, no. 1, pp. 42–51, 2012.

[48] S. N. Tabrizi, M. Unemo, D. Golparian et al., "Analytical evaluation of GeneXpert CT/NG, the first genetic point-of-care assay for simultaneous detection of Neisseria gonorrhoeae and Chlamydia trachomatis," Journal of Clinical Microbiology, vol. 51, no. 6, pp. 1945–1947, 2013.

[49] S. Cho, T. S. Park, T. G. Nahapetian, and J. Yoon, "Smartphone-based, sensitive μPAD detection of urinary tract infection and gonorrhea," Biosensors and Bioelectronics, vol. 74, pp. 601–611, 2015.

[50] A. Samarawickrama, S. Alexander, and C. Ison, "A laboratory-based evaluation of the BioStar Optical ImmunoAssay point-of-care test for diagnosing Neisseria gonorrhoeae infection," Journal of Medical Microbiology, vol. 60, no. 12, pp. 1779–1781, 2011.

[51] D. M. Pearce, D. N. Styles, J. P. Hardick, and C. A. Gaydos, "A new rapid molecular point-of-care assay for Trichomonas vaginalis: preliminary performance data," Sexually Transmitted Infections, vol. 89, no. 6, pp. 495–497, 2013.

[52] W. H. Su, T. S. Tsou, C. S. Chen et al., "Diagnosis of Chlamydia infection in women," Taiwanese Journal of Obstetrics and Gynecology, vol. 50, no. 3, pp. 261–267, 2011.

[53] C. Gaydos and J. Hardick, "Point of care diagnostics for sexually transmitted infections: perspectives and advances," Expert Review of Anti-Infective Therapy, vol. 12, no. 6, pp. 657–672, 2014.

[54] C. L. McGowin, R. E. Rohde, and G. Redwine, "Trichomonas vaginalis: common, curable and in the diagnostic spotlight," Clinical Laboratory Science, vol. 27, no. 1, pp. 53–56, 2014.

[55] L. A. Watchirs Smith, R. Hillman, J. Ward et al., "Point-of-care tests for the diagnosis of Neisseria gonorrhoeae infection: a systematic review of operational and performance characteristics," Sexually Transmitted Infections, vol. 89, no. 4, pp. 320–326, 2013.

[56] A. Jain and C. A. Ison, "Chlamydia point-of-care testing: where are we now?" Sexually Transmitted Infections, vol. 89, no. 2, pp. 88–89, 2013.

[57] G. Brook, "The performance of non-NAAT point-of-care (POC) tests and rapid NAAT tests for chlamydia and gonorrhoea infections. An assessment of currently available assays," Journal of Medical Ethics, vol. 91, pp. 539–544, 2015.

9

Factors Associated with Hormonal and Intrauterine Contraceptive Use among HIV-Infected Men and Women in Lilongwe, Malawi

Jennifer H. Tang,[1,2] Sam Phiri,[3,4] Wingston Ng'ambi,[3] Jamie W. Krashin,[2] Linly Mlundira,[3] Thom Chaweza,[3] Bernadette Samala,[3] Hannock Tweya,[3,5] Mina C. Hosseinipour,[1,4] and Lisa B. Haddad[6]

[1] UNC Project-Malawi, Kamuzu Central Hospital, 100 Mzimba Road, Private Bag Box A-104, Lilongwe, Malawi
[2] University of North Carolina School of Medicine, Department of Obstetrics & Gynecology,
 University of North Carolina at Chapel Hill, 101 Manning Drive, CB No. 7570, Chapel Hill, NC 27599-7570, USA
[3] The Lighthouse Trust, Kamuzu Central Hospital, 100 Mzimba Road, Lilongwe, Malawi
[4] University of North Carolina School of Medicine, Department of Medicine, Chapel Hill, NC 27599-3368, USA
[5] The International Union against Tuberculosis and Lung Disease, 75006 Paris, France
[6] Emory University School of Medicine, Department of Gynecology and Obstetrics, Emory University,
 49 Jesse Hill Jr. Drive, Atlanta, GA 30303, USA

Correspondence should be addressed to Jennifer H. Tang; jennifer_tang@med.unc.edu

Academic Editor: Maria Gallo

Background. Understanding the factors associated with the use of hormonal and intrauterine contraception among HIV-infected men and women may lead to interventions that can help reduce high unintended pregnancy rates. *Materials and Methods.* This study is a subanalysis of a cross-sectional survey of 289 women and 241 men who were sexually active and HIV-infected and were attending HIV care visits in Lilongwe, Malawi. We estimated adjusted prevalence ratios (PRs) to evaluate factors associated with hormonal and intrauterine contraceptive use for men and women in separate models. *Results and Discussion.* 39.8% of women and 33.2% of men ($p = 0.117$) reported that they were using hormonal or intrauterine contraception at last intercourse. Having greater than 3 children was the only factor associated with hormonal and intrauterine contraceptive use among men. Among women, younger age, not wanting a pregnancy in 2 years, being with their partner for more than 4 years, and being able to make family planning decisions by themselves were associated with hormonal and intrauterine contraceptive use. *Conclusions.* The men and women in our study population differed in the factors associated with hormonal and intrauterine contraceptive use. Understanding these differences may help decrease unmet FP needs among HIV-infected men and women.

1. Background

At the end of 2014, an estimated 36.9 million people were living with HIV. Seventy percent (25.8 million) of these HIV-infected people lived in Sub-Saharan Africa [1]. Malawi has one of the highest HIV prevalence rates in the world, with an estimated 1.1 million people living with HIV [2]. Its overall prevalence rate is 10.6%, although the prevalence rate is almost 5% higher among women (12.9%) than among men

(8.1%) due to their increased vulnerability to HIV acquisition [3].

In July 2011, Malawi initiated a four-pronged strategy for prevention of maternal-to-child transmission of HIV. Prong 2 focuses on the reduction of unplanned or unintended pregnancies among HIV-infected women and included the integration of family planning (FP) provision into HIV care via HIV provider-initiated FP [4]. The strategy emphasized dual protection, stating that "condoms alone are not enough for family planning as they have to be used very consistently." More recently, Malawi published its HIV Prevention Strategy for 2015–2020, which has set a target of reducing unplanned or unintended pregnancies among HIV-infected women from 42,645/year in 2015 to 39,565/year by 2020, a 7.2% reduction [5]. It aims to meet this goal by increasing the contraceptive prevalence rate (CPR) and eliminating unmet need for FP among all women, which are currently at 35% and 18.5%, respectively [3]. The unmet need for FP is likely to be even higher among HIV-infected women, as a recent survey of HIV-infected women found that 68% of their last pregnancies were unintended, compared with the national unintended pregnancy rate of 45% [3, 6].

To increase contraceptive use among HIV-infected couples, we must first understand the characteristics of HIV-infected persons who are and are not using contraceptives in their relationship. Multiple studies in Sub-Saharan Africa have assessed factors associated with modern contraceptive use among HIV-infected women, which include the following: younger age [7, 8], higher education [7, 9, 10], higher income or socioeconomic status [7, 10], being married or in a committed relationship [8, 10], living in an urban setting [9], having more children [7–12], both partners not wanting more children [13], current use of antiretroviral therapy (ART) [12, 14, 15], disclosure to partner about HIV-infected status [8, 12, 16], having a regular sexual partner [9, 10, 17], talking with the partner about FP [9, 10], and being healthier by assessment by either CD4+ count or hemoglobin levels [8].

However, all the previously cited studies except for Polis et al.'s study included condoms as a contraceptive in their analyses. As condoms require very consistent use to be effective, they are considered to be only "moderately effective" or Tier 3 in their contraceptive effectiveness, as compared to oral contraceptives (OC) and the depot medroxyprogesterone acetate (DMPA) injection, which are "effective" or Tier 2, and the subdermal implant and the copper intrauterine device (IUD), which are "very effective" or Tier 1 [18]. In addition, condom use may be primarily used to decrease acquisition or transmission of HIV or sexually transmitted infections rather than being used for contraceptive purposes. Finally, none of these studies surveyed HIV-infected men about their contraceptive use. Therefore, the objective of this study was to evaluate factors that are associated with hormonal or intrauterine contraceptive use (the most effective nonpermanent contraceptive methods) among both HIV-infected women and men.

2. Materials and Methods

This cross-sectional study was approved by Malawi National Health Sciences Research Committee, the Emory University Institutional Review Board, and the University of North Carolina Institutional Review Board. It enrolled participants over three months at two Lighthouse Trust clinics in Lilongwe, Malawi, from 26 September 2013 to 20 December 2013. The Lighthouse Trust is a registered public trust that works closely with the Malawi Ministry of Health to operate two large integrated HIV testing, treatment, and care clinics in Lilongwe.

One clinic (Lighthouse) is based in the campus of Kamuzu Central Hospital and the other (Martin Preuss Clinic or MPC) is based at Bwaila Hospital under the Lilongwe District Health Office. Together, the two clinics care for over 23,000 patients on ART and over 2,000 patients who are not yet clinically eligible for ART. The Lighthouse began integrating FP services into its clinics in 2010, and, by the time of this study, it offered the following contraceptives on-site: condoms, OC, the DMPA injection, subdermal implants, and the copper IUD. MPC began its integration in February 2013 and offered condoms, OC, and DMPA on-site during the time of the study; for implant and IUD, it referred women to the Bwaila FP Clinic, which is located in building adjacent to MPC. Since male and female sterilization were not available at either clinic, referrals were made by both clinics for these services [19].

Study participants were recruited from the general waiting rooms of both clinics. Those who were interested in the study were invited into a private room, where they would be screened for eligibility into the study by a study research assistant. Potential participants were eligible if they (1) were between the ages of 18 and 45 years, (2) spoke Chichewa (the most commonly spoken local language) fluently, (3) had a sexual partner within the past 6 months, (4) had a documented HIV positive status, and (5) were a registered client at either Lighthouse or MPC. After confirming study eligibility, a research assistant would then undergo the informed consent process with the potential participant and obtain written consent if they agreed to enroll. Of note, the men and women in the study may have had partners who were also enrolled in the study, but these participants were not enrolled as couple dyads and completed their surveys independently of their partners.

Once enrolled, the study participant completed a face-to-face paper-based questionnaire administered by one of our two research assistants, with 160 questions for women and 130 questions for men. The questionnaire included information on the following: (1) demographics, (2) HIV and STI history, (3) condom use, (4) sexual history and current sexual behavior, (5) fertility preferences and pregnancy history, (6) contraceptive knowledge, attitudes, and use, (7) communication, and (8) ART knowledge and use. Questions were a compilation of original study questions and questions used in the Malawi 2010 Demographic and Health Survey [3]. Focus group discussions among men and women at the clinic conducted prior to this study also helped inform questionnaire development [manuscript under review].

A study database in Microsoft Access 2007 (Microsoft, Redmond, WA, USA) was created for the data entry and management. All data were double-entered and validated using predetermined queries. Stata 11.1 (StataCorp LP, College Station, TX, USA) was used for the statistical analysis. Based on the attendance numbers at the two clinics and our budget, we determined that we could enroll a convenience sample of up to 600 participants during our 3 months of recruitment. For this analysis, we excluded participants who had missing data on contraceptive use or who had used a permanent method of contraception (bilateral tubal ligation or vasectomy) at last intercourse.

Multivariable modified Poisson regression analysis with robust variance was used to estimate the unadjusted and adjusted prevalence ratios (PRs) and 95% confidence intervals (CIs) for all exposure variables selected for inclusion in our models [20, 21]. Our outcome variable was use of hormonal or intrauterine methods (OC, DMPA injection, implant, and the IUD) at last intercourse. Since we hypothesized that the factors that influence hormonal and intrauterine contraceptive use would differ by gender, we ran two separate models: one for female participants and one for male participants. To select our exposure variables for both models, we reviewed the literature and identified 18 potential variables from our questionnaire that we hypothesized might be associated with our outcome variable (Table 1). To help guard against obtaining unreliable estimates of parameters due to overfitting, we aimed to reduce our list of 18 variables so that no more than $m/10$ predictor terms would be included in each model, where m is the minimum of the number in either category of the outcome variable [22]. (Note that a variable with k categories would contribute $k - 1$ predictor terms to the model.)

To avoid bias and inflation of type I error rates, reduction of the characteristics was carried out before we examined any bivariate (or any other) relationships between the potential exposure variables and the outcome variable. Reduction of the characteristics was based on our prior knowledge of the subject matter (prioritizing variables previously found to be associated with the outcome variable), observed distributions (variables with narrow distributions in which >90% of the responses were in one category or variables with >10% missing data were excluded), multicollinearity diagnostics (a variance inflation factor >2.5 was interpreted as evidence of collinearity between two exposure variables, so we chose the variable that had the stronger association with the outcome variable), and evaluation for confounding.

Based on this analysis plan, we reduced our list of 18 potential exposure variables to 8 variables (represented by 8 predictor terms, Table 2) for the analysis with men as there were 80 men whose most recent sexual partner was using hormonal or intrauterine contraception (Table 1). For our model for women, we reduced our list of 18 potential variables to 11 variables (represented by 11 predictor terms, Table 3) as there were 115 women using hormonal or intrauterine contraception at last intercourse.

3. Results and Discussion

We screened 349 women and 274 men and enrolled a total of 562 (308 women and 254 men) participants. We excluded 19 women from this analysis: 16 had undergone bilateral tubal ligation and 3 had missing contraceptive data (none had a partner who had undergone vasectomy). We also excluded 13 men from our analysis, all of whom had a partner who had undergone bilateral tubal ligation (no men enrolled in the study had undergone vasectomy). Therefore, our final analysis population included 289 women and 241 men.

The men and women in our study population significantly differed in seven out of the 17 variables that we examined (Table 1). The men had more children and were older, but they were less likely to report a history of an unplanned pregnancy and that the female made decisions about FP alone. However, the men were more likely to report that neither they nor their partner wanted to have more children, that they knew their most recent partner was HIV positive, that they had talked to their partner about which contraceptive to use, and that they had used a condom at last intercourse. Thirty-nine percent of women reported that they were using hormonal or intrauterine contraception at last intercourse, compared with 33.2% of men, which was not significantly different ($p = 0.117$). The men and women also did not significantly differ in education level, religion, current relationship status, residence, desire for another pregnancy in two years, length of time since HIV diagnosis, use of antiretroviral therapy, disclosure of HIV status to most recent partner, length of time with most recent partner, frequency of sex in the past month, use of other specific FP methods (excluding condoms), or use of hormonal or intrauterine contraception.

In the model for men, the only variable that was found to be predictive of hormonal or intrauterine contraceptive use by their most recent partner was the man having 3 or more children (Table 2, adjusted PR: 1.69; 95% CI: 1.11–2.59; $p = 0.014$). In the model for women, four variables were found to be predictive of hormonal or intrauterine contraceptive use at last intercourse (Table 3). Women using hormonal or intrauterine contraception were more likely to be younger (adjusted PR: 0.96; 95% CI: 0.94–0.98), less likely to want a pregnancy in two years (adjusted PR: 0.47; 95% CI: 0.31–0.72), more likely to have been with their most recent partner for four or more years (adjusted PR: 1.46; 95% CI: 1.02–2.09), and more likely to report that they alone made decision about FP (adjusted PR: 1.91, 95% CI: 1.32–2.77).

Some of the results for our analyses with women were similar to the findings from other studies, even though most of them include condom use as a contraceptive in their models. Younger age was also found to be associated with modern contraceptive use in two studies [7, 8]; these findings may suggest that younger women are more open to using modern contraceptives than previous generations. Having a regular partner (defined in our study as having sex more than four times a week) was also found to be associated with modern contraceptive use in three studies [9, 10, 17], which suggests that women who consider themselves to be of higher risk for pregnancy are more likely to use effective contraception. However, unlike other studies, we did not find higher education level, having three or more children, ART use, or disclosure of HIV status to partner to be associated with hormonal or intrauterine contraceptive use [7–12, 14–16]. The differences in findings may be due to the inclusion of condoms and permanent methods in some of the other studies or due to differences in our study populations.

It was encouraging to see that pregnancy intention for the next two years was associated with hormonal and intrauterine contraceptive use, suggesting that women who want to limit or delay future childbearing are getting the appropriate contraceptive counseling and access they need to meet their fertility goals. It was also reassuring to find that ART use was not associated with a decrease in hormonal

TABLE 1: Baseline characteristics of participants (by sex).

Characteristic	Women (N = 289) n (%)	Men (N = 241) n (%)	p value*
Age**			<0.001***
18–24 years	36 (12.5)	1 (0.4)	
25–34 years	151 (52.1)	84 (34.9)	
≥35 years	102 (35.3)	155 (64.3)	
Education			0.806
Completed primary school or less	141 (48.8)	115 (47.7)	
Completed some secondary school or more	148 (51.2)	126 (52.3)	
Religion**			0.509
Catholic	60 (20.8)	52 (21.7)	
Protestant	204 (70.6)	166 (69.2)	
Muslim	23 (8.0)	18 (7.5)	
No religion	1 (0.4)	4 (1.7)	
Current relationship status			0.910
Married/committed relationship with 1 partner	281 (97.2)	236 (98.0)	
Dating one or more persons	5 (1.7)	3 (1.2)	
Not currently dating	3 (1.0)	2 (0.8)	
Residence**			0.154
Urban	260 (90.0)	208 (86.3)	
Rural	28 (9.7)	33 (13.7)	
Number of children			0.014***
0	23 (7.0)	9 (3.7)	
1-2	138 (47.8)	98 (40.7)	
3-4	100 (34.6)	95 (39.4)	
5 or more	28 (9.7)	39 (16.2)	
History of unplanned pregnancy**			0.032***
No	146 (50.5)	143 (59.3)	
Yes	143 (49.5)	96 (39.8)	
Wants pregnancy within the next 2 years**			0.159
No	202 (69.9)	178 (73.9)	
Yes	87 (30.1)	58 (24.1)	
Neither you nor partner wants more kids**			0.010***
No	142 (49.1)	92 (38.2)	
Yes	144 (49.8)	147 (61.0)	
Length of time since HIV diagnosis**			0.223
≤5 years	135 (46.7)	101 (41.9)	
>5 years	151 (52.2)	140 (58.1)	
On antiretroviral therapy			0.516
No	33 (11.4)	32 (13.3)	
Yes	256 (88.6)	209 (86.7)	
HIV status of most recent partner**			0.044***
Negative	56 (19.4)	44 (18.3)	
Positive	184 (63.7)	173 (71.8)	
Do not know	48 (16.6)	23 (9.5)	
Most recent partner knows your HIV status**			0.790
No	18 (6.2)	12 (5.0)	
Yes	270 (93.4)	227 (94.2)	
Do not know	1 (0.4)	1 (0.4)	

TABLE 1: Continued.

Characteristic	Women ($N = 289$) n (%)	Men ($N = 241$) n (%)	p value[*]
Length of time with most recent partner[**]			0.994
≤4 years	92 (31.8)	78 (32.4)	
>4 years	189 (65.4)	160 (66.4)	
In the past month, frequency of sex[**]			0.370
≤4 times (once a week or less)	56 (19.4)	55 (22.8)	
>4 times (more than once a week)	129 (44.6)	103 (42.7)	
Talk to most recent partner about which FP method to use[**]			0.008[***]
Yes	19 (6.6)	191 (79.3)	
No	203 (70.2)	5 (2.1)	
Who makes decisions about family planning[*]			<0.001[***]
Female only	189 (65.4)	84 (34.9)	
Male only	38 (13.1)	66 (27.4)	
Both	40 (13.8)	62 (25.7)	
Have you ever learned about family planning from a healthcare provider?[**]			N/A
No	17 (5.9)	N/A	
Yes	271 (94.8)	N/A	
Contraceptive(s) used at last intercourse			
No method	77 (26.6)	52 (21.6)	0.176
Natural family planning	1 (0.3)	0 (0)	N/A
Withdrawal	1 (0.3)	1 (0.4)	1.000
Condoms	167 (57.8)	161 (66.8)	0.033[***]
Condoms only	96 (33.2)	108 (44.8)	0.006[***]
Condoms plus another method	71 (24.6)	53 (22.0)	0.001[***]
Oral contraceptive	14 (4.8)	10 (4.1)	0.689
Injection	67 (23.1)	43 (17.8)	0.121
Implant	31 (10.7)	25 (10.4)	0.874
Intrauterine device	3 (1.0)	2 (0.8)	0.582
Emergency contraception	0 (0)	0 (0)	N/A
Hormonal or intrauterine contraception	115 (39.8)	80 (33.2)	0.117

[*] p value calculated using Pearson's chi-squared test or Fisher's exact test.
[**] Contains missing data so percentages may not add up to 100%.
[***] Statistically significant with $p < 0.05$.

and intrauterine contraceptive use, despite concerns about drug-drug interactions between certain ART with pills and implants [23]. However, this study was performed before several of the more recent studies related to ART-implant interactions were published, so it may not be reflective of current hormonal and intrauterine contraceptive use among women using ART in Malawi [24–27]. Ongoing evaluation of the impact of ART on contraceptive choice is warranted.

The differing results for variables associated with hormonal and intrauterine contraceptive use among the men and women in our study may be a result of the differences in their study population. As noted earlier, the men were significantly older than the women, with only one man below 25 years of age. Similarly, they were almost twice as likely to already have five or more children compared to women; ideal family size for both men and women in Malawi has been reported to be around 4 children [3].

Strengths of our study include our relatively large sample size, which allowed us to assess many variables in our models,

and the fact that we surveyed both men and women and were able to compare the differences between them. However, the men and women in our survey were not necessarily couples and were not interviewed as couple dyads, so we could not corroborate the responses that the participants gave with their partners. This limitation is particularly important for the men who may not always be aware of what contraceptive methods their partner is using and may only have been reporting their perceptions rather than actual use. In addition, social desirability bias may have led both men and women to overreport modern contraceptive use or other variables such as decision-making in FP use. Using the variable "FP use at last intercourse" instead of current FP use also has its limitations as the participants may no longer be in a relationship and using that contraceptive. However, since we only included men and women who had been sexually active within the past six months, we felt that the participants' contraceptive behavior at last intercourse was more indicative of future contraceptive practices, particularly

TABLE 2: Unadjusted and adjusted prevalence ratios for hormonal or intrauterine contraceptive use at last intercourse among 241 HIV-infected men.

Variable (N)	n (%) using modern FP	Unadjusted PR[a] (95% CI)	Adjusted PR[b] (95% CI)	p value[c]
Age (N = 240, continuous)	N/A	1.00 (0.97–1.04)	0.97 (0.94–1.01)	0.117
Education (N = 241)				0.366
Completed primary school or less	43 (37.4)	—	—	
Completed some secondary school or more	37 (29.4)	0.79 (0.55–1.13)	0.84 (0.58–1.22)	
Religion (N = 241)				0.919
Not Catholic (Protestant/Muslim/none)	63 (33.3)	—	—	
Catholic	14 (32.7)	0.98 (0.63–1.52)	1.02 (0.67–1.55)	
Number of children (N = 241)				0.014*
0–2	26 (24.3)	—	—	
3 or more	54 (40.3)	1.65 (1.12–2.46)	1.69 (1.11–2.59)	
History of unplanned pregnancy (N = 239)				0.121
No	50 (35.0)	—	—	
Yes	29 (30.2)	0.86 (0.59–1.26)	0.74 (0.50–1.08)	
Wants pregnancy within the next 2 years (N = 236)				0.081
No	67 (37.6)	—	—	
Yes	13 (22.4)	0.60 (0.36–1.00)	0.61 (0.35–1.06)	
HIV status of most recent partner (N = 240)				0.914
Negative	14 (31.8)	—	—	
Positive/do not know	66 (33.7)	1.06 (0.66–1.70)	1.03 (0.64–1.66)	
Length of time with most recent partner (N = 238)				0.108
≤4 years	19 (24.4)	—	—	
>4 years	61 (38.1)	1.57 (1.01–2.43)	1.44 (0.92–2.23)	

[a] Unadjusted results from modified Poisson regression models.
[b] Adjusted results from modified Poisson regression model (N = 232 observations with nonmissing values on all independent variables), adjusting for all other variables in Table 2.
[c] p value from Poisson regression model adjusting for all variables in Table 2.
* Statistically significant with p < 0.05.

for those who were not currently in a relationship. Finally, given that our study was limited only to men and women who were attending HIV testing and treatment clinic in Lilongwe and who were mostly urban dwellers, the results may not be generalizable to other populations outside of Malawi or in more rural places in Malawi where access to hormonal and intrauterine contraception may be more limited. Even so, this analysis is the first to examine potential factors that are related to hormonal and intrauterine contraceptive use among men.

The findings from our study can help Malawi to meet its goals for Prong 2 of its HIV Prevention Strategy, which focuses on the reduction of unplanned or unintended pregnancies among HIV-infected women and HIV provider-initiated FP [5]. Integrating FP counseling and provision into HIV care is a challenge for many HIV providers given the high volume of HIV clients, limited number of providers, and extra time required to individually counsel all clients about their fertility desires and FP needs [19]. Understanding that HIV-infected men with 3 or more children may be more interested in using hormonal and intrauterine contraception in their relationship can encourage HIV providers to target these men and their partners for discussions about their desired family size and using effective contraceptive methods to prevent unwanted pregnancy. Similarly, providers should be encouraged to talk to HIV-infected women about their

pregnancy intentions for the next 2 years, with the knowledge that those who do not want another pregnancy within 2 years may be particularly receptive to initiating hormonal or intrauterine contraception and should undergo targeted FP counseling.

Future studies could consider interviewing both members of a couple separately and then matching and comparing their responses to evaluate if they reported similar behaviors and perceptions within the couple and assess which questions were answered differently. They could also further explore the complex role that male partners play in FP decision-making, given the strong association found for our variable about FP decision-making in our model for women. Our study found that women who made FP decisions alone were more likely to be using hormonal or intrauterine contraception compared to women who involved the male partner or had a male partner who made all the FP decisions. Because of a large amount of missing data for our variable about talking to the partner about which FP method to use, we were not able to include it in our models. But the interplay between FP decision-making and the role of discussing hormonal and intrauterine contraceptive use needs to be better understood, particularly since two other studies found that it was associated with modern contraceptive use [9, 10].

TABLE 3: Unadjusted and adjusted prevalence ratios for hormonal or intrauterine contraceptive use at last intercourse among 289 HIV-infected women.

Variable (N)	% using modern family planning	Unadjusted PR[a] (95% CI)	Adjusted PR[b] (95% CI)	p value[c]
Age (N = 289, continuous)	N/A	0.98 (0.96–1.01)	0.96 (0.94–0.98)	0.001[*]
Education (N = 289)				0.301
Completed primary school or less	50 (35.5)	—	—	
Completed some secondary school or more	65 (43.9)	1.24 (0.93–1.65)	1.16 (0.87–1.55)	
Religion (N = 289)				0.385
Not Catholic (Protestant/Muslim/none)	89 (38.9)	—	—	
Catholic	26 (43.3)	1.11 (0.80–1.55)	1.10 (0.81–1.48)	
Number of children (N = 289)				0.385
0–2	61 (37.9)	—	—	
3 or more	54 (42.2)	1.11 (0.84–1.48)	1.15 (0.84–1.55)	
History of unplanned pregnancy (N = 289)				0.643
No	61 (41.8)	—	—	
Yes	54 (37.8)	0.90 (0.68–1.20)	0.94 (0.71–1.24)	
Wants pregnancy in next 2 years (N = 289)				<0.001[*]
No	96 (47.5)	—	—	
Yes	19 (21.8)	0.46 (0.30–0.70)	0.47 (0.31–0.72)	
Length of time since HIV diagnosis (N = 286)				0.528
≤5 years	54 (40.0)	—	—	
>5 years	60 (39.7)	0.99 (0.75–1.32)	0.91 (0.69–1.21)	
On antiretroviral therapy (N = 289)				0.498
No	13 (39.4)	—	—	
Yes	102 (39.8)	1.01 (0.64–1.59)	0.87 (0.58–1.30)	
HIV status of most recent partner (N = 289)				0.595
Negative	22 (39.3)	—	—	
Positive/do not know	93 (40.1)	1.02 (0.71–1.47)	0.92 (0.66–1.26)	
Length of time with most recent partner (N = 281)				0.037[*]
≤4 years	28 (30.4)	—	—	
>4 years	85 (45.0)	1.48 (1.04–2.09)	1.46 (1.02–2.09)	
Who makes decisions about family planning (N = 289)				0.001[*]
Female only	89 (47.1)	1.81 (1.26–2.61)	1.91 (1.32–2.77)	
Male only/both female and male	26 (26.0)	—	—	

[a]Unadjusted results from modified Poisson regression models.
[b]Adjusted results from modified Poisson regression model (N = 277 observations with nonmissing values on all independent variables), adjusting for all other variables in Table 3.
[c]p value from Poisson regression model adjusting for all variables in Table 3.
[*]Statistically significant with $p < 0.05$.

4. Conclusions

Among men, use of hormonal and intrauterine contraception in their most recent relationship was associated with having 3 or more children, whereas, among women, younger age, not wanting a pregnancy in 2 years, being with their partner for more than 4 years, and being able to make family planning decisions by themselves were associated with hormonal and intrauterine contraceptive use. Knowledge of these associations may help providers to better understand the contraceptive needs and preferences of HIV-infected men and women and improve their FP uptake through targeted FP counseling.

Competing Interests

The authors declare that they have no competing interests.

Authors' Contributions

Lisa B. Haddad conceived of the study and drafted the survey with Jennifer H. Tang and Hannock Tweya. Jennifer H. Tang oversaw its operational aspects with Sam Phiri, Hannock Tweya, Thom Chaweza, Bernadette Samala, and Linly Mlundira. Jennifer H. Tang conducted data analysis with Jamie W. Krashin and drafted the initial paper. All authors read and approved the final paper.

Acknowledgments

This study was supported by a grant from the Society in Family Planning [SFPR no. 11–14, PI: Lisa B. Haddad]. The authors would like to thank the study participants, the study research assistants (Justin Milonde and Felix Mtunga), and the staff of the Lighthouse Trust clinics for their assistance and support of the study. The authors would also like to thank Dr. Joanne Garrett for her statistical advice during analyses.

References

[1] World Health Organization, *WHO HIV/AIDS Fact Sheet, #360*, World Health Organization, Geneva, Switzerland, 2015, http://www.who.int/mediacentre/factsheets/fs360/en/.

[2] UNAIDS, *UNAIDS Malawi HIV/AIDS Estimates (2014)*, UNAIDS, Geneva, Switzerland, 2014, http://www.unaids.org/en/regionscountries/countries/malawi.

[3] National Statistical Office (NSO) and ICF Macro, *Malawi Demographic and Health Survey 2010*, NSO and ICF Macro, Zomba, Malawi, 2011.

[4] Ministry of Health, *Clinical Management of HIV in Children and Adults*, Ministry of Health, Malawi, Lilongwe, Malawi, 2011.

[5] National AIDS Commission, *National HIV Prevention Strategy, 2015–2020*, National AIDS Commission, Lilongwe, Malawi, 2014.

[6] L. Haddad, S. Phiri, C. Cwiak et al., "Fertility preferences, unintended pregnancy and contraceptive use among HIV-positive women desiring family planning in Lilongwe, Malawi," *Contraception*, vol. 84, no. 3, p. 325, 2011.

[7] W. Muyindike, R. Fatch, R. Steinfield et al., "Contraceptive use and associated factors among women enrolling into HIV care in southwestern Uganda," *Infectious Diseases in Obstetrics and Gynecology*, vol. 2012, Article ID 340782, 9 pages, 2012.

[8] C. J. Chibwesha, M. S. Li, C. K. Matoba et al., "Modern contraceptive and dual method use among HIV-infected women in Lusaka, Zambia," *Infectious Diseases in Obstetrics and Gynecology*, vol. 2011, Article ID 261453, 8 pages, 2011.

[9] Y. A. Melaku and E. G. Zeleke, "Contraceptive utilization and associated factors among HIV positive women on chronic follow up care in tigray region, northern ethiopia: a cross sectional study," *PLoS ONE*, vol. 9, no. 4, Article ID e94682, 2014.

[10] C. B. Polis, R. H. Gray, T. Lutalo et al., "Trends and correlates of hormonal contraceptive use among HIV-infected women in Rakai, Uganda, 1994–2006," *Contraception*, vol. 83, no. 6, pp. 549–555, 2011.

[11] A. Polisi, E. Gebrehanna, G. Tesfaye, and F. Asefa, "Modern contraceptive utilization among female ART attendees in health facilities of Gimbie town, West Ethiopia," *Reproductive Health*, vol. 11, no. 1, article 30, 2014.

[12] H. M. Asfaw and F. E. Gashe, "Contraceptive use and method preference among HIV positive women in Addis Ababa, Ethiopia: a cross sectional survey," *BMC Public Health*, vol. 14, no. 1, article 566, 2014.

[13] C. I. Nieves, A. Kaida, G. R. Seage et al., "The influence of partnership on contraceptive use among HIV-infected women accessing antiretroviral therapy in rural Uganda," *Contraception*, vol. 92, no. 2, pp. 152–159, 2015.

[14] I. Andia, A. Kaida, M. Maier et al., "Highly active antiretroviral therapy and increased use of contraceptives among HIV-positive women during expanding access to antiretroviral therapy in Mbarara, Uganda," *American Journal of Public Health*, vol. 99, no. 2, pp. 340–347, 2009.

[15] A. Kaida, F. Laher, S. A. Strathdee et al., "Contraceptive use and method preference among women in Soweto, South Africa: the influence of expanding access to HIV care and treatment services," *PLoS ONE*, vol. 5, no. 11, Article ID e13868, 2010.

[16] D. O. Laryea, Y. A. Amoako, K. Spangenberg, E. Frimpong, and J. Kyei-Ansong, "Contraceptive use and unmet need for family planning among HIV positive women on antiretroviral therapy in Kumasi, Ghana," *BMC Women's Health*, vol. 14, no. 1, article 126, 2014.

[17] E. C. Ezugwu, P. O. Nkwo, P. U. Agu, E. O. Ugwu, and A. O. Asogwa, "Contraceptive use among HIV-positive women in Enugu, southeast Nigeria," *International Journal of Gynecology & Obstetrics*, vol. 126, no. 1, pp. 14–17, 2014.

[18] World Health Organization, Department of Reproductive Health and Research (WHO/RHR), Johns Hopkins Bloomberg School of Public Health, and Center for Communication Programs (CCP), *Knowledge for Health Project. Family Planning: A Global Handbook for Providers (2011 update)*, CCP and WHO, Baltimore, Md, USA, 2011.

[19] S. Phiri, C. Feldacker, T. Chaweza et al., "Integrating reproductive health services into HIV care: strategies for successful implementation in a lowresource HIV clinic in Lilongwe, Malawi," *Journal of Family Planning and Reproductive Health Care*, vol. 42, no. 1, pp. 17–23, 2016.

[20] G. Y. Zou, "A modified poisson regression approach to prospective studies with binary data," *American Journal of Epidemiology*, vol. 159, no. 7, pp. 702–706, 2004.

[21] L. M. S. Coutinho, M. Scazufca, and P. R. Menezes, "Methods for estimating prevalence ratios in cross-sectional studies," *Revista de Saúde Pública*, vol. 42, no. 6, pp. 1–6, 2008.

[22] F. E. Harrell, *Regression Modeling Strategies: With Applications to Linear Models, Logistic Regression, and Survival Analysis*, Springer, New York, NY, USA, 2001.

[23] World Health Organization, *Medical Eligibility Criteria*, WHO, Geneva, Switzerland, 5th edition, 2015.

[24] S. H. Perry, P. Swamy, G. A. Preidis, A. Mwanyumba, N. Motsa, and H. N. Sarero, "Implementing the Jadelle implant for women living with HIV in a resource-limited setting: concerns for drug interactions leading to unintended pregnancies," *AIDS*, vol. 28, no. 5, pp. 791–793, 2014.

[25] M. Pyra, R. Heffron, N. R. Mugo et al., "Effectiveness of hormonal contraception in HIV-infected women using antiretroviral therapy," *AIDS*, vol. 29, no. 17, pp. 2353–2359, 2015.

[26] R. C. Patel, M. Onono, M. Gandhi et al., "Pregnancy rates in HIV-positive women using contraceptives and efavirenz-based or nevirapine-based antiretroviral therapy in Kenya: a retrospective cohort study," *The Lancet HIV*, vol. 2, no. 11, pp. e474–e482, 2015.

[27] K. K. Scarsi, K. M. Darin, S. Nakalema et al., "Unintended pregnancies observed with combined use of the levonorgestrel contraceptive implant and efavirenz-based antiretroviral therapy: a three-arm pharmacokinetic evaluation over 48 weeks," *Clinical Infectious Diseases*, vol. 62, no. 6, pp. 675–682, 2016.

10

Human Papillomavirus Infection as a Possible Cause of Spontaneous Abortion and Spontaneous Preterm Delivery

Lea Maria Margareta Ambühl,[1] Ulrik Baandrup,[1] Karen Dybkær,[2] Jan Blaakær,[3] Niels Uldbjerg,[3] and Suzette Sørensen[1]

[1]Center for Clinical Research, North Denmark Regional Hospital and Department of Clinical Medicine, Aalborg University, Bispensgade 37, 9800 Hjørring, Denmark
[2]Department of Hematology, Aalborg University Hospital, Søndre Skovvej 15, 9000 Aalborg, Denmark
[3]Department of Obstetrics and Gynecology, Aarhus University Hospital, Palle Juul-Jensens Boulevard 99, 8200 Aarhus N, Denmark

Correspondence should be addressed to Suzette Sørensen; suzette.soerensen@rn.dk

Academic Editor: Susan Cu-Uvin

Based on the current literature, we aimed to provide an overview on Human Papillomavirus prevalence in normal pregnancies and pregnancies with adverse outcome. We conducted a systematic literature search in PubMed and Embase. Data extracted from the articles and used for analysis included HPV prevalence, pregnancy outcome, geographical location, investigated tissue types, and HPV detection methods. The overall HPV prevalence in normal full-term pregnancies was found to be 17.5% (95% CI; 17.3–17.7) for cervix, 8.3% (95% CI; 7.6–9.1) for placental tissue, 5.7% (95% CI; 5.1–6.3) for amniotic fluid, and 10.9% (95% CI; 10.1–11.7) for umbilical cord blood. Summary estimates for HPV prevalence of spontaneous abortions and spontaneous preterm deliveries, in cervix (spontaneous abortions: 24.5%, and preterm deliveries: 47%, resp.) and placenta (spontaneous abortions: 24.9%, and preterm deliveries: 50%, resp.), were identified to be higher compared to normal full-term pregnancies ($P < 0.05$ and $P < 0.0001$). Great variation in HPV prevalence was observed between study populations of different geographical locations. This review demonstrates an association between spontaneous abortion, spontaneous preterm delivery, and the presence of HPV in both the cervix and the placenta. However, a reliable conclusion is difficult to draw due to the limited number of studies conducted on material from pregnancies with adverse outcome and the risk of residual confounding.

1. Introduction

Intrauterine infection by bacteria is well established as a pathway leading to spontaneous abortion and spontaneous preterm birth [1, 2]. Other pathways, however, may be equally important including decidual hemorrhage, cervical disorders, genetic components, and environmental exposures like smoking [3]. Much less is known about viral infection and adverse pregnancy outcome. Human Papillomavirus (HPV), which is known as a well-established cause for cervical cancer, does though constitute a candidate. The over 180 known HPV-types are small, double-stranded DNA viruses with a circular genome of nearly 8,000 base pairs. HPV infections are common, but about 90% of all infections can be cleared within less than 2 years by unknown mechanisms [4–6].

HPV-6 and HPV-11 are the most common low-risk types and are found to be causative for genital warts [6]. The cancer associated high-risk types include HPV-16 and HPV-18 [6] and there is growing evidence of HPV infections playing a relevant role in other anogenital and head and neck cancers [7–9]. Worth to mention is also the morbidity of cutaneous HPV lesions, particularly in immunosuppressed people [9].

Pregnancy has previously proven to be a state of mild immunosuppression due to the decrease in the number of natural killer cells [10], possibly making pregnant women more prone to infections with, for example, HPV. Various immunological theories have been discussed to explain the possibility for pregnancy and the survival of the "semiallogeneic" fetus. Theories include immunological privilege in the uterus, antigenic immaturity of the fetus, and maternal immunosuppression during pregnancy [11]. While attempting to explain the immunological basis of normal pregnancy, the argumentation may have implications for the generation of immune responses to pathogens infecting the placenta, as viruses seem to face similar confrontations like the invading trophoblast [11]. Thus, it is not surprising that viruses take up some of the same strategies to avoid immune detection as do trophoblast cells [12]. Also there is some evidence that elevated steroid hormone levels during pregnancy influence the increase of HPV virus replication by interacting with hormone response elements in the viral genome, thereby giving another possible explanation for the higher incidence of HPV infection during pregnancy [13, 14]. In 2014, Liu et al. [15] conducted a systematic review on HPV prevalence in pregnant and nonpregnant women and reported an increased risk of HPV infection in pregnant women, thereby supporting the debate of how far HPV may be involved in adverse pregnancy outcomes. Various authors report an infection with HPV during pregnancy to be associated with the risk of spontaneous abortion, spontaneous preterm delivery, and placental abnormalities [16–21]. HPV DNA has been detected in the cervix [13, 21–23], fetal membranes [24], amniotic fluid [25], umbilical cord blood [26, 27], and the placenta [13, 18, 27–29]. HPV detection rates range however widely from 6 to 65% and the results are controversial [13, 18, 20, 22, 23, 27, 30–32].

It is therefore of great interest to examine how widespread HPV infections are among pregnant women and whether or not there is an association between HPV infection and spontaneous abortion or spontaneous preterm delivery. Moreover, nowadays there exists a successful vaccination to prevent infection and disease caused by infection with HPV-6, HPV-11, HPV-16, and HPV-18. Thus, there might be a chance to minimize the risk for pregnancy complications by applying the same or a modified version of vaccination. Our group studies the impact of placental HPV infection on spontaneous abortion and preterm delivery. In this context the aim of this study is to provide an overview of the existing literature by doing a systematic review on HPV prevalence in pregnancy. We focused on pregnancies with adverse outcome and included a discussion of possible factors influencing or explaining the reported differences in HPV detection rates.

2. Material and Methods

PRISMA and MOOSE guidelines were used where applicable [33].

2.1. Search Strategy. A systematic literature search was conducted in the PubMed and Embase databases and search terms were used as follows: (1) "Human papillomavirus AND pregnancy"; (2) "Human papillomavirus AND preterm delivery"; (3) "Human papillomavirus AND preterm birth"; (4) "Human papillomavirus AND abortion". The search was restricted to articles in English, on humans and published between January 1995 and October 2014. The search was carried out on October 28, 2014.

2.2. Study Selection. In order to identify relevant articles for whole-paper revision, duplicates were removed and titles and abstracts were screened based on the following exclusion criteria: studies investigating cell lines only, HPV vaccines, or sperm-related aspects, as well as guideline articles, general articles describing public health, and literature reviews. The remaining articles were assigned to subsequent whole-paper revision. These articles were systematically reviewed in accordance with the inclusion and exclusion criteria. The inclusion criteria were set to the following: studies on asymptomatic healthy pregnant women and women experiencing a spontaneous preterm delivery or spontaneous abortion; investigation of HPV infection within cervix, placenta, amniotic fluid, or umbilical cord blood; HPV detection test directly linkable to index pregnancy. Studies restricted to nonpregnant women or HPV positive women only, case reports, follow-up and association studies, and *in vitro* fertilization studies were excluded.

Studies including women with history of HPV-related lesions were not excluded, as this will be the case in any normal study population. There was no restriction for studies of different geographical origins, the time point of sample collection, methods of sample collection, and HPV testing method. Information on the latter was included in Table 1, characteristics of included studies.

2.3. Data Extraction and Statistics. Data, which includes information about the investigated tissue types, country where the study was performed, sample size, sampling time point, HPV prevalence, and HPV detection method, was extracted and analyzed using MatLab (version R2011b). Data from all studies was pooled and women were grouped according to their pregnancy outcome or the pregnancy status at time point of sample collection. An overall HPV prevalence was calculated including 95% confidence interval (CI) in normal pregnancies and in pregnancies with adverse outcome. This was done for various tissue types, geographical origins, time points of sample collection, and HPV detection methods used. Studies from Mexico and Brazil have been grouped into "Latin America." Statistical significance between two proportions was tested using "Two-sample test of proportions." All P values were two-sided and $P < 0.05$ was considered significant.

3. Results

3.1. Study Selection. The initial PubMed database search resulted in the identification of a total of 650 articles (Figure 1). After removal of duplicates and screening of titles and abstracts, the remaining 57 articles were subjected to whole-paper revision (Figure 1). Of these, 42 articles met the final inclusion criteria and were used for data extraction and quantitative analyses (Figure 1). The supplementary search in Embase database was conducted in the same way and three additional articles were included for data extraction and quantitative analysis. The 45 articles included investigated 14 470 pregnant women in total, of which 13 757 underwent normal full-term pregnancies, 145 experienced spontaneous preterm deliveries, 536 experienced spontaneous abortions, and 32 had performed an induced abortion. The study populations were from Europe ($n = 4639$) [13, 22, 27, 28,

TABLE 1: Characteristics of included studies.

References	Country	Inclusion criteria	Gestational age at sample collection (weeks)	Examined tissue type	Sample size	HPV prevalence%	HPV detection method	Study strengths	Study quality Potential biases
[34]	Korea	Pregnant women healthy, ≥18 years of age, sonographically confirmed intrauterine pregnancy	1st, 2nd, or 3rd trimester or postpartum	Cervix	Total: 960 1st trimester: 380 2nd trimester: 193 3rd trimester: 195 Postpartum: 192	Total: 24.3 1st trimester: 20.5 2nd trimester: 34.2 3rd trimester: 23.1 Postpartum: 22.9	DNA chip	Large cohort, multivariant logistic regression analysis, separate analysis for trimesters	Sample collection at different time points, including women with abnormal pap smear
[35]	Korea	PD healthy, <37 weeks of gestation	6-week postpartum	Cervix	45	15.6	HCA	Multivariant logistic regression analysis	Small sample size, postpartum sampling only, HCA sensitivity limited to 13 HPV-types
[36]	Mexico	SA: healthy, curettage up to week 20 ND: healthy, attending for delivery at term with viable products	SA: <20 ND: before delivery	Cervix	SA: 139 ND: 138	SA: 24.4 ND: 15.2	PCR	Large cohort, risk analysis	Comparison of SA (first trimester) with ND (at term). HPV-related disease history unclear
[37]	Korea	Pregnant women healthy, singleton, in first trimester	Cervix: 1st, 2nd, and 3rd trimester, postpartum Placenta, umbilical cord blood: at birth	Cervix, placenta, umbilical cord blood	Cervix: 153 Placenta: 152	Cervix: 24 Placenta: 3.3 Umbilical cord blood: 1.3	DNA chip	Large cohort, longitudinal follow-up, multivariant logistic regression analysis	Sample collection from cervix at different time points
[38]	Poland	Pregnant women singleton, normal cervical smear	33–41	Cervix	135	16.3	PCR	Large cohort, multivariant logistic regression analysis, confirmation by sequencing	Vaginal and cesarean deliveries included, potential contamination problem (HPV11 present in all positive samples)
[23]	Korea	Pregnant women healthy, over 36 weeks of gestation	>36	Cervix, placenta, umbilical cord blood	469	Cervix: 15.4 Placenta: 0 Umbilical cord blood: 0	DNA chip	Large cohort, confirmation by in situ hybridization	Vaginal and cesarean deliveries included Umbilical cord blood and placenta were collected from HPV positive mothers
[39]	China	Pregnant women healthy, asymptomatic	22.5–26.7	Cervix	3139	13.4	DNA chip	Large cohort, logistic regression analysis	Vaginal and cesarean deliveries included, women with abnormal cervical cytology included
[40]	Netherlands	Pregnant women NA	1st, 2nd, and 3rd trimester, postpartum	Cervix	51	21.6	PCR	Matched groups, detection method with high analytical sensitivity	Small sample size, self-sampling, sample collection at different time points
[41]	Korea	Pregnant women healthy, over 36 weeks of gestation	>36	Cervix	291	18.9	DNA chip	Large cohort, stratified analysis to test for confounding	Women with abnormal cervical cytology included, vaginal and cesarean deliveries included

TABLE 1: Continued.

References	Country	Inclusion criteria	Gestational age at sample collection (weeks)	Examined tissue type	Sample size	HPV prevalence%	HPV detection method	Study quality Study strengths	Potential biases
[42]	Finland	Pregnant women healthy, in third trimester	3rd trimester, at birth	Cervix, placenta, umbilical cord blood	Cervix: 329 Placenta: 306 Umbilical cord: 311	Cervix: 16.4 Placenta: 4.2 Umbilical cord blood: 3.5	PCR	Large cohort, regression analysis, multimetrix assay for HPV detection, pap smear at baseline	—
[43]	Poland	SA: healthy ND: healthy; delivering at term	SA: 6–16 ND: at birth	Aborted products of conception, placenta	SA: 51 ND: 78	SA: 17.7 ND: 24.4	PCR	—	Small sample size, comparison of SA with ND, HPV-related disease history unclear
[44]	Mexico	Pregnant women healthy, in third trimester, delivering at term	3rd trimester	Cervix, placenta	72	Cervix: 75 Placenta: 47.2	PCR	PCR process was blinded	Potential contamination problem (HPV18 present in all positive placenta samples), vaginal and cesarean deliveries included
[45]	Lithuania	Pregnant women NA	1st and 3rd trimester	Cervix	1st trimester: 213 3rd trimester: 146	1st trimester: 17.8 3rd trimester: 10.3	PCR	Large cohort, risk analysis, separate analysis for trimesters	Big proportion with history of gynecological diseases, exclusion of 67 women due to change of residency/miscarriage/premature delivery, no inclusion and exclusion criteria, commercial HPV PCR kit
[46]	Japan	Pregnant women NA	1st, 2nd, or 3rd trimester or postpartum	Cervix	151	35.8	PCR	Large cohort, pap smear at study entry	Sample collection at different time points, unclear how and when women deliver
[21]	USA	PD <37 weeks of gestation, available HPV-test results	NA	Cervix	70	67.1	HCA	Risk analysis (age, race), data from over 11 years	Sampling method and time point not mentioned, study including African Americans, HCA restricted to 13 HPV-types only
[47]	Turkey	Pregnant women NA	18–22	Cervix	134	2.2	PCR	Large cohort	22 with abnormal ultrasound findings, other virus types being in focus, HPV-related disease history unclear, no inclusion and exclusion criteria, outpatient clinic (low socioeconomic group)

TABLE 1: Continued.

References	Country	Inclusion criteria	Gestational age at sample collection (weeks)	Examined tissue type	Sample size	HPV prevalence%	HPV detection method	Study quality Study strengths	Potential biases
[32]	Belgium	Pregnant women assigned for abdominal CVS, mainly due to high risk for chromosomal abnormalities	11–13	Placenta	35	5.7	PCR	Transabdominal sampling (no birth canal contamination), highly sensitive detection method, confirmation by sequencing	Small sample size, highly selected group of women, limited amount of placenta material (actual HPV prevalence higher?), HPV-related disease history unclear
[48]	USA	Pregnant women healthy, in third trimester, 18 and above	3rd trimester	Cervix	333	28	PCR	Large cohort, logistic regression analysis, confirmation by sequencing	Vaginal and cesarean deliveries included, unclear if deliveries are at term, 25% of women with history of HPV-related lesions
[49]	Brazil	Pregnant women NA	2–37	Cervix	371	35.3	HCA	Large cohort, multivariant logistic regression analysis	Inclusion at ambulatories for patients suspected to infectious diseases, no inclusion and exclusion criteria, sample collection at different time points, women with genital warts included
[50]	Brazil	Pregnant women NA	NA	Cervix	40	25	PCR	—	Small sample size, inclusion at outpatient clinic (low socioeconomic group), no inclusion and exclusion criteria, HPV-related disease history unclear, sampling time point not mentioned
[51]	Spain	Pregnant women unselected	29–33	Cervix	828	6.5	PCR	Large cohort, multivariant logistic regression analysis	Goal to find HPV positive women for prospective cohort study on mother-to-child transmission, HPV-related disease history unclear, no inclusion and exclusion criteria, vaginal and cesarean deliveries

TABLE 1: Continued.

References	Country	Inclusion criteria	Gestational age at sample collection (weeks)	Examined tissue type	Sample size	HPV prevalence%	HPV detection method	Study quality Study strengths	Potential biases
[27]	Finland	Pregnant women third trimester	31.6–42.5	Placenta, Umbilical cord blood	Placenta: 306 Umbilical cord blood: 311	Placenta: 4.2 Umbilical cord blood: 3.5	PCR	Large cohort, multivariant regression analysis, pap smear at study entry, confirmation by sequencing	Included women delivering before week 37, part of women showing genital warts or cervical lesions, no HPV status examination before recruitment
[20]	USA	PD: spontaneous, <37 weeks of gestation ND: delivering at term	PD: 21–36 ND: 37–42	Placenta	PD: 30 ND: 30	PD: 50 ND: 20	PCR	Comparison of PD to ND (best possible control), confirmation by sequencing	Small sample size, study including mostly African Americans, HPV-related disease history unclear, type-specific PCR only
[29]	USA	SA: singleton, in second trimester IA: singleton, for congenital anomalies or maternal medical indications	16.7–23.6	Placenta	SA: 84 IA: 16	SA: 57 IA: 31	PCR	Multivariable logistic regression analysis, comparison of SA to IA (best possible control), confirmation by sequencing	Small sample size, imbalance between cases and controls, study including African Americans, HPV-related disease history unclear, gestational age of controls being greater
[52]	Japan	Pregnant women healthy, unselected	1st, 2nd, or 3rd trimester	Cervix	1183	12.5	PCR	Large cohort	HPV-related disease history unclear, sample collection at different time points
[53]	USA	Pregnant women clinically indicating amniocentesis, intact membranes	NA	Amniotic fluid	142	0	PCR	Large cohort, transabdominal sampling (no birth canal contamination)	HPV-related disease history unclear, sampling time point not mentioned, highly selected group of women, unclear how/when they deliver
[54]	Mexico	Pregnant women healthy	1st, 2nd, or 3rd trimester	Cervix	274	37.1	HCA	Large cohort, unconditional/conditional logistic regression	Self-sampling, HPV-related disease history unclear, sample collection at different time points, HCA restricted to 13 HR-types
[55]	China	Pregnant women asymptomatic (cervical)	1st, 2nd, or 3rd trimester	Cervix, amniotic fluid, umbilical cord blood	116	Cervix: 36.2	PCR	Large cohort	Sample collection at different time points

TABLE 1: Continued.

References	Country	Inclusion criteria	Gestational age at sample collection (weeks)	Examined tissue type	Sample size	HPV prevalence%	HPV detection method	Study quality Study strengths	Potential biases
[13]	Austria	Pregnant women healthy, uncomplicated pregnancy, undergoing cesarean section	37.1–40.2	Cervix, placenta, amniotic fluid, umbilical cord blood	153	Cervix: 36.6 Placenta:5.2 Amniotic fluid: 0 Umbilical cord blood: 0	HCA, PCR	Large cohort, univariant/multivariant logistic regression analysis	Highly selected group of women, placenta swabs (quality of material)
[56]	USA	Pregnant women unselected	35 and 39	Cervix	577	29	PCR	Large cohort, logistic regression analysis, confirmation by sequencing, pap smear at study entry	No inclusion and exclusion criteria, women with history of HPV-related lesions included
[28]	Croatia	SA normal cervix	4–19	Placenta	108	7.4	PCR	Large cohort, only women with normal cervix	49.1% having a miscarriage before, 35.2% having abnormal karyotype, possible contamination due to curettage, positive results only with HPV16 and 18 specific primers
[57]	China	Pregnant women unselected, regardless of sexual history or cervical disease	1st, 2nd, or 3rd trimester	Cervix	308	10.1	PCR	Large cohort, confirmation by sequencing, age-matched controls	Sample collection at different time points, inclusion of women regardless of sexual history or cervical diseases
[22]	Austria	Pregnant women assigned for CVS or placental biopsy	9.6–31.3	Cervix, placenta	Cervix: 179 Placenta: 147	Cervix: 24.6 Placenta: 0	HCA, PCR	Large cohort, univariant/multivariant logistic regression analysis, transabdominal sampling (no birth canal contamination)	Highly selected group of women, unusual PCR primers (E6), unclear how/when they delivered, analysis of placenta by PCR, cervix by HCA
[58]	France, Switzerland, Germany	Pregnant women assigned for amniocentesis due to maternal or fetal abnormalities	14–25	Amniotic fluid	238	12	PCR, Southern blot	Large cohort, transabdominal sampling (no birth canal contamination), confirmation by Study strength	Highly selected group of women, HPV-related disease history unclear, samples collected in three countries, unclear how/when they deliver
[59]	Italy	Pregnant women healthy, negative pap smear at first trimester	36–39	Cervix	711	5.2	PCR	Large cohort, pap smear at study entry, no history of HPV-related lesions	Sampling method not mentioned, vaginal and cesarean deliveries

TABLE 1: Continued.

References	Country	Inclusion criteria	Gestational age at sample collection (weeks)	Examined tissue type	Sample size	HPV prevalence%	HPV detection method	Study quality Study strengths	Potential biases
[60]	Greece	SA <20 weeks of gestation	6–20	Aborted product of conception	102	0	PCR	Large cohort	11 women have had previous SA, 3 cases with other diseases, GP5/6 primer (low sensitivity?), HPV-related disease history unclear
[61]	China	Pregnant women singleton	36–40	Cervix	301	22.6	PCR	Large cohort, confirmation by Study strength	Study including vaginal and cesarean deliveries, women with abnormal pap smear included, used specific E6 PCR primers only
[62]	France, Germany	SA: NA IA: for social indication	NA	Aborted product of conception	SA: 27 IA: 1	SA: 70.4 IA: 100	PCR	—	Small sample size, HPV-related disease history unclear, sampling time point not mentioned, no inclusion and exclusion criteria, PCR primer with low sensitivity
[63]	Italy	Pregnant women healthy, negative pap smear at entry	36–39	Cervix	752	5.4	PCR	Large cohort, control for confounders, logistic regression analysis, confirmation by Study strength	Sampling method not mentioned
[64]	Finland	Pregnant women healthy	At birth	Cervix	86	30.2	PCR	Confirmation by Study strength and sequencing	Possible sampling error, contamination, multiple HPV infection, inclusion of women with signs of cervical HPV infection, vaginal and cesarean deliveries
[18]	USA	SA and IA first trimester	1st trimester	Aborted product of conception	SA: 25 IA: 15	SA: 60 IA: 20	PCR	Comparison of SA to IA (best possible control), confirmation by dot blot hybridization	Small sample size, possible contamination from cervix and vagina, HPV-related disease history unclear
[65]	USA	Pregnant women healthy	NA	Cervix	114	34.2	Southern blot	Large cohort, logistic regression analysis	History of CIN not used as exclusion criteria, sampling time point not mentioned, study mostly including African Americans and Hispanics, Bronx → low socioeconomic group, Southern Blot (HPV11, 16, 18 only), unclear how/when they deliver

TABLE 1: Continued.

References	Country	Inclusion criteria	Gestational age at sample collection (weeks)	Examined tissue type	Sample size	HPV prevalence%	HPV detection method	Study quality	
								Study strengths	Potential biases
[66]	Germany	Pregnant women uncomplicated pregnancies	1st, 2nd, and 3rd trimester, postpartum	Cervix	108	13.9	HCA	Large cohort, logistic regression analysis, age-frequency matched controls	Specimens instead of patients, sample collection at different time points, commercial HPV detection kit (6 HPV-types only)
[67]	Hungary	Pregnant women cytologically and colposcopically healthy	1st, 3rd trimester, postpartum	Cervix	39	31	PCR	Cytologically and colposcopically healthy women	Small sample size, 8 deliveries being preterm, HPV-related disease history unclear, sample collection at different time points, outpatient clinic → low socioeconomic group
[68]	USA	Pregnant women healthy, in first trimester, ≥18 years of age	1st trimester	Cervix	245	31	HCA	Large cohort, univariant risk analysis/multiple logistic regression analysis, confirmation by Study strength	Study including African-Americans, HCA sensitivity limited to 14 HPV-types

ND = normal deliveries, PD = preterm deliveries, IA = induced abortion, SA = spontaneous abortion.

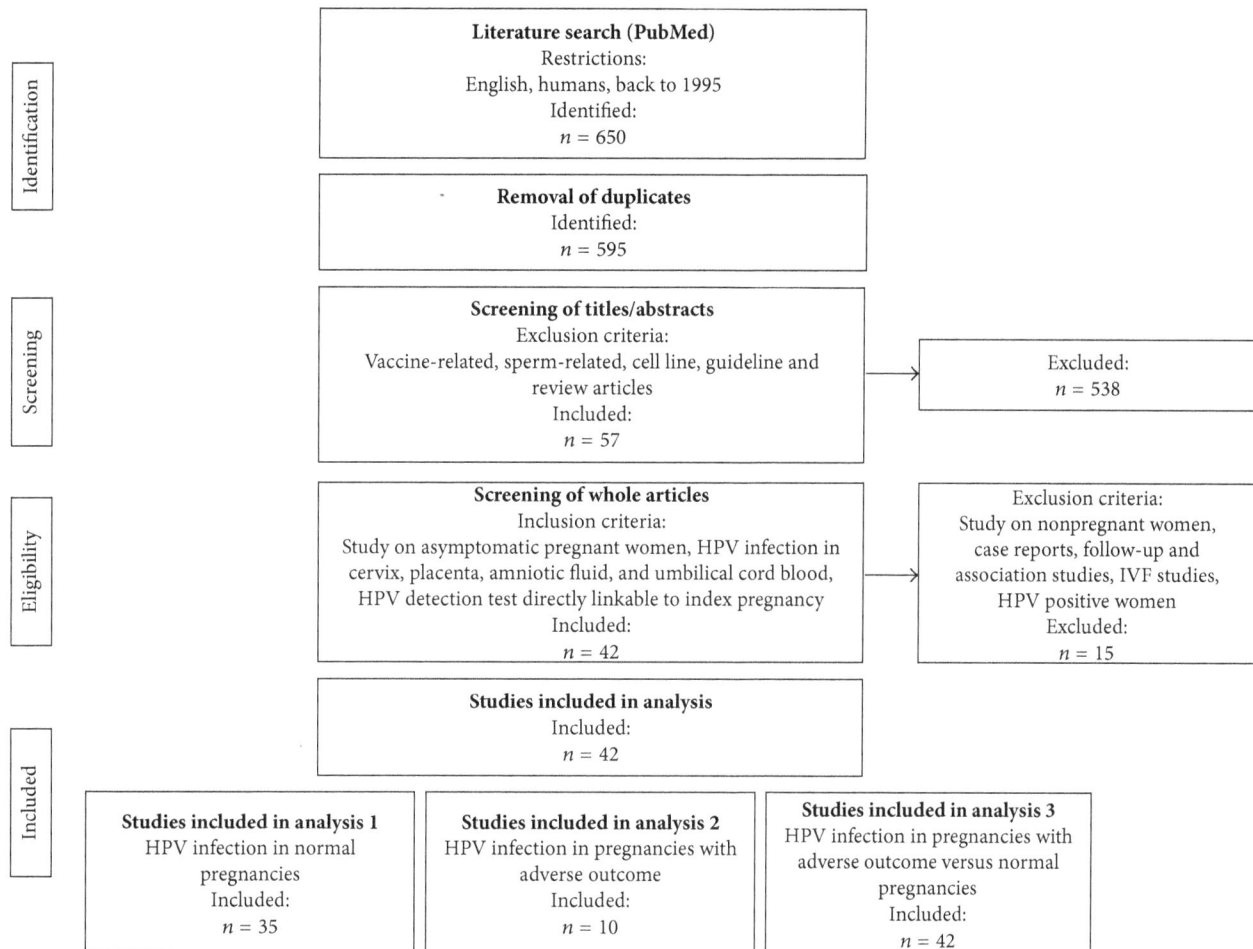

FIGURE 1: Flow diagram of literature search. The flow diagram shows the search in the PubMed database. A supplementary search in the Embase database was conducted in the same way and resulted in three additional articles for data extraction and quantitative analysis.

32, 38, 40, 42, 43, 45, 47, 51, 58–60, 62–64, 66, 67], Asia ($n = 7116$) [23, 34, 35, 37, 39, 41, 46, 52, 55, 57, 61], USA ($n = 1681$) [18, 20, 21, 29, 48, 53, 56, 65, 68], and Latin America ($n = 1034$) [36, 44, 49, 50, 54]. Table 1 shows demographic characteristics, key aspects of study design, and study strength and potential biases of all included studies.

3.2. HPV Prevalence in Different Tissue Types of Normal Full-Term Pregnancies. HPV prevalence in healthy pregnant women giving birth at term was investigated in 38 of the 45 included studies and provided data on 13 757 pregnant women. HPV prevalence appears to be highly dependent on the tissue type tested (Figure 2). In all studies included, HPV prevalence varied between 2.2% and 75% in cervical tissue, with a summary estimate of 17.5% (95% CI; 17.3–17.7). In placental tissue and abortion products, 8.3% (95% CI; 7.6–9.1) of the analyzed pregnancies were found to be HPV positive and varied between 0% and 47.2%. HPV prevalence in amniotic fluid varied between 0% and 25%, with a summary estimate of 5.7% (95% CI; 5.1–6.3). Finally, umbilical cord blood was calculated to be HPV positive in 10.9% (95% CI; 10.1–11.7) of all cases and varied between 0% and 57.9%. The

difference between all proportions was significant ($P < 0.05$, $P < 0.001$, and $P < 0.0001$, resp.).

3.3. HPV Prevalence in Pregnancies with Adverse Outcome and Comparison to Normal Pregnancies. HPV prevalence in pregnancies with adverse outcome, including spontaneous abortion and spontaneous preterm delivery, was investigated in 10 of the 45 included studies and provided data on 681 pregnancies. Three studies were investigating cervical HPV infection and seven studies looking at HPV prevalence in placental tissue. Details are given in Table 2. Only one study analyzed HPV prevalence in cervical tissue of spontaneous abortions and found 24.5% of all cervical samples to be HPV positive (Table 2). Placental HPV prevalence in spontaneous abortions varied between 0% and 70.4%, with a summary estimate of 24.9% (95% CI; 22.4–27.5) (Table 2). HPV prevalence in spontaneous preterm deliveries was found to be 47% (95% CI; 42.3–51.6) in cervix, with a variation between 15.6% and 67.1% (Table 2). Placental tissue of spontaneous preterm deliveries was only investigated in one study where a HPV prevalence of 50% was observed (Table 2).

The overall HPV prevalence in cervical tissue of normal pregnancies was found to be 17.5% (95% CI; 17.3–17.7)

TABLE 2: HPV prevalence in pregnancies with adverse outcome. Studies investigating HPV prevalence in pregnancies with adverse outcome. (a) Spontaneous abortion. (b) Spontaneous preterm delivery.

(a) HPV prevalence in spontaneous abortion

	Cervix			Placenta			Geographical origin	HPV detection method	References
	n	HPV positive cases	%	n	HPV positive cases	%			
	139	34	24.5	84	48	57.1	USA	PCR	Srinivas et al. 2006 [29]
				51	9	17.7	Latin America	PCR	Conde-Ferráez et al. 2013 [36]
Spontaneous abortion				108	8	6.5	Europe	PCR	Skoczyński et al. 2011 [43]
				102	0	0	Europe	PCR	Matovina et al. 2004 [28]
				27	19	70.4	Europe	PCR	Sifakis et al. 1998 [60]
				25	15	60.0	Europe	PCR	Malhomme et al. 1997 [62]
							USA	PCR	Hermonat et al. 1997 [18]
Total	**139**	**34**	**24.5**	**397**	**99**	**24.9**			

(b) HPV prevalence in spontaneous preterm delivery

	Cervix			Placenta			Geographical origin	HPV detection method	References
	n	HPV positive cases	%	n	HPV positive cases	%			
	45	7	15.6				Asia	Hybrid capture assay	Cho et al. 2013 [35]
Spontaneous preterm delivery				30	15	50.0	USA	PCR	Gomez et al. 2008 [20]
	70	47	67.1				USA	Hybrid capture assay	Zuo et al. 2011 [21]
Total	**115**	**54**	**47.0**	**30**	**15**	**50.0**			

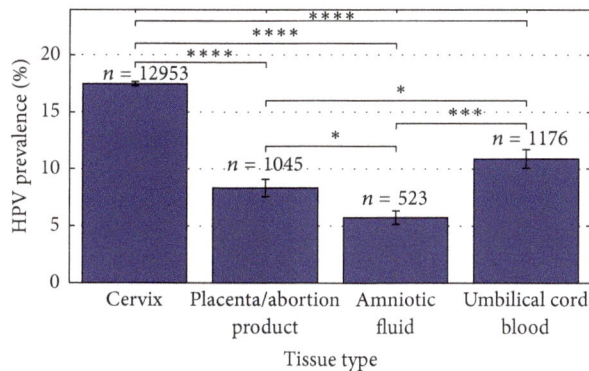

FIGURE 2: HPV prevalence depends on the investigated tissue type. HPV prevalence in different tissue types of normal pregnancies in %. 38 studies have been included in the present analysis, N_{cervix} = 32, $N_{placenta/abortion\ product}$ = 9, $N_{amniotic\ fluid}$ = 4, and $N_{umbilical\ cord\ blood}$ = 7. N indicates number of studies included. n indicates number of cases included. $^*P < 0.05$, $^{***}P < 0.001$, and $^{****}P < 0.0001$.

(Figure 2). This is significantly lower than in spontaneous preterm deliveries (47%, $P < 0.0001$) and spontaneous abortions (24.5%, $P < 0.05$) (Figure 3). An even bigger contrasting picture is seen in placental tissue. Here normal pregnancies are found to be HPV positive in 8.3% (95% CI; 7.6–9.1) of all cases (Figure 2), whereas placental tissues of spontaneous preterm deliveries and spontaneous abortions are found to be positive in 50% ($P < 0.0001$) and 24.9% ($P < 0.0001$) of cases, respectively (Figure 3).

3.4. HPV Prevalence in Normal Pregnancies Depends on Geographical Location. Information on geographical distribution of the investigated studies was collected to see if ethnicity might be a contributing factor to the great variation in HPV prevalence observed. The goal of the investigation was to determine whether women from different countries may be differentially exposed to HPV and some may thereby have a higher risk for possible HPV-induced pregnancy deficiencies.

Figure 4 shows the geographical distribution of HPV prevalence in cervical specimens from women with normal full-term pregnancies. Here it is clear that pregnant women from USA and Latin America have a significantly higher ($P < 0.0001$) HPV prevalence compared to European and Asian women (Figure 4). Latin America is represented by Mexico and Brazil and the summary estimate for HPV prevalence was 35.5% (95% CI; 34.6–36.5). HPV prevalence found in the included studies varied between 15.2% and 75%. The analysis of the population from USA found a HPV prevalence of 29.6% (95% CI; 29.5–29.7). Here a variation of 28% to 34.2% has been reported. The Asian population is represented by China, Japan, and Korea. The cervical HPV prevalence in Asia varied between 10.1% and 36.2%, with a summary estimate of 16.4% (95% CI; 16.3–16.6). The European population is represented by Spain, France, Italy, Germany, Belgium, Netherlands, Finland, Switzerland, Austria, Hungary, Greece, Croatia, Turkey, Poland, and Lithuania and the HPV prevalence varied between 2.2% and 36.6%, with a

summary estimate of 11% (95% CI; 10.7–11.3). The difference between all proportions was highly significant ($P < 0.01$ and $P < 0.0001$, resp.), meaning that HPV prevalence in pregnant women is dependent on geographical or ethnical parameters, with pregnant women from USA and Latin America having the highest HPV prevalence reported. The same tendency can be observed in placenta, amniotic fluid, and umbilical cord blood, but numbers were insufficient for proper analyses.

Variation of HPV prevalence between studies conducted on different continents can also be observed in studies investigating pregnancies with adverse outcome (Table 2), but a proper analysis is difficult due to the small number of studies. However, it can be stated that studies from USA consistently report a significantly higher HPV prevalence in spontaneous abortions and spontaneous preterm deliveries compared to normal pregnancies, in both cervical and placental tissue [18, 20, 21, 29]. European studies vary a lot in their HPV prevalence found in placenta, which makes it difficult to estimate the risk of a HPV infection for European pregnant women. There are no studies conducted on cervical specimens of spontaneous abortions or spontaneous preterm deliveries in Europe. Asian and Latin American studies are also limited [35, 36] and a conclusion of the risk of HPV infection for pregnant women is not possible. It can though be speculated whether the relatively high HPV prevalence found in the Latin American population of normal pregnancies (Figure 4) may influence the pregnancy outcome in those countries.

3.5. Influence of the Time Point of Sample Collection and the HPV Detection Method on HPV Prevalence. There are multiple factors that may influence HPV prevalence. For the present analysis, data on the time point of sample collection and the HPV detection methods used were collected. Figure 5(a) shows cervical HPV prevalence in relation to the time point of sample collection. Samples from the first trimester of pregnancy were found to be HPV positive in 23.9% (95% CI; 23.4–24.4) of all cases and showed a variation between 1.1% and 41.2%. Samples taken at birth were tested positive in 21.7% (95% CI; 21.3–22.2) of all cases. Here HPV prevalence varied between 12.6% and 30.2%. The second and third trimester as well as postpartum samples showed a HPV prevalence of 16.7% (95% CI; 16.5–17.0), 15.2% (95% CI; 14.9–15.6), and 17.3% (95% CI; 16.7–17.9). HPV prevalence varied between 2.2% and 40%, 5.2% and 75%, and 6.2% and 27%. The difference between proportions was significant ($P < 0.05$, $P < 0.01$, $P < 0.001$, and $P < 0.0001$ resp.). Not significant was the difference between the proportions for the first trimester and at birth samples ($P = 0.12$), the second trimester and the third trimester, respectively, and the postpartum period ($P = 0.07$ and $P = 0.39$), and the third trimester and the postpartum period ($P = 0.14$).

Also the HPV detection methods used may influence the found HPV prevalence. Figure 5(b) shows the analysis of HPV prevalence according to the HPV detection method used. Hybrid capture assay identified HPV in 26.4% (95% CI; 25.6–27.2) of all analyzed samples. The HPV prevalence found varied between 0% and 67.1%. The summary estimate for HPV prevalence by PCR was calculated to be 15.5% (95% CI; 15.3–15.8) and varied between studies from 0% to 100%.

(a) Cervix

(b) Placenta

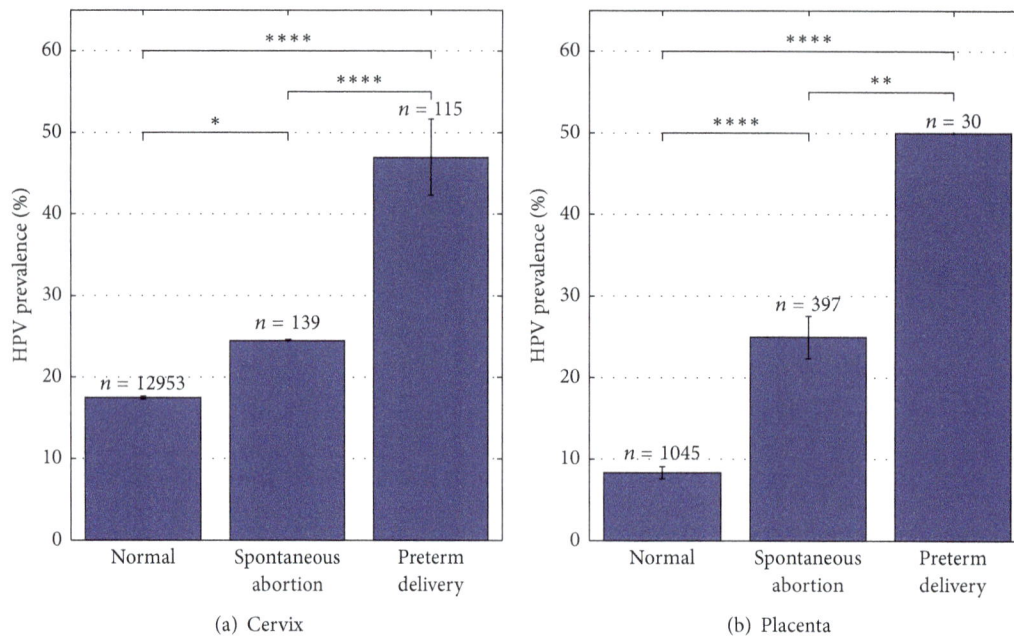

FIGURE 3: Higher HPV prevalence detected in pregnancies with adverse outcome compared to normal pregnancies. HPV prevalence in normal pregnancies, spontaneous abortions, and spontaneous preterm deliveries in %. (a) In cervix. 34 studies have been included in the present analysis, $N_{Normal} = 32$, $N_{Spontaneous\ abortion} = 1$, and $N_{Preterm\ delivery} = 2$. (b) In placenta. 14 studies have been included in the present analysis, $N_{Normal} = 9$, $N_{Spontaneous\ abortion} = 6$, and $N_{Preterm\ delivery} = 1$. N indicated number of studies included. n indicates number of cases included. $^{*}P < 0.05$, $^{**}P < 0.01$, and $^{****}P < 0.0001$.

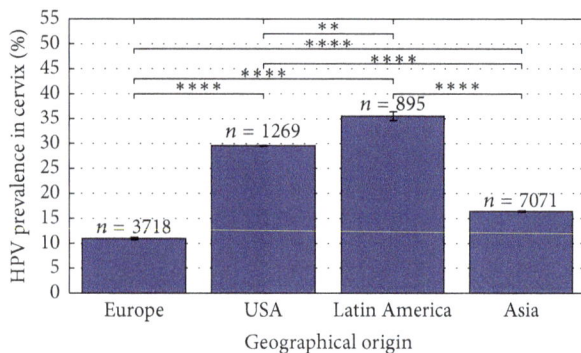

FIGURE 4: HPV prevalence in normal pregnancies depends on geographical location. HPV prevalence in cervix of normal pregnancies in %. 32 studies have been included in the present analysis, $N_{Europe} = 13$, $N_{USA} = 4$, $N_{Latin\ America} = 5$, and $N_{Asia} = 10$. N indicated number of studies included. n indicates number of cases included. $^{**}P < 0.01$, $^{****}P < 0.0001$.

HPV prevalence identified by DNA chip varied between 0% and 24.3%, with a summary estimate of 15.1% (95% CI; 15.0–15.3). Southern blotting was only used in two studies and a HPV prevalence of 19.9% (95% CI; 18.7–21.0) has been found. HPV positivity varied between studies from 12% to 34.2%. The difference between all but one of the proportions was significant ($P < 0.05$, $P < 0.01$, and $P < 0.0001$, resp.). Not significant was the difference between proportions for PCR and DNA chip ($P = 0.25$). The HPV detection method used most widely was PCR with $n = 9674$ followed by DNA chip with $n = 5461$.

4. Discussion

In this quantitative analysis on the prevalence of HPV infection in normal pregnancies and pregnancies with adverse outcome, 45 studies were included and data on 14 470 pregnant women were analyzed and summarized. HPV prevalence in normal pregnancies was found to vary between tissue types and study populations of different geographical locations. The highest HPV prevalence could be reported in cervix (17.5%; 95% CI; 17.3–17.7) and in the population from Latin America (35.5% (95% CI; 34.6–36.5)) and USA (29.6% (95% CI; 29.5–29.7)). In comparison to HPV prevalence found in normal pregnancies, spontaneous abortions and spontaneous preterm deliveries were found to have higher HPV positive detection rates ($P < 0.05$ and $P < 0.0001$), in both placenta (spontaneous abortions: 24.9%, and preterm deliveries: 50% versus 8.3%, resp.) and cervix (spontaneous abortions: 24.5%, and preterm deliveries: 47% versus 17.5%, resp.). Beyond the geographical location, the time point of sample collection in pregnancy as well as the HPV detection methods used may influence the results on HPV prevalence.

The present work has some weaknesses. First, heterogeneity between studies is a problem. Due to the limited number of studies conducted within the field of HPV infections and adverse pregnancy outcomes, inclusion criteria were set relatively widely. This results in a higher number of pregnancies to analyze but possibly more heterogeneous study groups and thereby inflict restricted options to compare directly between studies. The possibility of forming totally homogenous study groups is limited by the study quality and information given,

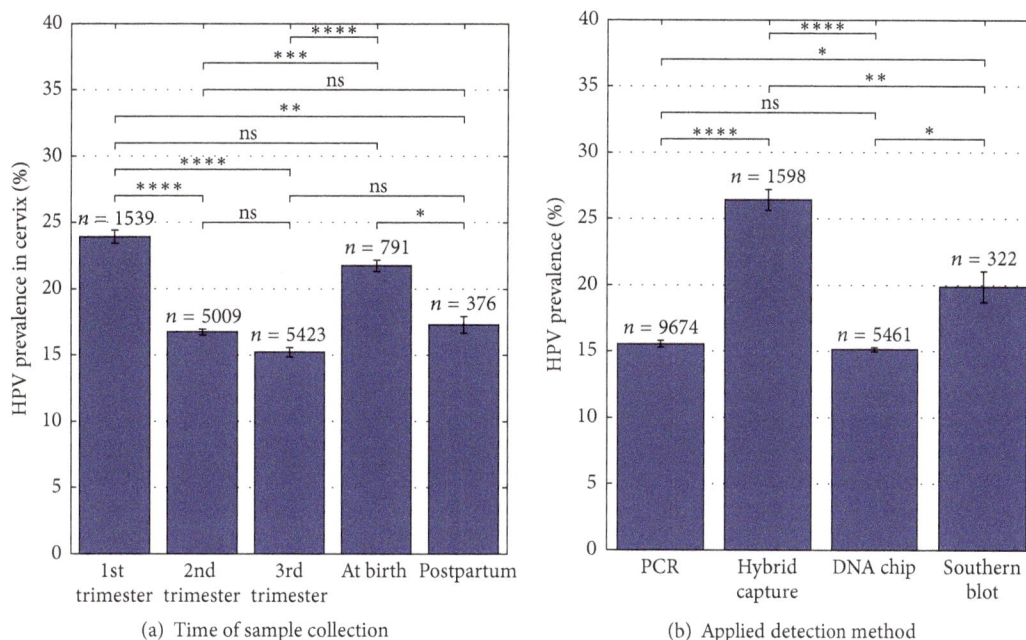

(a) Time of sample collection

(b) Applied detection method

FIGURE 5: HPV prevalence depends on time of sample collection and on the applied HPV detection method. (a) Cervical HPV prevalence in % at different time points of sample collection of normal pregnancies. 25 studies have been included in the present analysis, $N_{\text{1st trimester}} = 10$, $N_{\text{2nd trimester}} = 10$, $N_{\text{3rd trimester}} = 18$, $N_{\text{at birth}} = 4$, and $N_{\text{postpartum}} = 4$. (b) HPV prevalence in % in relation to the detection method used. Note that only two studies were using Southern blot as their main detection method. 45 studies have been included in the present analysis, $N_{\text{PCR}} = 34$, $N_{\text{hybrid capture}} = 8$, $N_{\text{DNA chip}} = 5$, and $N_{\text{Southern blot}} = 2$. N indicated number of studies included. n indicates number of cases included. $^{*}P < 0.05$, $^{**}P < 0.01$, $^{***}P < 0.001$, and $^{****}P < 0.0001$; ns: not significant.

and data on patient-level is missing in most, if not all, of the included studies, which makes controlling for all potential biases difficult. Table 1 contains potential biases and study strength for every single study. Potential biases may include some of the following: unclear inclusion and exclusion criteria for participating women, missing information on ethnicity/method of sample collection/time point of sample collection/mode of delivery, study on highly selected group of women (cesarean sections, amniocentesis, and CVS) or group from low socioeconomically regions, and so forth. The interconnection between HPV infection and pregnancy outcome is complex and will therefore most probably not be explainable by a single parameter analyzed in the present work. The analyses done can however point towards a possible explanation by pregnancy outcome, geographical location, or HPV detection method. Second, studies vary in their inclusion of women with histories of HPV-related diseases. Approximately one-third excludes women with HPV-related lesions, whereas one-third does not exclude but report it and in the last third of studies this information is missing. Genital warts and cervical lesions are known to be HPV-related and a higher percentage of HPV infection would be expected. Third, studies of adverse pregnancies were few. The actual HPV prevalence may therefore be higher or lower than the ones reported in this paper. On the other hand, the present quantitative analysis includes over 14 000 pregnancies and covers many different factors possibly influencing HPV prevalence, thereby providing a broad overview. Fourth, only studies published in English were included, which might limit the results. However, English is the primary common scientific language and the selection criterion "publications in English" is therefore considered to be acceptable.

HPV prevalence in pregnant women has been reported to be higher compared to nonpregnant women [54, 68, 69]. Our analysis of normal pregnancies, including 38 studies from 19 different countries on four continents, yields an overall HPV prevalence in the cervix for pregnant women of 17.5% (95% CI: 17.3–17.7). A worldwide meta-analysis by de Sanjosé et al. from 2007 reported a prevalence of cervical HPV infections in nonpregnant women with normal cytology of 10.4% [70]. The difference between the proportions is noticeable and it can therefore be speculated if a higher HPV prevalence in pregnant women can lead to various pregnancy complications. Pregnancy has previously been described as a state of immune suppression, facilitating the survival of the "semiallogeneic" fetus [52]. The inhibition of the host immune response may simultaneously increase the susceptibility to HPV and make it more difficult to clear HPV infections [54, 69, 71–74]. Higher incidences of HPV infection during pregnancy may though possibly be explained by the presence of hormone response elements in the HPV gene that could be triggered through high steroid levels [13, 14].

An infection with HPV during pregnancy has been associated with risk for spontaneous abortion and spontaneous preterm delivery as well as placental abnormalities [16–21]. Our analysis of 10 studies investigating HPV infection in pregnancies with adverse outcome found HPV prevalence in cervix and placenta to be higher than in normal full-term pregnancies, supporting the hypothesis of HPV infection being a risk for pregnancy outcome. Typically the placenta is a relatively effective barrier guarding against many microbes [75, 76] and the fetus *in utero* is therefore well protected. Nevertheless, multiple studies indicate that viral infection can impair trophoblast function, potentially contributing to pregnancy loss or abnormal implantation [76, 77]. Furthermore, upper genital tract infection was found to be an important cause of preterm birth [78].

As previously mentioned, the wide range of HPV prevalence found is related to several factors including study design, geographic and demographic characteristics, choice of detection method, and risk factor profiles, such as maternal age, gestational age, and history of cesarean section [31, 35, 70, 79]. The present work underlines the importance to consider geographical and demographic variances. The HPV prevalence around the world was found to differ significantly (11–35.5%) with Latin America having the highest cervical HPV prevalence in pregnant women. This is well in line with the previous literature where Latin America and Africa are reported as the geographical areas with the highest cervix cancer rate in the world [8]. North American studies do in general report a relatively high HPV prevalence [20, 48, 56, 65, 68] and our analysis found a HPV prevalence of 29.6% (95% CI; 29.5–29.7) for USA. This may be a bit puzzling since the population in North America due to historical reasons is expected to resemble the population in Europe. It can therefore be speculated that studies conducted in North America include a distinct number of the Latin American and African American population as has been stated by Gomez et al. in 2008 [20]. Unfortunately information of ethnicity of participating women is not available for many of the included studies, providing a potential bias to the results presented on geographical origin.

The time point of sample collection during pregnancy is thought to have an influence on HPV prevalence as differences in HPV prevalence regarding the trimester tested have been published [80–83]. Our analysis involved over 13 000 samples and summarized many of the studies investigating the topic. Hereby the first trimester was found to have the highest overall HPV prevalence, closely followed by the samples taken at birth. Analyzed samples collected in the second and third trimester as well as in the postpartum period showed lower HPV prevalence. This is contradictory to studies reporting highest HPV prevalence during the second [34] and third [54, 65, 68] trimester. On the other hand, multiple HPV infections were observed in the first trimester by Yamasaki et al. in 2011 and high-risk HPV-types were found to be selectively increased in the first trimester as well [46, 68]. It is however important to keep in mind that all those time points in reality are time intervals, thereby making a comparison very difficult. To reduce potential bias due to uncertainty about the time point of sample collection, we have chosen to include only studies providing information on the time point of sample collection. This is the case for 25 of the 45 included studies.

Finally, we compared HPV prevalence with respect to choice of HPV detection methods, since studies have shown that HPV DNA detectable and the HPV-genotypes identified largely depend on this [42]. Our analysis of HPV prevalence in regard to the applied detection methods revealed hybrid capture assay as the method detecting most HPV positive cases (Figure 5(b)). PCR is thought to be the most sensitive method, detecting less than 10 copies of HPV DNA [46, 84, 85]. In our analysis the HPV prevalence detected by PCR was found to be 15.5% (95% CI; 15.3–15.8). Currently an increasing number of studies use broad spectrum primers [26, 31, 56] instead of type-specific primers. These are designed to detect various HPV-types at the same time, hereby giving a broader picture of the HPV-types present. The downside of high sensitivities allowed by PCR is the risk of false-positives due to contamination [84]. It is therefore crucial to evaluate tissue samples on different molecular levels, confirming the detected virus to be correctly localized and active, thus being able to explain the causality of adverse pregnancy outcome or diseases in general.

Functional studies investigating HPV infection in relation to pregnancy are limited. Following the detection of HPV in placental tissue [17, 18, 62] most research is focused on the study of HPV infections in trophoblast cell lines. Being one of the most critical tissues of the placenta, the trophoblast layer plays an important role in contacting maternal tissues and serves multiple roles during gestation. Several lines of evidence point towards the trophoblasts as being the target cells of placental HPV infection. First, it was shown that HPV is able to undergo a complete life cycle in trophoblast cell lines [86, 87]. Second, trophoblast morphology and behavior during HPV infection have been investigated, reporting a higher rate of apoptosis and lower invasion capabilities, agreeing with possible placental dysfunction and adverse pregnancy outcome [20]. Third, studies analyzing trophoblast cells transfected with the HPV genes E5, E6, and E7 report effects on trophoblastic adhesion and increased migratory and invasive properties and may eventually explain potential abnormal implantation due to inappropriate trophoblast spreading [88]. However, a convincing role for HPV infection in connection with spontaneous abortion and spontaneous preterm delivery, at the molecular level, has still to be demonstrated.

5. Conclusion

Based on the present quantitative analyses it can be concluded that HPV prevalence is higher in pregnancies with adverse outcome, such as spontaneous abortion or spontaneous preterm delivery, compared to women experiencing a normal full-term pregnancy. HPV infection may therefore be constituted as a risk for the present pregnancy.

HPV prevalence has been shown to be dependent on the tissue type tested and the geographical location of the study population analyzed. However, the number of studies investigating HPV infection on material from spontaneous abortions and spontaneous preterm deliveries is very limited and study groups are heterogeneous which makes a reliable conclusion difficult. It can be stated that study design is important, the selection of proper controls is essential, and, for a valuable comparison between studies, similarity in samples/patients needs to be controlled as strictly as possible. Furthermore, one should keep in mind that the simple detection of a virus never is equal to a real causative role in the adverse outcome of a pregnancy or diseases in general. It is therefore inevitable to study the viral activity and cellular localization to be able to conclude on the impact for a given situation. Therefore we recommend including an investigation of the molecular mechanism of HPV infections in material of pregnancies with adverse outcome and inviting researchers to conduct new studies to clarify HPV's impact on spontaneous abortion and spontaneous preterm delivery. As a consequence of the aforementioned limitations our study group has initiated a prospective study addressing the complexity of HPV in pregnancy.

Competing Interests

The authors have no competing interests in connection with this paper. However, Jan Blaakær has received lecture fees and advisory board fees from Merck, Sanofi Pasteur MSD, and Glaxo Smith Kline.

Acknowledgments

The authors acknowledge Innovation Fund Denmark for the support of the present work. This work is financially supported by Center for Clinical Research, North Denmark Regional Hospital, and Department of Clinical Medicine, Aalborg University. Furthermore, the project has received funding of 180,000 DKK from "Region Nordjyllands Forskningsfond" and "Marie Pedersen og Jensine Heibergs Legat" to cover running expenses.

References

[1] G. G. Donders, B. Van Bulck, J. Caudron, L. Londers, A. Vereecken, and B. Spitz, "Relationship of bacterial vaginosis and mycoplasmas to the risk of spontaneous abortion," *American Journal of Obstetrics & Gynecology*, vol. 183, no. 2, pp. 431–437, 2000.

[2] J. A. Robertson, L. H. Honore, and G. W. Stemke, "Serotypes of ureaplasma urealyticum in spontaneous abortion," *Pediatric Infectious Disease Journal*, vol. 5, no. 6, pp. S270–S272, 1986.

[3] M. G. Gravett, C. E. Rubens, and T. M. Nunes, "Global report on preterm birth and stillbirth (2 of 7): discovery science," *BMC Pregnancy and Childbirth*, vol. 10, supplement 1, p. S2, 2010.

[4] H.-U. Bernard, R. D. Burk, Z. Chen, K. van Doorslaer, H. Z. Hausen, and E.-M. de Villiers, "Classification of papillomaviruses (PVs) based on 189 PV types and proposal of taxonomic amendments," *Virology*, vol. 401, no. 1, pp. 70–79, 2010.

[5] J. Doorbar, "The papillomavirus life cycle," *Journal of Clinical Virology*, vol. 32, supplement, pp. 7–15, 2005.

[6] M. A. Stanley, "Epithelial cell responses to infection with human papillomavirus," *Clinical Microbiology Reviews*, vol. 25, no. 2, pp. 215–222, 2012.

[7] P. Aggarwal, "Cervical cancer: can it be prevented?" *World Journal of Clinical Oncology*, vol. 5, no. 4, pp. 775–780, 2014.

[8] L. Bruni, L. Barrionuevo-Rosas, G. Albero et al., *Human Papillomavirus and Related Diseases in the World. Summary Report 2014*, 2014.

[9] H. A. Cubie, "Diseases associated with human papillomavirus infection," *Virology*, vol. 445, no. 1-2, pp. 21–34, 2013.

[10] E. D. Weinberg, "Pregnancy-associated depression of cell-mediated immunity," *Reviews of Infectious Diseases*, vol. 6, no. 6, pp. 814–831, 1984.

[11] G. Entrican, "Immune regulation during pregnancy and host-pathogen interactions in infectious abortion," *Journal of Comparative Pathology*, vol. 126, no. 2-3, pp. 79–94, 2002.

[12] H. Huddleston and D. J. Schust, "Immune interactions at the maternal-fetal interface: a focus on antigen presentation," *American Journal of Reproductive Immunology*, vol. 51, no. 4, pp. 283–289, 2004.

[13] C. Worda, A. Huber, G. Hudelist et al., "Prevalence of cervical and intrauterine human papillomavirus infected in the third trimester in asymptomatic women," *Journal of the Society for Gynecologic Investigation*, vol. 12, no. 6, pp. 440–444, 2005.

[14] R. Mittal, A. Pater, and M. M. Pater, "Multiple human papillomavirus type 16 glucocorticoid response elements functional for transformation, transient expression, and DNA-protein interactions," *Journal of Virology*, vol. 67, no. 9, pp. 5656–5659, 1993.

[15] P. Liu, L. Xu, Y. Sun, and Z. Wang, "The prevalence and risk of human papillomavirus infection in pregnant women," *Epidemiology & Infection*, vol. 142, no. 8, pp. 1567–1578, 2014.

[16] C. C. Pao, J. J. Hor, C.-J. Wu, Y.-F. Shi, X. Xie, and S.-M. Lu, "Human papillomavirus type 18 DNA in gestational trophoblastic tissues and choriocarcinomas," *International Journal of Cancer*, vol. 63, no. 4, pp. 505–509, 1995.

[17] B. Sikstroöm, D. Hellberg, S. Nilsson, C. Brihmer, and P.-A. Mårdh, "Contraceptive use and reproductive history in women with cervical human papillomavirus infection," *Advances in Contraception*, vol. 11, no. 4, pp. 273–284, 1995.

[18] P. L. Hermonat, L. Han, P. J. Wendel et al., "Human papillomavirus is more prevalent in first trimester spontaneously aborted products of conception compared to elective specimens," *Virus Genes*, vol. 14, no. 1, pp. 13–17, 1997.

[19] M. Rabreau and J. Saurel, "Presence of human papilloma viruses in the deciduous membranes of early abortion products," *La Presse medicale*, vol. 26, p. 1724, 1997.

[20] L. M. Gomez, Y. Ma, C. Ho, C. M. McGrath, D. B. Nelson, and S. Parry, "Placental infection with human papillomavirus is associated with spontaneous preterm delivery," *Human Reproduction*, vol. 23, no. 3, pp. 709–715, 2008.

[21] Z. Zuo, S. Goel, and J. E. Carter, "Association of cervical cytology and HPV DNA status during pregnancy with placental abnormalities and preterm birth," *American Journal of Clinical Pathology*, vol. 136, no. 2, pp. 260–265, 2011.

[22] W. Eppel, C. Worda, P. Frigo, M. Ulm, E. Kucera, and K. Czerwenka, "Human papillomavirus in the cervix and placenta," *Obstetrics and Gynecology*, vol. 96, no. 3, pp. 337–341, 2000.

[23] H. S. Hahn, M. K. Kee, H. J. Kim et al., "Distribution of maternal and infant human papillomavirus: risk factors associated with vertical transmission," *European Journal of Obstetrics Gynecology and Reproductive Biology*, vol. 169, no. 2, pp. 202–206, 2013.

[24] X. Wang, Q. Zhu, and H. Rao, "Maternal-fetal transmission of human papillomavirus," *Chinese Medical Journal*, vol. 111, no. 8, pp. 726–727, 1998.

[25] E. Armbruster-Moraes, L. M. Ioshimoto, E. Leao, and M. Zugaib, "Detection of human papillomavirus deoxyribonucleic acid sequences in amniotic fluid during different periods of pregnancy," *American Journal of Obstetrics and Gynecology*, vol. 169, no. 4, pp. 1074–1075, 1993.

[26] R. L. Rombaldi, E. P. Serafini, J. Mandelli, E. Zimmermann, and K. P. Losquiavo, "Transplacental transmission of human papillomavirus," *Virology Journal*, vol. 5, article 106, 2008.

[27] M. E. Sarkola, S. E. Grénman, M. A. M. Rintala, K. J. Syrjänen, and S. M. Syrjänen, "Human papillomavirus in the placenta and umbilical cord blood," *Acta Obstetricia et Gynecologica Scandinavica*, vol. 87, no. 11, pp. 1181–1188, 2008.

[28] M. Matovina, K. Husnjak, N. Milutin, S. Ciglar, and M. Grce, "Possible role of bacterial and viral infections in miscarriages," *Fertility and Sterility*, vol. 81, no. 3, pp. 662–669, 2004.

[29] S. K. Srinivas, Y. Ma, M. D. Sammel et al., "Placental inflammation and viral infection are implicated in second trimester pregnancy loss," *American Journal of Obstetrics & Gynecology*, vol. 195, no. 3, pp. 797–802, 2006.

[30] E. M. Smith, J. M. Ritchie, J. Yankowitz et al., "Human papillomavirus prevalence and types in newborns and parents: concordance and modes of transmission," *Sexually Transmitted Diseases*, vol. 31, no. 1, pp. 57–62, 2004.

[31] L. R. Medeiros, A. B. de Moraes Ethur, J. B. Hilgert et al., "Vertical transmission of the human papillomavirus: a systematic quantitative review," *Cadernos de Saúde Pública*, vol. 21, no. 4, pp. 1006–1015, 2005.

[32] C. Weyn, D. Thomas, J. Jani et al., "Evidence of human papillomavirus in the placenta," *Journal of Infectious Diseases*, vol. 203, no. 3, pp. 341–343, 2011.

[33] D. Moher, A. Liberati, J. Tetzlaff, and D. G. Altman, "Preferred reporting items for systematic reviews and meta-analyses: the PRISMA statement," *BMJ*, vol. 339, no. 7716, pp. 332–336, 2009.

[34] Y. H. Kim, J. S. Park, E. R. Norwitz et al., "Genotypic prevalence of human papillomavirus infection during normal pregnancy: a cross-sectional study," *Journal of Obstetrics and Gynaecology Research*, vol. 40, no. 1, pp. 200–207, 2014.

[35] G. Cho, K.-J. Min, H.-R. Hong et al., "High-risk human papillomavirus infection is associated with premature rupture of membranes," *BMC Pregnancy and Childbirth*, vol. 13, article 173, 2013.

[36] L. Conde-Ferráez, A. D. A. Chan May, J. R. Carrillo-Martínez, G. Ayora-Talavera, and M. D. R. González-Losa, "Human papillomavirus infection and spontaneous abortion: a case-control study performed in Mexico," *European Journal of Obstetrics Gynecology and Reproductive Biology*, vol. 170, no. 2, pp. 468–473, 2013.

[37] S. M. Lee, J. S. Park, E. R. Norwitz et al., "Risk of vertical transmission of human papillomavirus throughout pregnancy: a prospective study," *PLoS ONE*, vol. 8, no. 6, Article ID e66368, 2013.

[38] M. Skoczyński, A. Goździcka-Józefiak, and A. Kwaśniewska, "Risk factors of the vertical transmission of human papilloma virus in newborns from singleton pregnancy—preliminary report," *Journal of Maternal-Fetal & Neonatal Medicine*, vol. 27, no. 3, pp. 239–242, 2014.

[39] Y. Hong, S.-Q. Li, Y.-L. Hu, and Z.-Q. Wang, "Survey of human papillomavirus types and their vertical transmission in pregnant women," *BMC Infectious Diseases*, vol. 13, no. 1, article 109, 2013.

[40] C. E. Schmeink, W. J. G. Melchers, J. C. M. Hendriks, W. G. V. Quint, L. F. Massuger, and R. L. M. Bekkers, "Human papillomavirus detection in pregnant women: a prospective matched cohort study," *Journal of Women's Health*, vol. 21, no. 12, pp. 1295–1301, 2012.

[41] H. Park, S. W. Lee, I. H. Lee et al., "Rate of vertical transmission of human papillomavirus from mothers to infants: relationship between infection rate and mode of delivery," *Virology Journal*, vol. 9, article 80, 2012.

[42] H.-M. Koskimaa, T. Waterboer, M. Pawlita, S. Grénman, K. Syrjänen, and S. Syrjänen, "Human papillomavirus genotypes present in the oral mucosa of newborns and their concordance with maternal cervical human papillomavirus genotypes," *Journal of Pediatrics*, vol. 160, no. 5, pp. 837–843, 2012.

[43] M. Skoczyński, A. Goździcka-Józefiak, and A. Kwaśniewska, "Prevalence of human papillomavirus in spontaneously aborted products of conception," *Acta Obstetricia et Gynecologica Scandinavica*, vol. 90, no. 12, pp. 1402–1405, 2011.

[44] O. Uribarren-Berrueta, J. Sánchez-Corona, H. Montoya-Fuentes, B. Trujillo-Hernández, and C. Vásquez, "Presence of HPV DNA in placenta and cervix of pregnant Mexican women," *Archives of Gynecology and Obstetrics*, vol. 285, no. 1, pp. 55–60, 2012.

[45] G. Domža, Ž. Gudlevičienė, J. Didžiapetrienė, K. P. Valuckas, B. Kazbarienė, and G. Drąsutienė, "Human papillomavirus infection in pregnant women," *Archives of Gynecology and Obstetrics*, vol. 284, no. 5, pp. 1105–1112, 2011.

[46] K. Yamasaki, K. Miura, T. Shimada et al., "Epidemiology of human papillomavirus genotypes in pregnant Japanese women," *Journal of Human Genetics*, vol. 56, no. 4, pp. 313–315, 2011.

[47] B. Dinc, G. Bozdayi, A. Biri et al., "Molecular detection of cytomegalovirus, herpes simplex virus 2, human papillomavirus 16–18 in Turkish pregnants," *Brazilian Journal of Infectious Diseases*, vol. 14, no. 6, pp. 569–574, 2010.

[48] E. M. Smith, M. A. Parker, L. M. Rubenstein, T. H. Haugen, E. Hamsikova, and L. P. Turek, "Evidence for vertical transmission of HPV from mothers to infants," *Infectious Diseases in Obstetrics and Gynecology*, vol. 2010, Article ID 326369, 7 pages, 2010.

[49] S. M. M. Pereira, D. Etlinger, L. S. Aguiar, S. V. Peres, and A. Longatto Filho, "Simultaneous Chlamydia trachomatis and HPV infection in pregnant women," *Diagnostic Cytopathology*, vol. 38, no. 6, pp. 397–401, 2010.

[50] L. B. Freitas, C. C. Pereira, R. Checon, J. P. G. Leite, J. P. Nascimento, and L. C. Spano, "Adeno-associated virus and human papillomavirus types in cervical samples of pregnant and non-pregnant women," *European Journal of Obstetrics Gynecology and Reproductive Biology*, vol. 145, no. 1, pp. 41–44, 2009.

[51] X. Castellsagué, T. Drudis, M. P. Cañadas et al., "Human Papillomavirus (HPV) infection in pregnant women and mother-to-child transmission of genital HPV genotypes: a prospective study in Spain," *BMC Infectious Diseases*, vol. 9, article 74, 2009.

[52] K. Takakuwa, T. Mitsui, M. Iwashita et al., "Studies on the prevalence of human papillomavirus in pregnant women in Japan," *Journal of Perinatal Medicine*, vol. 34, no. 1, pp. 77–79, 2006.

[53] M. T. Ruffin IV, J. M. Bailey, D. Roulston et al., "Human papillomavirus in amniotic fluid," *BMC Pregnancy and Childbirth*, vol. 6, article 28, 2006.

[54] C. Hernández-Girón, J. S. Smith, A. Lorincz, E. Lazcano, M. Hernández-Ávila, and J. Salmerón, "High-risk human papillomavirus detection and related risk factors among pregnant and nonpregnant women in Mexico," *Sexually Transmitted Diseases*, vol. 32, no. 10, pp. 613–618, 2005.

[55] D. Deng, L. Wen, W. Chen, and X. Ling, "Asymptomatic genital infection of human papillomavirus in pregnant women and the vertical transmission route," *Journal of Huazhong University of Science and Technology*, vol. 25, no. 3, pp. 343–345, 2005.

[56] E. M. Smith, J. M. Ritchie, J. Yankowitz, D. Wang, L. P. Turek, and T. H. Haugen, "HPV prevalence and concordance in the cervix and oral cavity of pregnant women," *Infectious Disease in Obstetrics and Gynecology*, vol. 12, no. 2, pp. 45–56, 2004.

[57] P. K. S. Chan, A. R. Chang, W.-H. Tam, J. L. K. Cheung, and A. F. Cheng, "Prevalence and genotype distribution of cervical human papillomavirus infection: comparison between pregnant women and non-pregnant controls," *Journal of Medical Virology*, vol. 67, no. 4, pp. 583–588, 2002.

[58] T. Burguete, M. Rabreau, M. Fontanges-Darriet et al., "Evidence for infection of the human embryo with adeno-associated virus in pregnancy," *Human Reproduction*, vol. 14, no. 9, pp. 2396–2401, 1999.

[59] P. Tenti, R. Zappatore, P. Migliora, A. Spinillo, C. Belloni, and L. Carnevali, "Perinatal transmission of human papillomavirus from gravidas with latent infections," *Obstetrics and Gynecology*, vol. 93, no. 4, pp. 475–479, 1999.

[60] S. Sifakis, M. Ergazaki, G. Sourvinos, M. Koffa, E. Koumantakis, and D. A. Spandidos, "Evaluation of Parvo B19, CMV and HPV viruses in human aborted material using the polymerase chain reaction technique," *European Journal of Obstetrics Gynecology and Reproductive Biology*, vol. 76, no. 2, pp. 169–173, 1998.

[61] C.-J. Tseng, C.-C. Liang, Y.-K. Soong, and C.-C. Pao, "Perinatal transmission of human papillomavirus in infants: relationship between infection rate and mode of delivery," *Obstetrics and Gynecology*, vol. 91, no. 1, pp. 92–96, 1998.

[62] O. Malhomme, N. Dutheil, M. Rabreau, E. Armbruster-Moraes, J. R. Schlehofer, and T. Dupressoir, "Human genital tissues containing DNA of adeno-associated virus lack DNA sequences of the helper viruses adenovirus, herpes simplex virus or cytomegalovirus but frequently contain human papillomavirus DNA," *Journal of General Virology*, vol. 78, no. 8, pp. 1957–1962, 1997.

[63] P. Tenti, R. Zappatore, P. Migliora et al., "Latent human papillomavirus infection in pregnant women at term: a case- control study," *Journal of Infectious Diseases*, vol. 176, no. 1, pp. 277–280, 1997.

[64] M. H. Puranen, M. H. Yliskoski, S. V. Saarikoski, K. J. Syrjanen, and S. M. Syrjanen, "Exposure of an infant to cervical human papillomavirus infection of the mother is common," *American Journal of Obstetrics and Gynecology*, vol. 176, no. 5, pp. 1039–1045, 1997.

[65] E. A. B. Morrison, M. D. Gammon, G. L. Goldberg, S. H. Vermund, and R. D. Burk, "Pregnancy and cervical infection with human papillomaviruses," *International Journal of Gynecology and Obstetrics*, vol. 54, no. 2, pp. 125–130, 1996.

[66] J. Chang-Claude, A. Schneider, E. Smith, M. Blettner, J. Wahrendorf, and L. Turek, "Longitudinal study of the effects of pregnancy and other factors on detection of HPV," *Gynecologic Oncology*, vol. 60, no. 3, pp. 355–362, 1996.

[67] G. L. Veress, G. Csiky-Mészáros, J. Kónya, J. Czeglédy, and L. Gergely, "Follow-up of human papillomavirus (HPV) DNA and local anti-HPV antibodies in cytologically normal pregnant women," *Medical Microbiology and Immunology*, vol. 185, no. 3, pp. 139–144, 1996.

[68] K. H. Fife, B. P. Katz, J. Roush, V. D. Handy, D. R. Brown, and R. Hansell, "Cancer-associated human papillomavirus types are selectively increased in the cervix of women in the first trimester of pregnancy," *American Journal of Obstetrics and Gynecology*, vol. 174, no. 5, pp. 1487–1493, 1996.

[69] Y. Aydin, A. Atis, T. Tutuman, and N. Goker, "Prevalence of human papilloma virus infection in pregnant Turkish women compared with non-pregnant women," *European Journal of Gynaecological Oncology*, vol. 31, no. 1, pp. 72–74, 2010.

[70] S. de Sanjosé, M. Diaz, X. Castellsagué et al., "Worldwide prevalence and genotype distribution of cervical human papillomavirus DNA in women with normal cytology: a meta-analysis," *Lancet Infectious Diseases*, vol. 7, no. 7, pp. 453–459, 2007.

[71] K. Kelley and S. H. Vermund, "Human papillomavirus in women: methodologic issues and role of immunosuppression," in *Reproductive and Perinatal Epidemiology*, pp. 158–159, 1990.

[72] K. H. Fife, B. P. Katz, E. J. Brizendine, and D. R. Brown, "Cervical human papillomavirus deoxyribonucleic acid persists throughout pregnancy and decreases in the postpartum period," *American Journal of Obstetrics and Gynecology*, vol. 180, no. 5, pp. 1110–1114, 1999.

[73] S. Sethi, M. Muller, A. Schneider et al., "Serologic response to the E4, E6, and E7 proteins of human papillomavirus type 16 in pregnant women," *American Journal of Obstetrics & Gynecology*, vol. 178, no. 2, pp. 360–364, 1998.

[74] M. A. E. Nobbenhuis, T. J. M. Helmerhorst, A. J. C. Van den Brule et al., "High-risk human papillomavirus clearance in pregnant women: trends for lower clearance during pregnancy with a catch-up postpartum," *British Journal of Cancer*, vol. 87, no. 1, pp. 75–80, 2002.

[75] A. Alanen, "Polymerase chain reaction in the detection of microbes in amniotic fluid," *Annals of Medicine*, vol. 30, no. 3, pp. 288–295, 1998.

[76] H. Koi, J. Zhang, and S. Parry, "The mechanisms of placental viral infection," *Annals of the New York Academy of Sciences*, vol. 943, pp. 148–156, 2001.

[77] F. Arechavaleta-Velasco, H. Koi, J. F. Strauss III, and S. Parry, "Viral infection of the trophoblast: time to take a serious look at its role in abnormal implantation and placentation?" *Journal of Reproductive Immunology*, vol. 55, no. 1-2, pp. 113–121, 2002.

[78] W. W. Andrews, R. L. Goldenberg, and J. C. Hauth, "Preterm labor: emerging role of genital tract infections," *Infectious Agents and Disease*, vol. 4, no. 4, pp. 196–211, 1995.

[79] S. Syrjänen and M. Puranen, "Human papillomavirus infections in children: the potential role of maternal transmission," *Critical Reviews in Oral Biology and Medicine*, vol. 11, no. 2, pp. 259–274, 2000.

[80] A. Schneider, M. Hotz, and L. Gissmann, "Increased prevalence of human papillomaviruses in the lower genital tract of pregnant women," *International Journal of Cancer*, vol. 40, no. 2, pp. 198–201, 1987.

[81] R. F. Rando, S. Lindheim, L. Hasty, T. V. Sedlacek, M. Woodland, and C. Eder, "Increased frequency of detection of human papillomavirus deoxyribonucleic acid in exfoliated cervical cells during pregnancy," *American Journal of Obstetrics and Gynecology*, vol. 161, no. 1, pp. 50–55, 1989.

[82] E. M. Smith, S. R. Johnson, D. Jiang et al., "The association between pregnancy and human papilloma virus prevalence," *Cancer Detection and Prevention*, vol. 15, no. 5, pp. 397–402, 1991.

[83] A. M. De Roda Husman, J. M. M. Walboomers, E. Hopman et al., "HPV prevalence in cytomorphologically normal cervical scrapes of pregnant women as determined by PCR: the age-related pattern," *Journal of Medical Virology*, vol. 46, no. 2, pp. 97–102, 1995.

[84] T. Iftner and L. L. Villa, "Chapter 12: human papillomavirus technologies," *Journal of the National Cancer Institute Monographs*, vol. 2003, no. 31, pp. 80–88, 2003.

[85] P. J. F. Snijders, A. J. C. van den Brule, and C. J. L. M. Meijer, "The clinical relevance of human papillomavirus testing:

relationship between analytical and clinical sensitivity," *The Journal of Pathology*, vol. 201, no. 1, pp. 1–6, 2003.

[86] Y. Liu, H. You, M. Chiriva-Internati et al., "Display of complete life cycle of human papillomavirus type 16 in cultured placental trophoblasts," *Virology*, vol. 290, no. 1, pp. 99–105, 2001.

[87] H. You, Y. Liu, N. Agrawal et al., "Infection, replication, and cytopathology of human papillomavirus type 31 in trophoblasts," *Virology*, vol. 316, no. 2, pp. 281–289, 2003.

[88] S. Boulenouar, C. Weyn, M. van Noppen et al., "Effects of HPV-16 E5, E6 and E7 proteins on survival, adhesion, migration and invasion of trophoblastic cells," *Carcinogenesis*, vol. 31, no. 3, pp. 473–480, 2010.

11

The Effects of Viral Load Burden on Pregnancy Loss among HIV-Infected Women in the United States

Jordan E. Cates,[1] Daniel Westreich,[1] Andrew Edmonds,[1] Rodney L. Wright,[2]
Howard Minkoff,[3] Christine Colie,[4] Ruth M. Greenblatt,[5] Helen E. Cejtin,[6]
Roksana Karim,[7] Lisa B. Haddad,[8] Mirjam-Colette Kempf,[9] Elizabeth T. Golub,[10]
and Adaora A. Adimora[1,11]

[1] Department of Epidemiology, The University of North Carolina at Chapel Hill, Chapel Hill, NC 27599, USA
[2] Department of Obstetrics & Gynecology and Women's Health, Albert Einstein College of Medicine, Montefiore Medical Center, Bronx, NY 10467, USA
[3] Department of Obstetrics & Gynecology, Maimonides Medical Center, Brooklyn, NY 11219, USA
[4] Department of Obstetrics & Gynecology, Georgetown University, Washington, DC 20007, USA
[5] Departments of Clinical Pharmacy, Medicine Epidemiology and Biostatistics, University of California, San Francisco, San Francisco, CA 94143, USA
[6] Department of Obstetrics and Gynecology, John H. Stroger Hospital of Cook County, Chicago, IL 60612, USA
[7] Department of Preventive Medicine, Keck School of Medicine, University of Southern California, Los Angeles, CA 90032, USA
[8] Department of Gynecology and Obstetrics, Emory University School of Medicine, Atlanta, GA 30322, USA
[9] Schools of Nursing and Public Health, Department of Health Behavior, University of Alabama at Birmingham, Birmingham, AL 35294, USA
[10] Department of Epidemiology, Johns Hopkins Bloomberg School of Public Health, Baltimore, MD 21205, USA
[11] School of Medicine, The University of North Carolina at Chapel Hill, Chapel Hill, NC 27516, USA

Correspondence should be addressed to Daniel Westreich; westreic@email.unc.edu

Academic Editor: Faustino R. Perez-Lopez

Background. To evaluate the effects of HIV viral load, measured cross-sectionally and cumulatively, on the risk of miscarriage or stillbirth (pregnancy loss) among HIV-infected women enrolled in the Women's Interagency HIV Study between 1994 and 2013. *Methods.* We assessed three exposures: most recent viral load measure before the pregnancy ended, $\log_{10}$ copy-years viremia from initiation of antiretroviral therapy (ART) to conception, and $\log_{10}$ copy-years viremia in the two years before conception. *Results.* The risk of pregnancy loss for those with $\log_{10}$ viral load >4.00 before pregnancy ended was 1.59 (95% confidence interval (CI): 0.99, 2.56) times as high as the risk for women whose $\log_{10}$ viral load was ≤ 1.60. There was not a meaningful impact of $\log_{10}$ copy-years viremia since ART or $\log_{10}$ copy-years viremia in the two years before conception on pregnancy loss (adjusted risk ratios (aRRs): 0.80 (95% CI: 0.69, 0.92) and 1.00 (95% CI: 0.90, 1.11), resp.). *Conclusions.* Cumulative viral load burden does not appear to be an informative measure for pregnancy loss risk, but the extent of HIV replication during pregnancy, as represented by plasma HIV RNA viral load, predicted loss versus live birth in this ethnically diverse cohort of HIV-infected US women.

1. Introduction

In 2013, women accounted for over half of the 35 million people living with human immunodeficiency virus (HIV) worldwide [1]. HIV-infected women who adhere to antiretroviral therapy (ART) are living longer, healthier lives [2, 3]. Due to improved maternal health and the low probability of mother-to-child transmission with effective and timely treatment [3–5], increasing numbers of HIV-infected women of reproductive age are deciding to become pregnant or expressing a desire for future childbearing [4–9].

Prior to the era of effective ART, HIV-infected women had a substantially higher risk of adverse birth outcomes [10–13], with one meta-analysis reporting that HIV-infected women had a risk of miscarriage or stillbirth four times as high as uninfected women [10]. ART has reduced but not removed this disparity in risk. While ART is effective at lowering viremia [3], several studies have shown that maternal HIV infection is associated with an increased risk of adverse birth outcomes even in the presence of ART [13–16], although not all studies have observed this association [17].

The pathogenesis of adverse birth outcomes, including the possible increased risk among HIV-infected women, is not well understood, though some mechanisms have been suggested. Successful live childbirth is a culmination of an inflammatory cascade, and it has been speculated that dysregulation of this cascade by viral antigens may lead to adverse birth outcomes [18–20]. Higher plasma viral load is a marker of maternal HIV disease severity and has been associated with adverse birth outcomes [16, 21, 22]. For example, in a study of African women, each $\log_{10}$ increase in maternal HIV RNA viral load measured during early pregnancy was associated with a 90% relative increase in the odds of stillbirth [21].

There are several limitations regarding the current literature on pregnancy loss in HIV-infected women. To date, no studies have investigated whether long-term immune system inflammation due to continuous viral load burden could have an effect on adverse pregnancy outcomes. One novel measure for quantifying cumulative viral load is copy-years viremia [22]. Copy-years viremia since ART initiation has been shown to be a predictor of mortality [23–25] and specific types of lymphoma among HIV-infected individuals [26]. Additionally, most studies are from low resource environments [14–16, 21, 22], with limited data addressing the impact of viremia on pregnancy outcomes in high resource settings [17]. Also, while there are some studies concerning the effect of viral load burden on infant outcomes, such as preterm birth and low birth weight, there are fewer and more contradictory studies assessing its relationship with pregnancy loss (miscarriage and stillbirth) [14–17, 21, 22].

To better understand the pathogenesis of pregnancy loss among HIV-infected women in the United States, we used three different specifications of viral load burden. Specifically, we assessed whether (1) a single measure of most recent viral load before the pregnancy ended, (2) cumulative viral load ($\log_{10}$ copy-years viremia from ART initiation to conception), or (3) short-term viral load ($\log_{10}$ copy-years in the two years preceding pregnancy) in HIV-infected women was associated with increased risks of pregnancy loss (miscarriage and stillbirth).

2. Methods

2.1. Study Population and Definitions. The Women's Inter-agency HIV Study (WIHS) is an ongoing, multicenter, prospective cohort study of HIV-uninfected and HIV-infected women enrolled across the United States. The WIHS, which includes a semiannual medical exam and interview, has been described in detail previously [27, 28]. Written informed consent was obtained after IRB approval of WIHS protocols at all participating institutions.

To assess our three exposures, we constructed three separate analytic populations from the WIHS population (Figure 1). For all three populations, we analyzed data from 514 HIV-infected women enrolled in the WIHS, who provided data between October 1, 1994, and March 31, 2013, with at least one self-reported singleton pregnancy following enrollment. Only first, second, and third reported pregnancies (90% of all pregnancies) were included to reduce possible confounding by extreme gravidity. We excluded pregnancies without at least one viral load measure within the year prior to pregnancy outcome (analysis 1) and without at least two viral load measures prior to conception (analyses 2 and 3) (Figure 1). Analyses 1 and 3 included both ART-naïve and ART-initiated women, while analysis 2 was restricted to ART initiators as it focused on viral load since ART initiation.

ART was defined as use of any antiretroviral drug but was categorized as mono-/dual therapy and highly active ART (HAART). In a sensitivity analysis, we repeated analysis 2 but restricted it to those who initiated HAART. HAART was defined according to the US Department of Health and Human Services/Kaiser Panel guidelines [29].

Pregnancies and pregnancy outcomes were self-reported. Participants were asked at every visit, "have you been pregnant since your last visit?" (yes or no) and "what was the outcome of the pregnancy?" Pregnancy outcomes were explained to study subjects by trained interviewers to help reduce errors: miscarriage was defined as the spontaneous loss of a pregnancy before 20 weeks/5 months of gestation, stillbirth was defined as a child born dead after that time, and live birth was defined as a baby born alive [28]. The main outcome of interest, pregnancy loss, was defined as either a self-reported miscarriage or stillbirth and was compared to live births. Ectopic pregnancies were infrequent and were therefore excluded, while elective abortions were considered to be a presumptively uninformative competing risk and were therefore also excluded (Figure 1).

For pregnancies in which the woman had a WIHS visit during the pregnancy, we estimated that her date of conception was two weeks after her last menstrual period [30]. For all other pregnancies, assumptions based on published literature were used to estimate the date of conception: the approximate date of conception was estimated as 38 weeks before a live birth, 32 weeks before a stillbirth, and 11 weeks before a miscarriage [31–33].

HIV RNA viral load (copies per milliliter of plasma) was ascertained at each semiannual study visit. There were two challenges regarding the lower limit of detection (LLD) for the viral load assays used. First, assays changed over time with differing limits of detection; secondly, the viral loads at the LLD cannot be assumed to truly be at this left-censored measurement limit. For example, the LLD for the most commonly used assay during the full study period was 80: a woman with a viral load of 80 was assumed to have a true viral load between 0 and 80 (rather than 80 exactly). To avoid differentially misclassifying the exposure due to changes in assay sensitivity and left-censoring, we set all viral loads at or below 80 to 40 (half of 80); in addition, we also set all viral loads at LLDs other than 80 to 40.

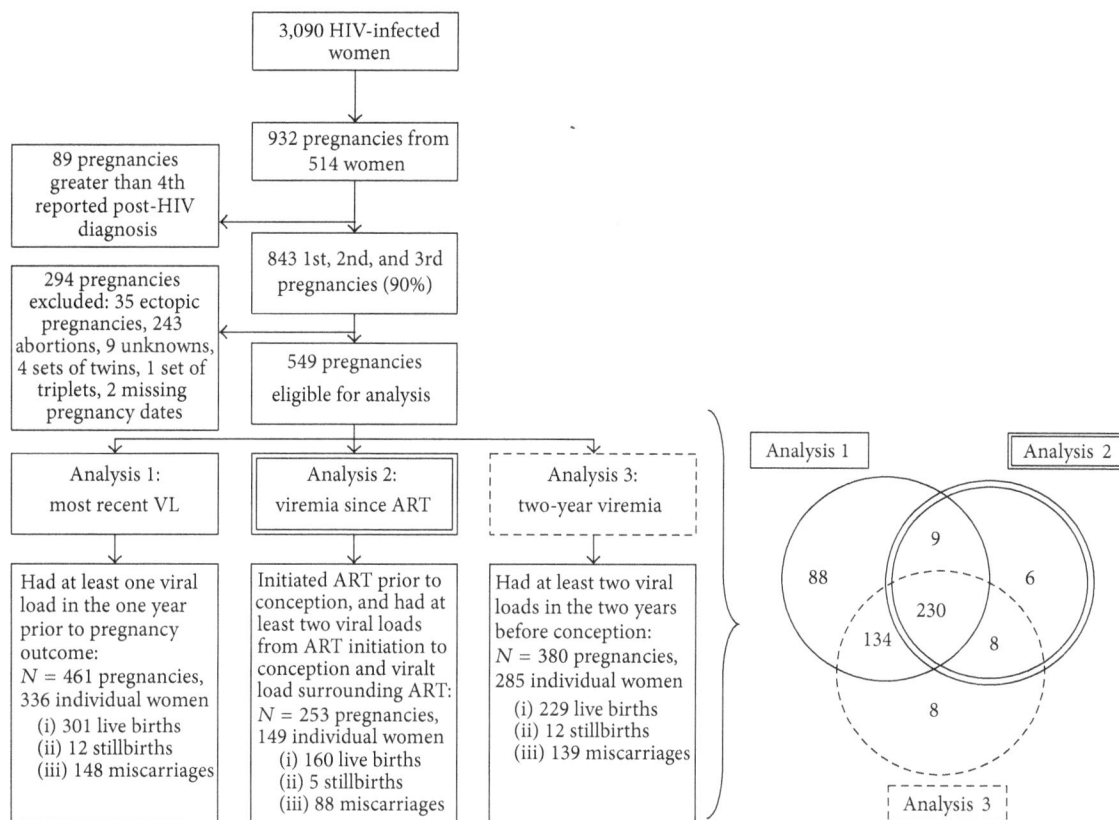

FIGURE 1: Flowchart and Venn diagram of women enrolled in the Women's Interagency HIV Study (WIHS) since 1994, illustrating the inclusion criteria for pregnancies included in analyses 1, 2, and 3. The Venn diagram illustrates the overlap between the three analytic populations.

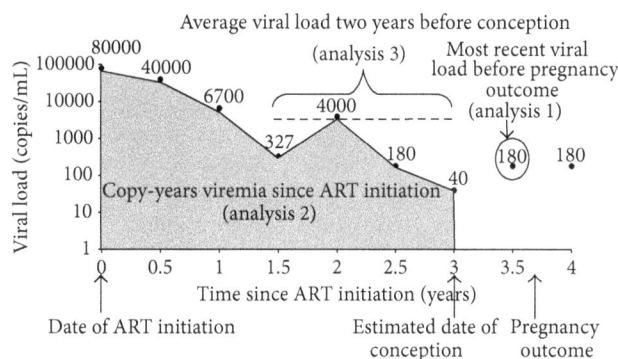

FIGURE 2: Construction of copy-years viremia, a calculation of the area under the longitudinal viral load curve from ART initiation to estimated date of conception (analysis 2). Also illustrated in the figure are the average viral load two years before conception (analysis 3), equivalent to copy-years viremia in two years before conception, and the most recent viral load measure proximal to pregnancy outcome (analysis 1).

For analysis 1, we used the exposure of most recent viral load before the pregnancy ended (Figure 2). For this analysis, the study population included all HIV-infected women with a viral load measure (whether during or before pregnancy, see Section 2.3) within one year before the pregnancy outcome.

For analysis 2, we used the exposure of $\log_{10}$ copy-years viremia from ART initiation to conception. For this analysis, the study population included all HIV-infected women with at least one self-reported pregnancy who initiated ART prior to their pregnancy. This analysis captured long-term ART users and did not include those who only initiated ART during pregnancy (however, these pregnancies were captured in analyses 1 and 3). Ideally, we would have liked to assess lifetime copy-years viremia since seroconversion; however because few WIHS participants seroconverted, these data were unavailable. Left-censoring copy-years viremia at a well-defined point, in this case ART initiation, was the next best option [24, 25]; controlling for CD4 count and other factors at time of ART initiation helped account for potential differences prior to ART initiation. Others have taken this approach and found that $\log_{10}$ copy-years viremia since ART initiation was predictive of mortality [24, 25].

$\log_{10}$ copy-years viremia from ART initiation to conception was defined as the area under a patient's longitudinal viral load curve from ART initiation to the estimated date of conception (Figure 2) [23]. Viral loads during pregnancy were not included to prevent differential misclassification by outcome, since women with a live birth would have more exposure time until their pregnancy outcome than a miscarriage or stillbirth. We conducted a complete case analysis, excluding women who did not have a viral load measure within a baseline window from 24 weeks prior to up to four weeks following ART initiation. A vast majority of women meeting this exclusion criterion enrolled in the WIHS after they initiated ART; thus this missing data was assumed to be uninformative.

For analysis 3, we used the exposure $\log_{10}$ copy-years viremia in the two years before conception and did not restrict it to ART initiators. For this analysis, we defined the study population as all HIV-infected women with at least two viral loads in the two years before conception. The calculation of this exposure was analogous to that for analysis 2, except this exposure only included those viral load values during the two years before conception (Figure 2). Since viral loads were not measured in the study exactly at conception and two years prior to conception, we imputed viral load values for these dates using the most proximal viral load to that time point. This enabled calculation of $\log_{10}$ copy-years viremia in the two years before conception using a homogeneous time frame for each woman.

2.2. Statistical Analysis. Demographic and clinical characteristics of women and their pregnancies were described using proportions for categorical variables and medians for continuous variables. Log-binomial and linear regression models were used to estimate the associations between the three exposures and the proportions of total pregnancy losses out of total pregnancies, using generalized estimating equations with an exchangeable correlation structure to account for within-subject correlation (multiple pregnancies per individual). For each analysis, we considered both continuous and categorical specifications of the viral load measures. Categories of cross-sectional viral load measures (analysis 1) were based on clinically informative cut-points (1.60, 3.00, and 4.00 $\log_{10}$ viral load), while the categories for cumulative viremia measures (analyses 2 and 3) were based on statistical quartiles since the meaningful cut-points of viremia in this context are unknown.

Multivariable models were used to adjust for covariates identified using posited causal directed acyclic graphs (DAGs). Based on our DAGs, confounders included for adjustment were maternal age, race/ethnicity, previous pregnancy loss, CD4 count, ART use, smoking, and injection and noninjection drug use (IDU and NIDU). CD4 counts and ART use were measured at baseline, which was defined as the beginning of exposure assessment: visit of viral load ascertainment before the pregnancy ended (analysis 1), visit when ART was initiated (analysis 2), and first visit during the two-year time period preceding pregnancy (analysis 3) (Figure 2). Smoking, IDU, and NIDU were measured at the WIHS visit prior to the pregnancy outcome. This measurement occurred during either the woman's pregnancy or the nearest measure to conception, representing the closest proxy to these covariates during pregnancy. We used a linear spline to flexibly control for maternal age. After exploring the frequencies of IDU among study participants (approximately 1-2% in all three populations), we excluded women with IDU from all analyses to reduce potential unmeasured confounding.

ART was controlled for in all analyses, through restriction in analysis 2 and through adjustment for ART use at baseline in analyses 1 and 3. We did not want to control for ART use after baseline, since ART use after the beginning of exposure assessment could be considered a downstream causal effect of viral load burden, and adjustment for it might bias estimates of the total effects of the exposures. Indicators variables were used to categorize ART use as mono-/dual therapy, HAART, or none. We did not adjust for duration of ART because we assumed that there was no independent effect of duration of ART on pregnancy loss external of its effect on our viral load burden.

2.3. Sensitivity Analyses. We conducted several analyses to assess the sensitivity of our results to key assumptions. For analyses 1 and 3, we restricted the analyses to pregnancies with exposure during 1998–2013. We altered the inclusion criterion for analysis 2 from ART initiation since 1994 to HAART initiation since 1998. For analyses 1 and 3, we also controlled for HAART instead of any ART. These sensitivity analyses were used to see if capturing slightly more modern study population and ART regimens changed the conclusions of the analyses. Ideally, we would have preferred to restrict the population to a more recent subgroup, but our sample size did not provide enough power for that analysis.

For analysis 1, we only included viral loads that were measured during pregnancy, since the original exposure allowed for measurements prior to pregnancy, as long as they were within one year of the pregnancy outcome. For analysis 2, we dropped the first viral load following ART initiation from the calculation of copy-years viremia to allow time for viral response to therapy. We also separately assessed the results for analysis 2 when adjusting for time on ART, to relax the assumption that the time on ART did not impact the effect of copy-years viremia (see Section 4). For analysis 3, we altered the baseline by varying the exposure period from two years prior to conception to one and three years prior to conception. For each analytic population, stillbirths were excluded from our definition of pregnancy loss to determine if focusing on miscarriages altered our results. Finally, we considered potential effect measure modification by CD4 count and adjustment for CD4 nadir instead of baseline CD4 count.

3. Results

3.1. Study Population. There were 932 self-reported singleton pregnancies from 514 HIV-infected women enrolled in the WIHS from October 1, 1994, to March 31, 2013 (Figure 1). The population for analysis 1, where the exposure was the most recent viral load before pregnancy outcome, comprised 461 pregnancies among 336 women; 160 (35%) of these pregnancies resulted in losses (148 miscarriages and 12 stillbirths). The population for analysis 2, where the exposure was $\log_{10}$ copy-years viremia from ART initiation to conception, comprised 253 pregnancies among 149 women; 93 (37%) of these pregnancies resulted in losses (88 miscarriages and 5 stillbirths). The population for analysis 3, where the exposure was

TABLE 1: Characteristics of HIV-infected women enrolled in the Women's Interagency HIV Study (WIHS) from October 1, 1994, to March 31, 2013, and their respective pregnancies meeting eligibility criteria for three analytic populations: (i) most recent viral load before pregnancy outcome, (ii) copy-years viremia since ART initiation, and (iii) copy-years viremia in the two years before conception.

Characteristic	Most recent VL (i)		Viremia since ART (ii)		Viremia in two years (iii)	
	Women ($n = 336$)	Pregnancies ($n = 461$)	Women ($n = 149$)	Pregnancies ($n = 253$)	Women ($n = 285$)	Pregnancies ($n = 380$)
Race						
Black	212 (63)	289 (63)	80 (54)	140 (55)	175 (61)	235 (62)
White	67 (20)	93 (20)	33 (22)	61 (24)	59 (21)	79 (21)
Other*	57 (17)	79 (17)	36 (24)	52 (21)	51 (18)	66 (17)
Income/year						
<$12,000	170 (53)	233 (53)	66 (46)	114 (47)	131 (48)	178 (49)
$12,001–$36,000	117 (36)	152 (35)	59 (41)	87 (36)	107 (39)	133 (37)
>$36,000	34 (11)	55 (13)	20 (14)	42 (17)	35 (13)	52 (14)
		Pregnancy dependent measures				
CD4 count[†]	—	438 (294–644)	—	369 (242–528)	—	445 (298–661)
IDU[‡]	—	7 (2)	—	3 (1)	—	4 (1)
Prior loss[§]	—	137 (30)	—	80 (32)	—	119 (31)
Smoking	—	166 (36)	—	87 (35)	—	138 (37)
Maternal age	—	32 (29–37)	—	34 (30–38)	—	33 (29–38)
ART initiated[†]	—	393 (85)	—	All	—	225 (59)
NIDU	—	84 (18)	—	36 (14)	—	66 (17)

Categorical variables expressed as number (% total); continuous variables as median (interquartile range). WIHS = Women's Interagency HIV Study, ART = antiretroviral therapy, VL = viral load, IDU = injection drug use, and NIDU = noninjection drug use.
* Unknown, Asian, Hispanic, Pacific Islander, Native American, and Alaskan.
[†] Measured at baseline, the visit at which the first viral load measure for each analysis occurred.
[‡] Injection drug users were excluded for the main analysis to reduce confounding.
[§] Self-reported previous miscarriage or stillbirth prior to and during WIHS enrollment.

$\log_{10}$ copy-years viremia in the two years before conception, comprised 380 pregnancies among 285 women; 151 (40%) of these pregnancies resulted in losses (139 miscarriages and 12 stillbirths).

3.2. Population and Pregnancy Characteristics. Most women in the study populations were black and low-income; the median maternal ages were in the early 30s (Table 1). A high percentage of women reported smoking at the visit prior to the pregnancy outcome (35–37% in all three populations). For analysis 1, the median most recent $\log_{10}$ viral load was 2.5 (interquartile range (IQR): 1.6, 3.8), with a median time from sample measurement to pregnancy outcome of 13 weeks (IQR: 6, 20). Of the 461 pregnancies eligible for analysis 1, 393 (85%) occurred among women who had ever initiated ART (Table 1). Of those 393 pregnancies, 324 occurred among women who reported currently taking ART at the visit of their viral load assessment, of whom 39 (11%) were on monotherapy, 36 (11%) were on combination therapy, and 249 (73%) were on HAART. Of note, 181 pregnancies included in analysis 1 (39%) had most recent viral load measures at or below the lower limit of detection. Also, for 356 pregnancies (77%) this viral load was measured during their pregnancy (see Section 2.3). For analysis 2, the median $\log_{10}$ copy-years viremia from ART initiation to conception was 4.4 (IQR: 3.8, 4.9), with a median time from ART initiation to conception

of 4.3 years (IQR: 2.2, 7.5). For analysis 3, the median $\log_{10}$ copy-years viremia in the two years before pregnancy was 5.7 (IQR: 4.3, 6.5). Univariate results indicated that prior pregnancy loss, maternal age, smoking, and noninjection drug use were all associated with pregnancy loss (Supplemental Table 1 in Supplementary Material available online at http://dx.doi.org/10.1155/2015/362357).

3.3. Effect Estimates. In analysis 1, the adjusted risk ratio (aRR) for the effect of a one-log increase in most recent viral load measure before pregnancy outcome on the risk of pregnancy loss was 1.17 (95% confidence interval (CI): 1.01, 1.35); the corresponding adjusted risk difference (aRD) was 0.04 (95% CI: −0.01, 0.08). Comparisons of categories of most recent viral load further suggest an increasing trend in both relative and absolute risk measures with increasing viral load (Table 2); notably, the absolute adjusted increase in risk was 0.14 (95% CI: −0.01, 0.28) for pregnancies whose viral load measurement was in the highest category (>4.00 $\log_{10}$) compared to those women whose final viral load was in the lowest category (≤1.60 $\log_{10}$). In analyses 2 and 3, the aRRs for the effect of a one-unit increase in $\log_{10}$ copy-years viremia from ART initiation to conception and viremia in the two years before conception on the risk of pregnancy loss were 0.80 (95% CI: 0.69, 0.92) and 1.00 (95% CI: 0.90, 1.11),

TABLE 2: Risk ratios and risk differences of the association of pregnancy loss with most recent cross-sectional viral load measure before the pregnancy ended ($N = 454$), $\log_{10}$ copy-years viremia from ART initiation to conception ($N = 250$), and $\log_{10}$ copy-years viremia in the two years prior to conception ($N = 376$).

	Pregnancy loss	Relative effect measures		Absolute effect measures	
	Losses/N	RR (95% CI)	aRR (95% CI)*	RD (95% CI)	aRD (95% CI)*
Analysis 1: most recent $\log_{10}$ viral load measure					
Continuous exposure	158/454	1.27 (1.13, 1.42)	1.17 (1.01, 1.35)	0.10 (0.06, 0.14)	0.04 (−0.01, 0.08)
Dichotomous exposure					
≤1.60	41/181	1.	1.	0.	0.
>1.60	117/273	1.89 (1.39, 2.58)	1.23 (0.87, 1.74)	0.20 (0.11, 0.29)	0.05 (−0.04, 0.14)[†]
Categorical[‡]					
Q1: ≤1.60	41/181	1.	1.	0.	0.
Q2: 1.61–3.00	30/91	1.47 (0.98, 2.19)	1.15 (0.79, 1.68)	0.10 (−0.01, 0.21)	0.03 (−0.06, 0.12)[†]
Q3: 3.01–4.00	39/90	1.87 (1.27, 2.75)	1.20 (0.77, 1.87)	0.19 (0.07, 0.32)	0.04 (−0.09, 0.17)[†]
Q4: >4.00	48/92	2.36 (1.68, 3.31)	1.59 (0.99, 2.56)	0.30 (0.18, 0.42)	0.14 (−0.01, 0.28)[†]
Analysis 2: $\log_{10}$ copy-years viremia since ART initiation					
Continuous exposure	92/250	0.83 (0.73, 0.95)	0.80 (0.69, 0.92)	−0.07 (−0.13, −0.02)	−0.10 (−0.14, −0.05)
Quartile of exposure[‡]					
Q1: 0–3.78	29/62	1.	1.	0.	0.
Q2: 3.79–4.38	24/63	0.84 (0.55, 1.30)	0.85 (0.56, 1.30)	−0.07 (−0.25, −0.11)	−0.05 (−0.21, 0.12)
Q3: 4.39–4.94	22/63	0.72 (0.45, 1.14)	0.70 (0.44, 1.13)	−0.13 (−0.31, −0.05)	−0.15 (−0.32, 0.03)
Q4: >4.94	17/62	0.61 (0.37, 1.00)	0.60 (0.36, 0.99)	−0.18 (−0.35, −0.01)	−0.18 (−0.36, −0.01)
Analysis 3: $\log_{10}$ copy-years viremia in two years before pregnancy					
Continuous exposure	149/376	1.12 (1.01, 1.24)	1.00 (0.90, 1.11)	0.05 (0.01, 0.09)	−0.01 (−0.05, 0.03)
Quartile of exposure[‡]					
Q1: 0–4.26	28/94	1.	1.	0.	NC
Q2: 4.27–5.73	34/94	1.19 (0.78, 1.81)	0.90 (0.61, 1.32)	0.06 (−0.08, 0.20)	NC
Q3: 5.74–6.49	46/94	1.57 (1.07, 2.29)	1.07 (0.72, 1.57)	0.17 (0.03, 0.31)	NC
Q4: >6.49	41/94	1.43 (0.97, 2.09)	0.92 (0.63, 1.35)	0.13 (−0.01, 0.26)	NC

ART = antiretroviral therapy, RR = risk ratio, aRR = adjusted risk ratio, RD = risk difference, and aRD = adjusted risk difference. NC = nonconvergence of model.

*Adjusted for maternal age (with a linear spline at age 35), race, income, noninjection drug use, prior pregnancy loss, smoking, CD4 count, and ART use (separately controlling for mono-/dual and HAART versus none) prior to viral load measurement (for analyses 1 and 3).

[†]Point estimates controlled for any ART instead of separately controlling for mono-/dual and HAART due to model nonconvergence.

[‡]Categories of cross-sectional viral load measures (analysis 1) were based on clinically informative cut-points, while the categories for cumulative viremia measures (analysis 2) were based on statistical quartiles.

respectively. The corresponding aRDs were −0.10 (95% CI: −0.14, −0.05) and −0.01 (95% CI: −0.01, 0.03).

Most of the different scenarios explored in the sensitivity analyses did not qualitatively alter the results (Table 3). The aRR for $\log_{10}$ copy-years viremia from ART initiation to conception when restricted to HAART initiators since 1998 moved closer to the null (Table 3). There did not appear to be any effect measure modification when comparing the effect measures among those with CD4 greater than 500 to those less than 500 for analyses 1 and 2 (Table 3). For analysis 3, the effect of two-year viremia remained close to the null among those with CD4 below 500, but the aRR for $\log_{10}$ copy-years viremia in two years was 1.16 (95% CI: 0.98, 1.36) among those with CD4 greater than 500.

4. Discussion

Previous research on the interplay between HIV infection, immune system inflammation, and pregnancy loss is both sparse and contradictory [13–17, 21, 22]. In this study, we found that the most recent viral load before birth outcome was associated with pregnancy loss among HIV-infected women (analysis 1). When controlling for confounding factors (maternal age, race, income, prior pregnancy loss, smoking, CD4 count, and ART use), a 14% absolute increase in risk of pregnancy loss was observed for the highest category compared to the lowest category of viral load. These results confirm the harmful effects of high maternal viral load on birth outcomes that others have observed in observational HIV cohorts [16, 21, 22].

In addition to benchmarking our work against the cross-sectional analyses of other studies, we also assessed two measures of cumulative viral load. The results of analysis 2 counterintuitively suggest a protective effect of higher $\log_{10}$ copy-years viremia from ART initiation to conception on pregnancy loss. There is no biological basis for the idea that increased cumulative viremia (and attendant inflammation) is protective against pregnancy loss: this apparently protective

TABLE 3: Sensitivity analyses; adjusted* risk ratios for a one-unit increase in exposure.

Sensitivity analysis description	aRR* (95% CI)		
	Most recent VL	Viremia since ART	Viremia in two years
Original	1.17 (1.01, 1.35)	0.80 (0.69, 0.92)	1.00 (0.90, 1.11)
Restricted to exposure after 1998 and adjusted for HAART	1.27 (1.07, 1.50)	0.99 (0.82, 1.17)	0.97 (0.83, 1.13)
Dropped VL at ART initiation	N/A	0.83 (0.68, 1.03)	N/A
Adjusted for time on ART	N/A	0.80 (0.68, 0.95)	N/A
Only included VL during pregnancy	1.10 (0.87, 1.39)	N/A	N/A
Time frame changed to one year	N/A	N/A	0.87 (0.75, 1.00)
Time frame changed to three years	N/A	N/A	0.97 (0.87, 1.09)
Excluded stillbirths	1.18 (1.01, 1.38)	0.80 (0.69, 0.93)	0.99 (0.88, 1.12)
Modification by CD4			
CD4 ≤ 500	1.15 (0.99, 1.33)	0.81 (0.68, 0.97)	0.94 (0.82, 1.07)
CD4 > 500	1.17 (0.95, 1.43)	0.81 (0.67, 0.98)	1.16 (0.98, 1.36)
Adjusted for CD4 nadir	1.18 (1.03, 1.35)	0.79 (0.69, 0.91)	1.02 (0.91, 1.14)

aRR = adjusted risk ratio, ART = antiretroviral therapy, HAART = highly active antiretroviral therapy, and VL = viral load.
*Adjusted for maternal age (with a linear spline at age 35), race, income, prior pregnancy loss, smoking, noninjection drug use, CD4 count at baseline, and ART use at baseline (separately controlling for mono-/dual and HAART versus none).

result should be interpreted cautiously and may be biased by residual confounding or measurement error. Women who became pregnant with elevated viral loads and higher cumulative viremia may have been treated aggressively with ART to reduce their viral burdens, which could be contributing to the protective effect of higher cumulative viremia. Additionally, if a woman was receiving ART for a longer period of time, she was potentially infected for a longer period of time and thus may have had larger copy-years viremia. In this instance, the protective effect of long-term ART could be outweighing any detrimental effects of cumulative inflammation and contributing to the protective effect we observed with this measure. Another issue that may come into play with this measure is the underlying assumption that the means of accumulating a specific amount of copy-years viremia did not impact the effect of that exposure. For example, we assumed that an exposure of three $\log_{10}$ copy-years viremia had the same impact on risk of pregnancy loss whether the exposure was accrued over 10 years, three years, or one year. Other cumulative measures, such as smoking pack-years, have faced similar scrutiny [34, 35], and future studies may wish to explore this issue further. To relax this assumption, we adjusted for time on ART in a sensitivity analysis and the effect estimates were unaffected (Table 3). Overall, analysis 2 indicates that copy-years viremia since ART initiation might not be a useful measure for reproductive outcomes, even though others have illustrated its utility for mortality [24, 25] and lymphoma [26].

In analysis 3, by constructing a time-constrained measure of viremia, we were focusing on comparisons of recent average viral load intensities before conception. The effect of viremia on pregnancy loss was no longer protective and now at the null, suggesting little harmful effect of copy-years viremia in the two years prior to conception. However, the results from our sensitivity analysis considering effect measure modification by CD4 count greater than 500 indicate that there is a potentially harmful effect of viremia in

the two years prior to conception among those with higher CD4 counts, but not among those with lower CD4 counts (Table 3). Although viral loads were not measured frequently enough to assess copy-years viremia during pregnancy, future studies may wish to explore this further given our cross-sectional results (analysis 1).

Our analyses had several limitations. First, the study covered a twenty-year period with secular changes over time, particularly in the use of antiretroviral therapy. We attempted to control for this potential lack of homogeneity over the study period by controlling for measured confounders and conducting a sensitivity analysis using only data from the "post-HAART" era, but we cannot discount the possibility of unmeasured confounding biasing our results. This limits any causal interpretations we might want to ascribe to our results. In addition, all pregnancy outcomes were self-reported, which may lead to bias. One particular concern is that some miscarriages might actually have become elective abortions if the pregnancy continued, or elective abortions might have become miscarriages, which would result in misclassification of miscarriage. As with all other retrospective studies on miscarriage, we were limited by the fact that many miscarriages occurring earlier in pregnancy were unrecognized by mothers, further limiting the accuracy of our outcome measurement [36]. Furthermore, the use of pregnancy loss as a composite outcome combines first-trimester miscarriage, late miscarriage, and stillbirth. Although the etiologic risk factors for these separate outcomes may vary, the study is underpowered to investigate these outcomes separately. We did exclude stillbirths in a sensitivity analysis to determine if focusing on miscarriages altered our results and found no differences. Also, while pregnancies were systematically ascertained through self-report at each biannual visit, there is still a possibility of biased detection by patient characteristics if certain individuals were more likely to report their pregnancies than others.

We also acknowledge other limitations specific to the exposures beyond those addressed above. Viral loads were collected semiannually; thus we were forced to assume that these measurements were representative of women's continuous viral load burdens. Another issue with cumulative exposure measures is that we were unable to account for within-person variation. For example, even if two pregnancies have similar cumulative viral load, the patterns of exposure leading to this composite measure are not captured [37]. Furthermore, our analysis provides no information regarding the effect of copy-years viremia on fertility. There is evidence from trials of low-dose aspirin that inflammation plays a role in impairing conception [38]; thus it is plausible that cumulative viremia may be impacting fertility.

Our analyses incorporated high-quality longitudinal measurements of viral load collected prospectively in an established clinical cohort. A main strength of this study is the utilization of two new constructs of viral load burden. As copy-years viremia has only recently been explored as an exposure for various prognoses [23–26], continued research on this exposure is valuable. We further add to the body of literature on HIV viral load burden and pregnancy loss by reporting risk differences in addition to risk ratios.

In conclusion, these results help elucidate the role of viral load burden in pregnancy loss among HIV-infected women. As this is the first study addressing cumulative viral load burden and pregnancy loss, future studies are needed to further investigate these findings. We addressed multiple constructs of viral load burden, including two new approaches to copy-years viremia as well as one cross-sectional measure of viral load for comparison to the literature. While cumulative viral load burden does not appear to be an informative measure for pregnancy loss risk in this setting, cross-sectional viral load proximal to pregnancy was associated with an increased risk of pregnancy loss on both the relative and absolute scales. These results emphasize the importance of early identification of pregnancy, initiation of or adjustment to more appropriate ART during pregnancy, and subsequent control of viral load to potentially reduce the risk of pregnancy loss.

Disclosure

Data in this paper were collected by the Women's Interagency HIV Study (WIHS), WIHS (Principal Investigators): UAB-MS WIHS (Michael Saag, Mirjam-Colette Kempf, and Deborah Konkle-Parker), U01-AI-103401; Atlanta WIHS (Ighovwerha Ofotokun and Gina Wingood), U01-AI-103408; Bronx WIHS (Kathryn Anastos), U01-AI-035004; Brooklyn WIHS (Howard Minkoff and Deborah Gustafson), U01-AI-031834; Chicago WIHS (Mardge Cohen), U01-AI-034993; Metropolitan Washington WIHS (Mary Young), U01-AI-034994; Miami WIHS (Margaret Fischl and Lisa Metsch), U01-AI-103397; UNC WIHS (Adaora Adimora), U01-AI-103390; Connie Wofsy Women's HIV Study, Northern California (Ruth Greenblatt, Bradley Aouizerat, and Phyllis Tien), U01-AI-034989; WIHS Data Management and Analysis Center (Stephen Gange and Elizabeth Golub), U01-AI-042590; Southern California WIHS (Alexandra Levine and Marek Nowicki), U01-HD-032632 (WIHS I–WIHS IV). The WIHS is funded primarily by the National Institute of Allergy and Infectious Diseases (NIAID), with additional cofunding from the Eunice Kennedy Shriver National Institute of Child Health and Human Development (NICHD), the National Cancer Institute (NCI), the National Institute on Drug Abuse (NIDA), and the National Institute on Mental Health (NIMH). Targeted supplemental funding for specific projects is also provided by the National Institute of Dental and Craniofacial Research (NIDCR), the National Institute on Alcohol Abuse and Alcoholism (NIAAA), the National Institute on Deafness and Other Communication Disorders (NIDCD), and the NIH Office of Research on Women's Health. WIHS data collection is also supported by UL1-TR000004 (UCSF CTSA) and UL1-TR000454 (Atlanta CTSA). Dr. D. Westreich participates in occasional, ad hoc consulting on epidemiologic methods with NICHD, with no overlap with the present work.

Disclaimer

The contents of this paper are solely the responsibility of the authors and do not represent the official views of the National Institutes of Health (NIH).

Conflict of Interests

The authors declare that there is no conflict of interests regarding the publication of this paper.

Acknowledgments

The authors thank the participants and staff of the Women's Interagency HIV Study. They would also like to thank Dr. Stephen R. Cole for his constructive suggestions on the use of copy-years viremia.

References

[1] WHO, "Reports on global HIV/AIDS situation," WHO, 2013, http://www.who.int/hiv/epiupdates/en/.

[2] What's New in the Guidelines?, Adult and Adolescent ARV Guidelines, AIDSinfo, https://aidsinfo.nih.gov/.

[3] E. L. Murphy, A. C. Collier, L. A. Kalish et al., "Highly active antiretroviral therapy decreases mortality and morbidity in patients with advanced HIV disease," *Annals of Internal Medicine*, vol. 135, no. 1, pp. 17–26, 2001.

[4] E. R. Cooper, M. Charurat, L. Mofenson et al., "Combination antiretroviral strategies for the treatment of pregnant HIV-1-infected women and prevention of perinatal HIV-1 transmission," *Journal of Acquired Immune Deficiency Syndromes*, vol. 29, no. 5, pp. 484–494, 2002.

[5] C. Giaquinto, E. Ruga, A. De Rossi et al., "Mother-to-child transmission of HIV infection in the era of highly active antiretroviral therapy," *Clinical Infectious Diseases*, vol. 40, no. 3, pp. 458–465, 2005.

[6] J. L. Chen, K. A. Philips, D. E. Kanouse, R. L. Collins, and A. Miu, "Fertility desires and intentions of HIV-positive men and

women," *Family Planning Perspectives*, vol. 33, no. 4, pp. 144–165, 2001.

[7] S. B. Kirshenbaum, A. E. Hirky, J. Correale et al., "'Throwing the dice': pregnancy decision-making among HIV-positive women in four U.S. cities," *Perspectives on Sexual and Reproductive Health*, vol. 36, no. 3, pp. 106–113, 2004.

[8] N. L. Stanwood, S. E. Cohn, J. R. Heiser, and M. Pugliese, "Contraception and fertility plans in a cohort of HIV-positive women in care," *Contraception*, vol. 75, no. 4, pp. 294–298, 2007.

[9] L. Rahangdale, A. Stewart, R. D. Stewart et al., "Pregnancy intentions among women living with HIV in the United States," *Journal of Acquired Immune Deficiency Syndromes*, vol. 65, no. 3, pp. 306–311, 2014.

[10] P. Brocklehurst and R. French, "The association between maternal HIV infection and perinatal outcome: a systematic review of the literature and meta-analysis," *British Journal of Obstetrics and Gynaecology*, vol. 105, no. 8, pp. 836–848, 1998.

[11] M. Temmerman, F. A. Plummer, N. B. Mirza et al., "Infection with HIV as a risk factor for adverse obstetrical outcome," *AIDS*, vol. 4, no. 11, pp. 1087–1093, 1990.

[12] A. Ross, L. Van der Paal, R. Lubega, B. N. Mayanja, L. A. Shafer, and J. Whitworth, "HIV-1 disease progression and fertility: the incidence of recognized pregnancy and pregnancy outcome in Uganda," *AIDS*, vol. 18, no. 5, pp. 799–804, 2004.

[13] C. D'Ubaldo, P. Pezzotti, G. Rezza, M. Branca, and G. Ippolito, "Association between HIV-1 infection and miscarriage: a retrospective study. DIANAIDS Collaborative Study Group. Diagnosi Iniziale Anomalie Neoplastiche AIDS," *AIDS*, vol. 12, no. 9, pp. 1087–1093, 1998.

[14] S. R. Schwartz, H. Rees, S. Mehta, W. D. F. Venter, T. E. Taha, and V. Black, "High incidence of unplanned pregnancy after antiretroviral therapy initiation: findings from a prospective cohort study in south africa," *PLoS ONE*, vol. 7, no. 4, Article ID e36039, 2012.

[15] J. Y. Chen, H. J. Ribaudo, S. Souda et al., "Highly active antiretroviral therapy and adverse birth outcomes among HIV-infected women in botswana," *Journal of Infectious Diseases*, vol. 206, no. 11, pp. 1695–1705, 2012.

[16] O. C. Ezechi, C. V. Gab-Okafor, D. A. Oladele et al., "Pregnancy, obstetric and neonatal outcomes in HIV positive Nigerian women," *African journal of reproductive health*, vol. 17, no. 3, pp. 160–168, 2013.

[17] L. S. Massad, G. Springer, L. Jacobson et al., "Pregnancy rates and predictors of conception, miscarriage and abortion in US women with HIV," *AIDS*, vol. 18, no. 2, pp. 281–286, 2004.

[18] J. E. Thaxton, T. A. Nevers, and S. Sharma, "TLR-mediated preterm birth in response to pathogenic agents," *Infectious Diseases in Obstetrics and Gynecology*, vol. 2010, Article ID 378472, 8 pages, 2010.

[19] S. K. Srinivas, Y. Ma, M. D. Sammel et al., "Placental inflammation and viral infection are implicated in second trimester pregnancy loss," *American Journal of Obstetrics and Gynecology*, vol. 195, no. 3, pp. 797–802, 2006.

[20] J. R. Challis, C. J. Lockwood, L. Myatt, J. E. Norman, J. F. Strauss III, and F. Petraglia, "Inflammation and pregnancy," *Reproductive Sciences*, vol. 16, no. 2, pp. 206–215, 2009.

[21] H.-Y. Kim, P. Kasonde, M. Mwiya et al., "Pregnancy loss and role of infant HIV status on perinatal mortality among HIV-infected women," *BMC Pediatrics*, vol. 12, no. 1, article 138, 2012.

[22] A. N. Turner, S. Tabbah, V. Mwapasa et al., "Severity of maternal HIV-1 disease is associated with adverse birth outcomes in Malawian women: a cohort study," *Journal of Acquired Immune Deficiency Syndromes*, vol. 64, no. 4, pp. 392–399, 2013.

[23] S. R. Cole, S. Napravnik, M. J. Mugavero, B. Lau, J. J. Eron Jr., and M. S. Saag, "Copy-years viremia as a measure of cumulative human immunodeficiency virus viral burden," *American Journal of Epidemiology*, vol. 171, no. 2, pp. 198–205, 2010.

[24] M. J. Mugavero, S. Napravnik, S. R. Cole et al., "Viremia copy-years predicts mortality among treatment-naive HIV-infected patients initiating antiretroviral therapy," *Clinical Infectious Diseases*, vol. 53, no. 9, pp. 927–935, 2011.

[25] S. T. Wright, J. Hoy, B. Mulhall et al., "Determinants of viremia copy-years in people with HIV/AIDS after initiation of antiretroviral therapy," *Journal of Acquired Immune Deficiency Syndromes*, vol. 66, no. 1, pp. 55–64, 2014.

[26] A. Zoufaly, H.-J. Stellbrink, M. an der Heiden, C. Kollan, C. Hoffmann, and J. van Lunzen, "Cumulative HIV viremia during highly active antiretroviral therapy is a strong predictor of AIDS-related lymphoma," *Journal of Infectious Diseases*, vol. 200, no. 1, pp. 79–87, 2009.

[27] S. E. Barkan, S. L. Melnick, S. Preston-Martin et al., "The women's interagency HIV study," *Epidemiology*, vol. 9, no. 2, pp. 117–125, 1998.

[28] M. C. Bacon, V. Von Wyl, C. Alden et al., "The women's interagency HIV study: an observational cohort brings clinical sciences to the bench," *Clinical and Diagnostic Laboratory Immunology*, vol. 12, no. 9, pp. 1013–1019, 2005.

[29] Panel on Clinical Practices for the Treatment of HIV Infection, *Guidelines for the Use of Antiretroviral Agents in HIV-Infected Adults and Adolescents*, US Department of Health and Human Services, Henry J. Kaiser Family Foundation, Oakland, Calif, USA, 2014.

[30] D. A. Savitz, I. Hertz-Picciotto, C. Poole, and A. F. Olshan, "Epidemiologic measures of the course and outcome of pregnancy," *Epidemiologic Reviews*, vol. 24, no. 2, pp. 91–101, 2002.

[31] E. Aaron, A. Bonacquisti, L. Mathew, G. Alleyne, L. P. Bamford, and J. F. Culhane, "Small-for-gestational-age births in pregnant women with HIV, due to severity of HIV disease, not antiretroviral therapy," *Infectious Diseases in Obstetrics and Gynecology*, vol. 2012, Article ID 135030, 9 pages, 2012.

[32] M. K. Goldhaber and B. H. Fireman, "The fetal life table revisited: spontaneous abortion rates in three Kaiser Permanente cohorts," *Epidemiology*, vol. 2, no. 1, pp. 33–39, 1991.

[33] U. M. Reddy, S. K. Laughon, L. Sun, J. Troendle, M. Willinger, and J. Zhang, "Prepregnancy risk factors for antepartum stillbirth in the United States," *Obstetrics and Gynecology*, vol. 116, no. 5, pp. 1119–1126, 2010.

[34] J. Peto, "That the effects of smoking should be measured in pack-years: misconceptions 4," *British Journal of Cancer*, vol. 107, no. 3, pp. 406–407, 2012.

[35] J. H. Lubin and N. E. Caporaso, "Misunderstandings in the misconception on the use of pack-years in analysis of smoking," *British Journal of Cancer*, vol. 108, no. 5, pp. 1218–1220, 2013.

[36] A. J. Wilcox and L. F. Horney, "Accuracy of spontaneous abortion recall," *American Journal of Epidemiology*, vol. 120, no. 5, pp. 727–733, 1984.

[37] D. B. Richardson, S. R. Cole, and B. Langholz, "Regression models for the effects of exposure rate and cumulative exposure," *Epidemiology*, vol. 23, no. 6, pp. 892–899, 2012.

[38] E. F. Schisterman, A. J. Gaskins, and B. W. Whitcomb, "Effects of low-dose aspirin in in-vitro fertilization," *Current Opinion in Obstetrics and Gynecology*, vol. 21, no. 3, pp. 275–278, 2009.

12

Extragenital Infections Caused by *Chlamydia trachomatis* and *Neisseria gonorrhoeae*

Philip A. Chan,[1] Ashley Robinette,[1] Madeline Montgomery,[1] Alexi Almonte,[1] Susan Cu-Uvin,[1] John R. Lonks,[1] Kimberle C. Chapin,[2] Erna M. Kojic,[1] and Erica J. Hardy[1]

[1]*Division of Infectious Diseases, Department of Medicine, Warren Alpert Medical School, Brown University, Providence, RI 02903, USA*
[2]*Department of Pathology, Rhode Island Hospital, Providence, RI 02903, USA*

Correspondence should be addressed to Philip A. Chan; pchan@lifespan.org

Academic Editor: Per Anders Mardh

In the United States, sexually transmitted diseases due to *Chlamydia trachomatis* and *Neisseria gonorrhoeae* continue to be a major public health burden. Screening of extragenital sites including the oropharynx and rectum is an emerging practice based on recent studies highlighting the prevalence of infection at these sites. We reviewed studies reporting the prevalence of extragenital infections in women, men who have sex with men (MSM), and men who have sex only with women (MSW), including distribution by anatomical site. Among women, prevalence was found to be 0.6–35.8% for rectal gonorrhea (median reported prevalence 1.9%), 0–29.6% for pharyngeal gonorrhea (median 2.1%), 2.0–77.3% for rectal chlamydia (median 8.7%), and 0.2–3.2% for pharyngeal chlamydia (median 1.7%). Among MSM, prevalence was found to be 0.2–24.0% for rectal gonorrhea (median 5.9%), 0.5–16.5% for pharyngeal gonorrhea (median 4.6%), 2.1–23.0% for rectal chlamydia (median 8.9%), and 0–3.6% for pharyngeal chlamydia (median 1.7%). Among MSW, the prevalence was found to be 0–5.7% for rectal gonorrhea (median 3.4%), 0.4–15.5% for pharyngeal gonorrhea (median 2.2%), 0–11.8% for rectal chlamydia (median 7.7%), and 0–22.0% for pharyngeal chlamydia (median 1.6%). Extragenital infections are often asymptomatic and found in the absence of reported risk behaviors, such as receptive anal and oral intercourse. We discuss current clinical recommendations and future directions for research.

1. Introduction

Sexually transmitted diseases (STDs) continue to be a significant cause of morbidity in the United States (US) with an estimated $15.9 billion spent annually on healthcare costs related to their diagnosis and treatment [1]. The two most common reportable bacterial STDs in the US are gonorrhea and chlamydia [2]. Chlamydia is caused by the bacterium *Chlamydia trachomatis* and is the most commonly reported STD. In 2014, over 1.4 million cases of chlamydia were diagnosed in the US [2], a 2.8% increase from the prior year and the greatest number of cases ever reported for an STD. Of chlamydia cases in 2014, the majority were among younger adults age 15–24 and women (70%). Despite overall higher prevalence of chlamydia infection among women in the US, diagnoses among men increased by 6.8% from 2013 to 2014. The difference in chlamydia diagnoses by

gender can likely be attributed to routine screening practices among women [2]. The major primary care guidelines in the US recommend annual chlamydia screening of all sexually active young women (age 24 years and younger) as part of annual routine reproductive healthcare services [3]. Similar to chlamydia, gonorrhea also disproportionately impacts younger populations. Gonorrhea is caused by the bacterium *Neisseria gonorrhoeae* with over 350,000 cases reported in 2014, a 5.1% increase from the prior year and a 10.5% increase since 2010 [2]. Unlike chlamydia, gonorrhea is now more prevalent among men than women. The number of gonorrhea cases among men increased by 27.9% from 2010 to 2014, whereas the number of cases among women decreased by 4.1% during that time. The rising number of new chlamydia and gonorrhea cases among men is likely due to increased diagnoses among gay, bisexual, and other men who have sex with men (MSM) [4, 5].

Gonorrhea and chlamydia are often asymptomatic in men as well as women. In men, only 14% infected with chlamydia and 40% infected with gonorrhea may be symptomatic [6, 7]. In women, urogenital chlamydia initially infects the cervix, causing symptoms of cervicitis which can then spread to the upper reproductive tract and cause pelvic inflammatory disease (PID). Untreated urogenital infections can lead to other serious complications such as chronic pain, ectopic pregnancy, and infertility [8]. The presence of gonorrhea or chlamydia at any site also increases the risk of acquiring HIV in both men and women [9, 10]. Complications specific to men include epididymitis, prostatitis, and proctitis. Both men and women with symptomatic urogenital infection most commonly present with urethritis, characterized by dysuria and urethral discharge. Reactive arthritis may also occur, often as part of a triad of other symptoms including urethritis and conjunctivitis [11].

N. gonorrhoeae and C. trachomatis can also be detected in the pharynx and rectum [2]. Gonorrhea and chlamydia infection in the rectum can cause rectal pain, bleeding, and discharge, as well as proctitis. In the pharynx, these infections can cause symptoms, such as pharyngitis and lymphadenitis, but are most often asymptomatic. Given that extragenital testing is not always part of routine STD screening, particularly in the absence of symptoms, many extragenital infections are undiagnosed and untreated. These untreated extragenital infections are a potential reservoir for ongoing transmission and may also lead to increased risk of HIV acquisition. Extragenital testing for N. gonorrhoeae and C. trachomatis is an emerging area that should be considered in both men and women. We review current screening recommendations and evidence to support extragenital testing for N. gonorrhoeae and C. trachomatis and discuss areas where future research is needed.

2. Materials and Methods

Current guidelines related to extragenital screening for N. gonorrhoeae and C. trachomatis in men and women were reviewed. A literature review was performed of all studies listed in PubMed evaluating extragenital gonorrhea and chlamydia infections through December 1, 2015. Studies included those describing extragenital infections by N. gonorrhoeae, C. trachomatis, or both, conducted in the US as well as internationally. The goal of the review was to describe the current epidemiology and prevalence of extragenital infections in the setting of the latest recommendations for screening. We specifically examined extragenital infections in separate subgroups of populations, including women, men who have sex only with women (MSW), and MSM. Only studies in English were included. The search terms "extragenital," "rectal," "pharyngeal," "chlamydia," and "gonorrhea" were used in combination and individually. References were reviewed and subsequently excluded if the study did not include findings of extragenital N. gonorrhoeae or C. trachomatis infection. Additionally, citations within these studies were reviewed and included if relevant. Full texts of relevant studies were retrieved and reviewed.

3. Results and Discussion

3.1. Current Screening Recommendations. The Centers for Disease Control and Prevention (CDC) currently recommends that all sexually active women less than 25 years of age, as well as older women who have specific risk factors (e.g., new or concurrent sex partners), be tested annually for urogenital chlamydia and gonorrhea infection [12]. Per the guidelines, the clinical significance of pharyngeal chlamydia infection is unclear and routine pharyngeal screening for chlamydia is not recommended [12–14]. The US Preventive Services Task Force (USPSTF), the preeminent primary care guidelines in the US, recommends screening for chlamydia and gonorrhea in all sexually active women of age 24 years and younger, and in older women who are at increased risk for infection (e.g., due to another current STD, a previous STD, new or concurrent sex partners, inconsistent condom use, drug use, commercial sex work, certain demographic characteristics, or high community prevalence of STDs). The American Congress of Obstetricians and Gynecologists (ACOG) recommends annual urogenital screening for gonorrhea and chlamydia for sexually active women age 25 years and younger, as well as for women over age 25 reporting risk factors for infection [15].

The CDC does not recommend routine chlamydia or gonorrhea screening in men [12], with the exception of "considering" screening in high-prevalence clinical settings such as STD clinics or among high-prevalence populations such as MSM. The CDC recommends that MSM be screened at least annually for chlamydia infection at sites of sexual contact, including the rectum and urethra; for gonorrhea, the guidelines recommend screening at the urethra, rectum, and pharynx. Per these guidelines, screening should be based on risk behaviors. MSM who report insertive sex should be screened for urogenital N. gonorrhoeae and C. trachomatis. MSM who report receptive anal sex should be screen for rectal N. gonorrhoeae and C. trachomatis. MSM who report receptive oral sex should be screened for pharyngeal N. gonorrhoeae only; screening for C. trachomatis pharyngeal infection is not recommended. The USPTF does not recommend screening for chlamydia or gonorrhea in MSW due to insufficient evidence to support this practice.

The majority of international STD treatment guidelines provide recommendations for extragenital testing in MSM. The International Union Against Sexually Transmitted Infections (IUSTI) recommends extragenital testing for both MSM and women at the rectum and pharynx if there is a reported history of sexual exposure [16, 17]. Similarly, the British Association for Sexual Health and HIV (BASHH) recommends that extragenital screening for chlamydia and gonorrhea infections be dependent on reported sexual behaviors among men and women [18]. The guidelines also recommend extragenital testing among specific groups of women, such as commercial sex workers [19, 20]. Other countries, such as South Africa, employ an algorithm-driven, syndromic approach to STD testing and treatment [21].

The group of women who have sex with women (WSW) encompasses a diverse set of individuals and sexual practices. The CDC addresses this unique group, recommending that screening for *N. gonorrhoeae* and *C. trachomatis* be based on a detailed history of sexual practices [12]. The CDC also specifically addresses transgender men and women and recommends STD risk assessment and testing be based on current anatomy and sexual behaviors in this group [12].

3.2. Overview of Existing Literature. A total of 80 studies were reviewed focusing on extragenital infection with *N. gonorrhoeae* or *C. trachomatis*. Studies were published between 1981 and 2015 and included sites in North America ($n = 37$), Europe ($n = 29$), Australia ($n = 9$), Asia ($n = 4$), and Africa ($n = 2$). Study settings included STD clinics ($n = 38$), other outpatient clinics ($n = 10$), genitourinary clinics ($n = 7$), HIV clinics ($n = 9$), gay men's health centers ($n = 3$), community-based and outreach settings ($n = 6$), and other settings ($n = 3$); a minority of studies presented findings from multiple sites ($n = 6$). Most studies evaluated a single population but some did include multiple populations of women, MSW, and MSM. The number of studies reporting specific populations included MSM ($n = 54$), women ($n = 33$), MSW ($n = 9$), and mixed populations ($n = 9$). The following sections describe extragenital *N. gonorrhoeae* and *C. trachomatis* infection in these different populations.

3.3. Extragenital Infections in Women. A total of 33 studies reported prevalence of extragenital infection in women due to *N. gonorrhoeae* or *C. trachomatis* infection [19, 22–52] (Table 1). The range of prevalence of extragenital infections reported was 0.6–35.8% for rectal gonorrhea (median 1.9%), 0–29.6% for pharyngeal gonorrhea (median 2.1%), 2.0–77.3% for rectal chlamydia (median 8.7%), and 0.2–3.2% for pharyngeal chlamydia (median 1.7%). Most study sites were STD clinics and other high-risk settings; few were primary care settings, clinics focusing on women's care, or centers focusing on transgender patient care.

Most extragenital infections in women are asymptomatic, with estimates including 93% of pharyngeal gonorrhea [39], 53–100% of rectal gonorrhea [39], 100% of pharyngeal chlamydia [39], and 36–100% of rectal chlamydia cases [29, 30, 39]. Furthermore, a significant number of women who test positive for rectal gonorrhea or chlamydia do not report anal sex [19, 29, 53]. Extragenital screening increases the yield of detection of either gonorrhea or chlamydia at pharyngeal or rectal sites by approximately 6–50% or greater in women compared to screening urogenital specimens alone [23–25, 27, 29–31, 39, 44–46]. Overall, reported risk factors for rectal infection in women include younger age ($n = 2$ studies), sex with an injection drug user ($n = 1$), exchanging sex for money ($n = 2$), anonymous partners ($n = 1$), a sex partner with gonorrhea or chlamydia ($n = 1$), and sex while under the influence of drugs or alcohol ($n = 1$) [23, 31, 48]. However, other studies have not found any associations with these risk factors [29, 30].

Based on prevalence data, universal screening for extragenital infection due to *N. gonorrhoeae* or *C. trachomatis* in settings which care for women who are at risk of these infections (e.g., those who are sexually active with concurrent or nonmutually monogamous partners, regardless of reported exposure sites) should be considered. Due to the frequency of asymptomatic extragenital infections and the inaccuracy of testing based on self-reported behavior [19], the evidence supports routine screening in high-risk settings such as STD clinics. Universal screening for extragenital infection will certainly increase case finding, which in turn will likely have both clinical and public health benefits such as avoiding reproductive health sequelae and limiting HIV transmission. However, extragenital screening protocols among sexually active women are not currently widespread, and further study is needed to evaluate the impact on sexual health outcomes. Additionally, given the paucity of extragenital infection studies in other settings (e.g., primary care clinics), prevalence in these settings is largely unknown and merits further study.

3.4. Extragenital Infections in MSM. A total of 53 studies evaluated the prevalence of extragenital infections due to *N. gonorrhoeae* or *C. trachomatis* in MSM [13, 19, 22, 25–27, 36, 38, 44, 45, 47–49, 54–93] (Table 2). Extragenital infections among MSM have been studied more extensively compared to women. MSM experience high rates of both extragenital gonorrhea and chlamydia. The prevalence of extragenital infection among MSM in these studies ranged from 0.2–24% for rectal gonorrhea (median 5.9%), 0.5–16.5% for pharyngeal gonorrhea (median 4.6%), 2.1–23% for rectal chlamydia (median 8.9%), and 0–3.6% for pharyngeal chlamydia (median 1.7%); the differences are due to different clinical settings and methods of diagnosis. Several studies have evaluated the national prevalence of extragenital infections among MSM in the US [12, 24, 29, 30, 35, 43, 59, 63–65, 69–71, 73, 74, 76–78, 80, 82, 83]. In a large cohort of 3,034 MSM who attended a STD clinic in Seattle, Washington in 2011, extragenital infections were common and included pharyngeal gonorrhea (6.5%) and chlamydia (2.3%), and rectal gonorrhea (9.7%) and chlamydia (11.9%) [57]. Fifty-seven percent of cases were found in only extragenital sites (nonurogenital).

Similarly, among 21,994 MSM screened as part of the CDC STD Surveillance Network, composed of 42 STD clinics across the US, the prevalence of infection was 7.9% for pharyngeal gonorrhea, 2.9% for pharyngeal chlamydia, 10.2% for rectal gonorrhea, and 14.1% for rectal chlamydia. Over 70% of extragenital infections in this sample would have been missed with urogenital screening alone. In summary, urogenital testing alone misses a significant percentage of gonorrhea and chlamydia infections among MSM; if MSM were screened for urogenital infections alone, 14% to 85% of rectal and oropharyngeal gonorrhea and chlamydia infections would have been missed [22, 57, 63, 64, 68, 79, 80].

The majority of extragenital infections among MSM are asymptomatic, with estimates ranging from 25% to 100% from reported studies [68, 76, 80, 89, 92, 94]. Men with extragenital gonorrhea may be more likely to be symptomatic than those with chlamydia [25, 62, 71, 95, 96]. For example, in one large study of MSM with extragenital infection, only 5.1% of pharyngeal and 11.9% of rectal infections were symptomatic with the most common pharyngeal symptoms being pharyngitis (65%), localized lymphadenopathy (16%), and inflammation of the oral cavity (10%). The most common

TABLE 1: Characteristics of studies reporting extragenital infections due to N. gonorrhoeae and C. trachomatis among women.

Author	Study year	Location	Time period	Risk	Setting	Sample	Gonorrhea Urogenital	Gonorrhea Rectal	Gonorrhea Pharyngeal	Chlamydia Urogenital	Chlamydia Rectal	Chlamydia Pharyngeal
Jones et al. [33]	1985	Indiana (US)	1985	Women	STD clinic	686/1,223	—	—	—	28.00%	5.20%	3.20%
Ostergaard et al. [38]	1997	Denmark	1995-1996	Women	STD clinic	196	—	—	—	3.60%	3.10%	1.50%
Linhart et al. [35]	2008	Tel Aviv, Israel	2008	Women	Sex worker outreach	300	5.00%	—	9.00%	6.30%	—	—
van der Helm et al. [49]	2009	Netherlands	2006-2007	Women	STD clinic	936	—	2.00%	—	—	9.00%	—
Barry et al. [24]	2010	California (US)	2007-2008	Women	STD clinic	1,308	1.80%	1.70%	—	5.40%	4.70%	—
Giannini et al. [28]	2010	Ohio (US)	2003-2007	Women	STD clinic, children's hospital	1,949	5.6–9.3%	2.9–13.4%	2.5–6.8%	—	—	—
Hunte et al. [30]	2010	Florida (US)	2007	Women	STD clinic	97	8.20%	13.40%	—	16.50%	17.50%	—
Raychaudhuri and Birley [41]	2010	United Kingdom	2005–2008	Women	Genitourinary clinic	120	27.50%	35.80%	—	—	—	—
Sethupathi et al. [42]	2010	United Kingdom	2006–2008	Women	Genitourinary clinic	152	—	—	—	11.90%	12.50%	—
Peters et al. [39]	2011	Netherlands	2007–2008	Women	STD clinic	4,299	1.10%	1.70%	0.80%	10.00%	8.70%	1.90%
Javanbakht et al. [31]	2012	California (US)	2008–2010	Women	STD clinic	2,084	3.30%	3.00%	—	12.00%	14.60%	—
Koedijk et al. [22]	2012	Netherlands	2006–2010	Women	STD clinic	207,134	1.00%	1.20%	1.20%	10.40%	9.30%	2.70%
Mayer et al. [36]	2012	US (4 cities)	2004–2006	Women (HIV+)	HIV clinic	119	1.00%	1.00%	2.00%	3.00%	2.00%	2.00%
Diaz et al. [26]	2013	Spain	2006–2010	Women	STD clinic	318	0.90%	3.10%	29.60%	—	—	—
Shaw et al. [43]	2013	United Kingdom	2013	Women	Genitourinary clinic	2,808	0.50%	0.60%	0.30%	6.70%	7.10%	1.30%
van Liere et al. [45]	2013	Netherlands	2010-2011	Women	STD clinic	1,321	1.30%	0.90%	2.30%	5.40%	4.80%	1.40%
Dimech et al. [102]	2014	Australia	2008–2010	Women	Surveillance system	415,069	—	—	—	6.7–10%	5.20%	1.70%
Jenkins et al. [32]	2014	Illinois (US)	2012-2013	Women	Emergency room	301	1.00%	—	0.70%	6.30%	—	0.70%
Ladd et al. [34]	2014	US (multiple cities)	2009-2011	Women	Mail	205	—	2.50%	—	—	11.10%	—
Peters et al. [40]	2014	South Africa	2011-2012	Women	Primary care clinic	604	10.00%	2.50%	0.00%	16.00%	7.10%	0.20%
van Liere et al. [46]	2014	Netherlands	2012-2013	Women	STD clinic	663	—	—	—	11.20%	8.40%	—
van Liere et al. [47]	2014	Netherlands	2010–2012	Women	STD clinic	1,321	1.30%	0.90%	2.30%	5.40%	4.80%	1.40%
Bazan et al. [23]	2015	Ohio (US)	2012-2013	Women	STD clinic	331	7.00%	6.00%	—	13.00%	13.00%	—

TABLE 1: Continued.

Author	Study year	Location	Setting	Time period	Risk	Sample	Gonorrhea Urogenital	Gonorrhea Rectal	Gonorrhea Pharyngeal	Gonorrhea Urogenital	Chlamydia Rectal	Chlamydia Pharyngeal
Danby et al. [25]	2016	Pennsylvania (US)	STD clinic	2014-2015	Women	175	2.90%	2.30%	2.30%	10.30%	11.40%	1.70%
Dukers-Muijrers et al. [19]	2015	Netherlands	STD clinic	2010–2013	Women	7,419	0.60%	0.70%	2.70%	10.20%	6.50%	1.40%
Garner et al. [27]	2015	United Kingdom	Sexual health clinic	2010	Women	649	0.80%	1.10%	0.60%	13.30%	6.60%	2.50%
Gratrix et al. [29]	2015	Canada	STD clinic	2012	Women	3055	—	—	—	9.40%	12.60%	—
Musil et al. [37]	2015	Australia	Sexual health clinic	2013-2014	Women	56	—	—	—	77.00%	57.00%	—
Trebach et al. [44]	2015	Maryland (US)	STD clinic	2011–2013	Women	4,402	2.80%	3.00%	2.10%	10.00%	8.60%	2.60%
van Liere et al. [48]	2015	Netherlands	STD clinic	2011-2012	Women	11,113	—	0.90%	—	—	9.50%	—
van Liere et al. [45]	2013	Netherlands	STD clinic	2010-2011	Women ("swingers")	461	—	1.08%	—	—	6.72%	—
Ding and Challenor [50]	2014	United Kingdom	STD clinic	2012-2013	Women	97	—	—	—	100%	77.3%	—
Cosentino et al. [51]	2012	Pennsylvania (US)	HIV clinic	2009-2010	Women	272	—	2.6%	—	—	7.7%	—
Bachmann et al. [52]	2010	US	STD clinic, HIV clinic	2003–2007	Women	99	20.30%	23.10–54.30%	8.20%	27.40%	5.60–19.20%	1.90%

Note. STD: sexually transmitted diseases; US: United States.

TABLE 2: Characteristics of studies reporting extragenital infections due to *N. gonorrhoeae* and *C. trachomatis* among men who have sex with men.

Author	Study year	Time period	Risk	Setting	Location	Sample	Gonorrhea Urogenital	Gonorrhea Rectal	Gonorrhea Pharyngeal	Chlamydia Urogenital	Chlamydia Rectal	Chlamydia Pharyngeal
McMillan et al. [73]	1981	1981	MSM	STD clinic	United Kingdom	150	—	—	—	6.70%	4.00%	1.30%
Rompalo et al. [83]	1986	1983	MSM	STD clinic	Washington (US)	1,429	—	8.00%	—	—	5.00%	—
Ostergaard et al. [38]	1997	1995–1996	MSM	STD clinic	Denmark	39	—	—	—	2.60%	2.60%	0.00%
Tabet et al. [87]	1998	1995	MSM	Community	Washington (US)	578	0.00%	0.20%	0.70%	0.00%	—	—
Kim et al. [69]	2003	2000	MSM (HIV+)	STD clinic	California (US)	564	—	7.10%	—	—	—	—
Manavi et al. [72]	2004	1999–2002	MSM	Genitourinary clinic	United Kingdom	443	—	—	—	—	7.20%	—
Kent et al. [68]	2005	2003	MSM	STD clinic, gay men's health center	California (US)	6,434	6.00%	6.90%	9.20%	5.20%	7.90%	1.40%
Currie et al. [60]	2006	2001–2003	MSM	Sexual health clinic	Australia	314	6.8% (Did not specify site)			9.6% (did not specify site)		
Hocking and Fairley [65]	2006	2002–2003	MSM	STD clinic	Australia	1,248	—	—	—	5.10%	6.20%	1.30%
Morris et al. [76]	2006	2001–2003	MSM	Community	California (US)	2,475	—	—	5.50%	—	—	—
Benn et al. [58]	2007	1999–2001	MSM	Genitourinary clinic	United Kingdom	613	7.20%	7.30%	7.30%	4.30%	6.50%	1.20%
Alexander et al. [54]	2008	2005–2007	MSM	Genitourinary clinic	United Kingdom	272	—	14.90%	6.50%	—	13.60%	—
Gunn et al. [64]	2008	1997–2003	MSM	STD clinic	California (US)	7,333	10.80%	9.80%	4.00%	—	—	—
Lister et al. [71]	2008	2002–2003	MSM	Sexual health clinic	Australia	366	—	5.00%	—	—	7.00%	—
Mimiaga et al. [74]	2008	2007	MSM	Gay men's health center	Massachusetts (US)	114	1.00%	1.70%	0.00%	2.60%	6.10%	—
Rieg et al. [82]	2008	2004–2006	MSM (HIV+)	HIV clinic	California (US)	212	1.50%	4.30%	3.30%	1.50%	2.90%	1.40%
Templeton et al. [89]	2008	2003	MSM	Community	Australia	1,427	—	—	—	—	—	1.10%
Annan et al. [55]	2009	2005–2006	MSM	HIV/genitourinary clinic	United Kingdom	3,076	—	4.10%	1.30%	5.40%	8.20%	—
Baker et al. [56]	2009	2006–2007	MSM	Outpatient clinic	Washington DC (US)	147	0.00%	1.40%	2.80%	0.00%	2.10%	0.70%
Dang et al. [61]	2009	2007–2008	MSM (HIV+)	HIV clinic	Switzerland	147	—	—	—	—	10.90%	—
Klausner et al. [70]	2009	2007–2008	MSM	Outpatient clinic	US (5 cities)	3,410/14,189	—	5.40%	5.30%	—	8.90%	1.60%
Mimiaga et al. [75]	2009	2003–2004	MSM	Gay men's health center	Massachusetts (US)	21,927	13.40%	8.80%	1.90%	5.70%	—	—
Ota et al. [77]	2009	2006–2008	MSM	Gay men's health center	Canada	248	—	11.70%	8.10%	—	7.70%	2.00%
van der Helm [49]	2009	2006–2007	MSM	STD clinic	Netherlands	1,458	—	7.00%	—	—	11.00%	—
Templeton et al. [90]	2010	2003	MSM	Community	Australia	1,427	—	—	0.60%	—	—	—
Marcus et al. [172]	2011	2008–2009	MSM	STD clinic	California (US)	3,398	0.40%	3.60%	5.00%	2.30%	7.80%	1.90%
Peters et al. [39]	2011	2007–2008	MSM	STD clinic	Netherlands	1,455	2.80%	6.00%	4.20%	4.00%	8.20%	1.50%
Soni and White [86]	2011	2009–2010	MSM (HIV+)	HIV clinic	United Kingdom	634	1.30%	4.20%	3.90%	2.60%	9.80%	1.70%
Vodstrcil et al. [93]	2011	2002–2009	MSM	Sexual health clinic	Australia	8,328/7,133	—	3.10%	1.80%	3.70%	5.40%	—
Koedijk et al. [22]	2012	2006–2010	MSM	STD clinic	Netherlands	69,506	3.40%	5.50%	3.90%	4.30%	10.10%	1.70%

Table 2: Continued.

Author	Study year	Location	Setting	Time period	Risk	Sample	Gonorrhea Urogenital	Gonorrhea Rectal	Gonorrhea Pharyngeal	Chlamydia Urogenital	Chlamydia Rectal	Chlamydia Pharyngeal
Mayer et al. [36]	2012	US (4 cities)	HIV clinic	2004–2006	MSM (HIV+)	365	0.00%	2.00%	3.00%	2.00%	7.00%	1.00%
Park et al. [78]	2012	California (US)	HIV/STD clinic, gay men's health center	2010	MSM	12,454	—	—	5.80%	—	—	1.70%
Pinsky et al. [81]	2012	New York (US)	University health center	2007–2010	MSM	200	—	0.50%	3.50%	—	3.00%	0.50%
Díaz et al. [26]	2013	Spain	STD clinic	2006–2010	MSM	1,320	58.30%	21.10%	5.20%	—	—	—
Jiménez et al. [66]	2013	Spain	HIV clinic	2011–2012	MSM (HIV+)	264	—	—	9.50%	—	—	—
Sexton et al. [85]	2013	Washington DC (US)	Primary care clinic, HIV/STD clinic	2009–2011	MSM	374	—	8.00%	9.30%	—	12.70%	1.30%
Turner et al. [92]	2013	Ohio (US)	STD clinic	2010-2011	MSM	125	—	24.00%	—	—	23.00%	—
Barbee et al. [57]	2014	Washington (US)	STD clinic	2011	MSM	3,034	5.50%	9.70%	6.50%	4.40%	11.90%	2.30%
Dudareva-Vizule et al. [62]	2014	Germany	STD clinic	2009-2010	MSM	2,247	1.90%	4.60%	5.50%	3.40%	8.00%	1.50%
Gratrix et al. [63]	2014	Canada	STD clinic	2012	MSM	972	2.40%	5.90%	—	4.30%	14.10%	—
Keaveney et al. [67]	2014	Ireland	HIV clinic	2012	MSM (HIV+)	121	0.00%	4.10%	3.30%	1.70%	6.60%	0.80%
Patton et al. [79]	2014	US (42 sites)	STD clinic	2011-2012	MSM	21,994	11.10%	10.20%	7.90%	8.40%	14.10%	2.90%
Sanders et al. [84]	2014	Kenya	Medical clinic	2011	MSM	244	1.60%	5.70%	—	6.10%	8.10%	—
van Liere et al. [47]	2014	Netherlands	STD clinic	2010–2012	MSM	2,436	1.50%	3.70%	3.40%	3.30%	7.90%	1.10%
Chow et al. [59]	2015	Australia	Sexual health clinic	2007–2013	MSM	12,873	2.30%	2.90%	1.70%	3.00%	5.60%	—
Danby et al. [25]	2016	Pennsylvania (US)	STD clinic	2014–2015	MSM	224	5.40%	11.60%	16.50%	4.50%	17.40%	2.20%
Dukers-Muijrers et al. [19]	2015	Netherlands	STD clinic	2010–2013	MSM	2,349	1.40%	4.00%	3.40%	3.20%	7.30%	0.70%
Garner et al. [27]	2015	United Kingdom	Sexual health clinic	2010	MSM	365	4.70%	9.00%	5.20%	5.30%	6.50%	2.20%
Taylor et al. [88]	2015	Arizona (US)	HIV clinic	2011–2013	MSM	1,591	—	19.60%	—	—	18.60%	—
Tongtoyai et al. [91]	2015	Thailand	Medical clinic	2006–2010	MSM	1,744	1.80%	6.10%	0.50%	4.50%	9.50%	3.60%
Trebach et al. [44]	2015	Maryland (US)	STD clinic	2011–2013	MSM	769	8.90%	17.90%	11.00%	1.50%	14.30%	2.50%
Van Liere et al. [167]	2015	Netherlands	STD clinic	2011–2012	MSM	9,549	—	4.20%	—	—	9.80%	—
van Liere et al. [45]	2013	Netherlands	STD clinic	2010-2011	MSM	926	—	3.46%	—	—	7.88%	—
Bachmann et al. [52]	2010	US	STD clinic, HIV clinic	2003–2007	MSM	297	5.10%	7.90%	8.30%	2.00%	10.30%	1.70%

Note. STD: sexually transmitted diseases; US: United States; MSM: men who have sex with men.

rectal symptoms were pruritus (36%) anal discharge (17%), burning (13%), inflammation (11%), pain (11%), and erythema around the anus (6%) [62]. Symptom-based screening may miss up to 60% of extragenital infections [30, 39, 45].

Extragenital infections may also be increasing in prevalence [59, 77, 95], as several studies have reported higher prevalence of extragenital infections among MSM in recent time periods. However, this could also reflect more thorough screening practices or improved testing methods [97, 98]. Extragenital infections among MSM are associated with concurrent partners, existing HIV infection ($n = 2$ studies), condomless anal sex ($n = 3$), and drug use during sex ($n = 1$) [62, 65, 69, 89, 91]. Concurrent infections with other STDs are common [99]. The overwhelming evidence indicates a high prevalence of extragenital N. gonorrhoeae and C. trachomatis infections among MSM, the asymptomatic nature of most of these infections, and the prevalence of extragenital infection without concurrent urogenital infection, all of which support the need for routine screening at extragenital sites.

3.5. Extragenital Infections in MSW. A total of nine studies evaluated the prevalence of extragenital infections due to N. gonorrhoeae or C. trachomatis in MSW [19, 26, 27, 33, 36, 38, 44, 45, 100] (Table 3). Overall, there are limited prevalence data of extragenital infections among MSW. The prevalence of extragenital infections among MSW in the studies reviewed ranged 0–5.7% for rectal gonorrhea (median 3.4%), 0.4–15.5% for pharyngeal gonorrhea (median 2.2%), 0–11.8% for rectal chlamydia (median 7.7%), and 0–22.0% for pharyngeal chlamydia (median 1.6%). These data represent studies that evaluated heterosexually identified men, some of whom may have engaged in sex with other men [44], a distinction which emphasizes the need to consistently focus on sexual behavior rather than identity. Other studies which did not evaluate for or stratify by specific risk behaviors further support the prevalence studies in individual populations [32, 100–107] (Table 3).

3.6. Diagnoses of Extragenital Infections. The gold standard for diagnosis of urogenital infection due to N. gonorrhoeae and C. trachomatis is the nucleic acid amplification test (NAAT). However, NAAT assays are not approved by the US Food and Drug Administration (FDA) for detecting N. gonorrhoeae and C. trachomatis from pharyngeal or rectal specimens [108]. Culture is still the only approved method for diagnosis at these sites. However, NAAT is the most sensitive test for detecting C. trachomatis and N. gonorrhoeae and is recommended for this purpose by the CDC [12]. NAAT has demonstrated higher sensitivity and specificity compared to culture for detecting extragenital infections [52, 74, 109, 110]. At the present time, laboratories must validate these tests in-house based on Clinical Laboratory Improvement Amendments (CLIA) regulatory requirements before performing NAAT testing on rectal and pharyngeal specimens; many large commercial laboratories have performed this validation and offer this testing option. The main disadvantages of performing NAAT testing over culture is the inability to determine antimicrobial susceptibilities and bacterial viability. Potentially lower sensitivity of NAAT for

N. gonorrhoeae in the pharynx and rectum may be linked to substantial colonization of these extragenital sites by a wide range of other organisms, including other Neisseria species, possibly leading to interference with N. gonorrhoeae isolation [111]. For suspected or documented treatment failure, N. gonorrhoeae cultures should be obtained and antimicrobial susceptibilities performed.

Extragenital specimens are collected via a swab of the rectum or pharynx, by either a clinician or a self-collected swab. Self-collected swab as a means of collecting pharyngeal and rectal specimens is supported by the CDC guidelines [12] and has been found to be an acceptable means of obtaining specimens among women [112, 113] and MSM [49, 54, 85, 114–117], which may lead to an increase in extragenital diagnoses [118] due to the noninvasive nature of the procedure. Self-collected swabs may also reduce the workload for clinic staff who obtain them and promote screening when clinicians are not available for collection.

3.7. Treatment of Extragenital Infections. Current US guidelines regarding treatment of extragenital infections due to N. gonorrhoeae and C. trachomatis are similar to those for the treatment of urogenital infections [12]. Treatment guidelines from the United Kingdom and Europe both recommend similar regimens for both urogenital and extragenital infections [17, 18, 119]. Extragenital pharyngeal and rectal gonorrhea and chlamydia infections may spontaneously clear even in the absence of treatment among MSM and high-risk women [120, 121]. If extragenital sites are a reservoir for ongoing transmission, then suboptimal treatment of extragenital infections could lead to the spread of any existing resistant organisms. Care should be taken with extragenital treatment and retesting should be performed if persistent infection or treatment failure is suspected.

The recommended treatment for urogenital chlamydia infection is azithromycin 1000 milligrams orally in a single dose or doxycycline 100 milligrams orally twice daily for seven days. Due to the ease of administration, the ability for directly observed therapy in a single dose, and the high rates of adherence, azithromycin is the usual treatment option in many clinics. Earlier reports demonstrated similar results with both regimens for treatment of urogenital infection, with high (>96%) cure rates [122]. In contrast, recent analyses have suggested a potential small advantage of doxycycline compared to azithromycin for urogenital chlamydia infection; the efficacy of doxycycline has been reported as being 100% compared to 97% for azithromycin [123, 124].

Efficacy of chlamydia treatments may differ for extragenital infections at rectal and pharyngeal sites [19]. Doxycycline may have slightly greater efficacy compared to azithromycin for both rectal [125–132] and pharyngeal [133] chlamydia infection, as single-dose azithromycin may not lead to sustained drug concentrations capable of curing extragenital infection [134]. For example, treatment failure was significantly more common with azithromycin (10% of patients) compared to doxycycline (2%) in a small study for treatment of pharyngeal chlamydia. In a meta-analysis of azithromycin and doxycycline for the treatment of rectal chlamydia, azithromycin was 83% effective compared to

TABLE 3: Characteristics of studies reporting extragenital infections due to *N. gonorrhoeae* and *C. trachomatis* among men who have sex with women and populations with mixed behaviors.

Author	Study year	Location	Setting	Time period	Risk	Sample	Gonorrhea			Chlamydia		
							Urogenital	Rectal	Pharyngeal	Urogenital	Rectal	Pharyngeal
Jones et al. [33]	1985	Indiana (US)	STD clinic	1985	MSW	706	—	—	—	21.00%	—	3.70%
Ostergaard et al. [38]	1997	Denmark	STD clinic	1995-1996	MSW	169	—	—	—	0.60%	0.00%	0.00%
Mayer et al. [36]	2012	US (4 cities)	HIV clinic	2004–2006	MSW (HIV+)	73	1.00%	0.00%	1.00%	0.00%	0.00%	1.00%
Wada et al. [173]	2012	Japan	Urology clinic	2007-2008	MSW	42	47.60%	—	11.90%	26.20%	—	2.40%
Diaz et al. [26]	2013	Spain	STD clinic	2006–2010	MSW	747	92.90%	0.00%	0.90%	—	—	—
Dukers-Muijrers et al. [19]	2015	Netherlands	STD clinic	2010–2013	MSW	5,007	0.60%	0.40%	2.20%	11.70%	0.90%	0.20%
Garner et al. [27]	2015	United Kingdom	Sexual health clinic	2010	MSW	553	0.90%	—	0.40%	12.40%	—	0.70%
Trebach et al. [44]	2015	Maryland (US)	STD clinic	2011–2013	MSW	5,218	4.30%	5.70%	2.50%	2.30%	9.10%	1.60%
van Liere et al. [45]	2013	Netherlands	STD clinic	2010–2012	MSW ("swingers")	303	—	0.33%	—	—	1.32%	—
Ivens et al. [103]	2007	United Kingdom	Genitourinary clinic	2003–2005	Mixed	1187	—	4.70%	—	—	8.50%	—
Tipple et al. [107]	2010	United Kingdom	Sexual health clinic	2006-2007	Mixed	2,406	—	—	—	—	—	1.90%
Chan et al. [100]	2012	Rhode Island (US)	Hospital system	2011-2012	Mixed	178/21,201	0.90%	5.30%	3.40%	5.70%	11.80%	1.70%
Rodriguez-Hart et al. [106]	2012	US	Primary care/adult film	2010	Mixed	168	2.40%	2.40%	1.20%	18.50%	11.30%	22.00%
Dimech et al. [102]	2014	Australia	Surveillance system	2008–2010	Men (mixed)	177,557	—	—	—	12.2-17.4%	5.20%	1.30%
Jenkins et al. [32]	2014	Illinois (US)	Emergency room	2012-2013	Men (mixed)	192	4.70%	—	2.10%	4.70%	—	1.00%
Oda et al. [104]	2014	Japan	Otorhinolaryngology clinic	2012	Mixed	225	—	—	2.20%	—	—	0.90%
Patterson et al. [105]	2014	US	Military STD clinic	2013-2014	Mixed (HIV+)	316	0.80%	4.30%	15.50%	1.00%	6.90%	6.50%
den Heijer et al. [101]	2016	Netherlands	gynecology, primary care clinic	2006–2010	Mixed	246/22,029	—	—	—	8.20%	10.10%	1.60%

Note. STD: sexually transmitted diseases; US: United States; MSW: men who have sex with women.

>99% efficacy of doxycycline [125]. Treatment guidelines in Europe [16] and Australia [135] recommend doxycycline as the treatment of choice for rectal infections. However, care should be taken when interpreting these smaller studies, and the potential small benefits must be weighed against the ease of administration, ability for directly observed therapy, and adherence for the single dose azithromycin therapy option. No randomized controlled trials have evaluated treatment regimens for extragenital chlamydia infection and further studies are needed to determine optimal management of these infections [136].

The current treatment recommendations for urogenital *N. gonorrhoeae* infections involve a dual regimen of ceftriaxone 250 milligrams intramuscularly as a single dose in addition to azithromycin 1000 milligrams orally in a single dose [12]. Uncomplicated rectal infections with *N. gonorrhoeae* should be treated in the same manner. Given that both ceftriaxone and azithromycin are administered as a single dose, these drugs should be administered together and under direct observation. These recommendations are based on a number of treatment failures with ceftriaxone alone and an increasing minimum inhibitory concentration (MIC) to oral cephalosporins which has been observed mostly outside of the US [137–148]. The dual therapy also has the advantage of treating *C. trachomatis* infection, which frequently accompanies *N. gonorrhoeae* infection. Doxycycline can be considered in place of azithromycin, but azithromycin is strongly preferred given increased resistance to doxycycline [144]. This regimen has a high (>98%) treatment efficacy for rectal infections [149, 150]. Pharyngeal infections with *N. gonorrhoeae* are more difficult to treat and have demonstrated ceftriaxone resistance and treatment failure in a number of countries outside the US [138–141, 143, 145, 146, 151, 152]. In both pharyngeal and rectal gonorrhea, persistence of the organism after treatment may be due to reinfection but can also reflect an elevated MIC to antibiotic regimens [153]. At this time, guidelines still recommend treating pharyngeal infection by *N. gonorrhoeae* with ceftriaxone and azithromycin [12]. The addition of azithromycin may improve treatment efficacy for pharyngeal infections [154, 155].

In general, test of cure is not recommended except in cases where there are persistent symptoms, therapy was not completed, or reinfection is suspected. Retesting for both urogenital and extragenital infections less than three weeks after treatment is not recommended and can result in false positive results due to the highly sensitive nature of NAAT and the possibility of detection of nonviable organisms [156, 157]. Furthermore, due to NAATs not being FDA-cleared at this time for the purpose of testing for cure, culture is the only retesting method that can be used to properly assess the efficacy of antibiotic treatments. The significance of positive NAAT at extragenital sites during this time is unclear and should be interpreted after a detailed clinical interview including presence or absence of symptoms, potential risk for reinfection, and adherence to treatment [158]. Men and women who are positive for *N. gonorrhoeae* and *C. trachomatis* should generally be tested for reinfection three to six months after treatment [12, 16].

4. Conclusions

Several key questions exist regarding screening for and management of extragenital infections. Urogenital screening for *N. gonorrhoeae* and *C. trachomatis* infection is generally performed to reduce complications in women and to decrease the risk of HIV infection in MSM [159–162]. However, there is a lack of data on clinical outcomes associated with rectal and pharyngeal infections, including impact on overall morbidity. Two major questions are whether routine screening and treatment for extragenital gonorrhea and chlamydia infections in women prevent sequelae observed in urogenital infection (such as PID, ectopic pregnancy, and infertility), and whether routine screening and treatment reduces the risk of HIV transmission in MSM. With regard to management, optimal treatment regimens for rectal and pharyngeal extragenital infections is unknown. Asymptomatic extragenital infections may be a reservoir of ongoing transmission and antibiotic resistant strains from these reservoir sites may go undetected and promote the spread of resistance.

The contribution of extragenital infections to overall transmission of gonorrhea and chlamydia, including the transmission potential between different anatomic sites, is also unclear. In women, evidence suggests that rectal infections can be spread to urogenital sites [163]. It is also likely that pharyngeal infections can be spread to the male urethra [13, 14, 164] and rectum [165]. Contributing to potential transmission risk may be bacterial load at different anatomic sites [166, 167]. These data suggest that the prevalence and associated morbidity of extragenital infections caused by *N. gonorrhoeae* and *C. trachomatis*, especially among women, may be reduced by thorough extragenital screening and early treatment of extragenital infections, although this is unproven. Screening and treatment for rectal infections, especially among populations at high risk of HIV (e.g., MSM), may be a cost-effective intervention to prevent HIV [168]. Optimal screening strategies for extragenital infections are largely unknown. Further studies are needed in settings other than reproductive health and STD clinics, especially in primary care clinics and resource-limited settings.

Extragenital infections due to *N. gonorrhoeae* and *C. trachomatis* are common, especially in settings which provide services to higher-risk men and women. In general, MSM demonstrate a higher prevalence of extragenital infection compared to women and MSW [22, 25–27, 44, 47–49]. Despite the accumulating data on the prevalence of these infections, screening at extragenital sites remains uncommon [101, 102, 169]. STD and other sexual health clinics should consider implementing routine, universal extragenital screening for *N. gonorrhoeae* and *C. trachomatis* infection among high-risk men and women. Importantly, guidelines suggest screening based on reported risk behaviors; however, this may miss a significant amount of extragenital infection [19, 22, 45, 47, 49, 52, 59, 62, 68, 77–79, 90, 103, 107, 120, 133, 170, 171]. In addition to targeting those with symptoms and those reporting condomless anal or oral sex, screening should also include those without symptoms and those who do not report condomless sex at a specific extragenital site, as the nature of the infections are often asymptomatic, and high-risk behaviors are not consistently reported by patients.

Competing Interests

The authors report no conflict of interests.

Acknowledgments

Philip A. Chan is supported by Grant K23AI096923 from the National Institutes of Health. Additional support was provided by the Lifespan/Tufts/Brown Center for AIDS Research, funded by the National Institute of Allergy and Infectious Diseases (P30AI042853).

References

[1] Office of Disease Prevention and Health Promotion, Sexually transmitted diseases [Internet]. Healthy People 2020. 2014, https://www.healthypeople.gov/2020/topics-objectives/topic/sexually-transmitted-diseases.

[2] Centers for Disease Control and Prevention, *Sexually Transmitted Disease Surveillance 2014*, U.S. Department of Health and Human Services, Atlanta, Ga, USA, 2015.

[3] D. Meyers, T. Wolff, K. Gregory et al., "USPSTF recommendations for STI screening," *American Family Physician*, vol. 77, no. 6, pp. 819–824, 2008.

[4] K. K. Fox, C. del Rio, K. K. Holmes et al., "Gonorrhea in the HIV era: a reversal in trends among men who have sex with men," *American Journal of Public Health*, vol. 91, no. 6, pp. 959–964, 2001.

[5] C. A. Rietmeijer, J. L. Patnaik, F. N. Judson, and J. M. Douglas Jr., "Increases in gonorrhea and sexual risk behaviors among men who have sex with men: a 12-year trend analysis at the Denver Metro Health Clinic," *Sexually Transmitted Diseases*, vol. 30, no. 7, pp. 562–567, 2003.

[6] R. Detels, A. M. Green, J. D. Klausner et al., "The incidence and correlates of symptomatic and asymptomatic *Chlamydia trachomatis* and *Neisseria gonorrhoeae* infections in selected populations in five countries," *Sexually Transmitted Diseases*, vol. 38, no. 6, pp. 503–509, 2011.

[7] J. A. Cecil, M. R. Howell, J. J. Tawes et al., "Features of *Chlamydia trachomatis* and *Neisseria gonorrhoeae* infection in male army recruits," *The Journal of Infectious Diseases*, vol. 184, no. 9, pp. 1216–1219, 2001.

[8] C. Mitchell and M. Prabhu, "Pelvic inflammatory disease: current concepts in pathogenesis, diagnosis and treatment," *Infectious Disease Clinics of North America*, vol. 27, no. 4, pp. 793–809, 2013.

[9] F. D. H. Koedijk, J. E. A. M. van Bergen, N. H. T. M. Dukers-Muijrers, A. P. van Leeuwen, C. J. P. A. Hoebe, and M. A. B. van der Sande, "The value of testing multiple anatomic sites for gonorrhoea and chlamydia in sexually transmitted infection centres in the Netherlands, 2006–2010," *International Journal of STD and AIDS*, vol. 23, no. 9, pp. 626–631, 2012.

[10] M. S. Cohen, "Sexually transmitted diseases enhance HIV transmission: no longer a hypothesis," *The Lancet*, vol. 351, pp. S5–S7, 1998.

[11] J. D. Carter and R. D. Inman, "Chlamydia-induced reactive arthritis: hidden in plain sight?" *Best Practice and Research: Clinical Rheumatology*, vol. 25, no. 3, pp. 359–374, 2011.

[12] K. A. Workowski and G. A. Bolan, "Sexually transmitted diseases treatment guidelines, 2015," *MMWR Recommendations and Reports*, vol. 64, no. 3, pp. 1–138, 2015.

[13] J. L. Marcus, R. P. Kohn, P. M. Barry, S. S. Philip, and K. T. Bernstein, "*Chlamydia trachomatis* and *Neisseria gonorrhoeae* transmission from the female oropharynx to the male urethra," *Sexually Transmitted Diseases*, vol. 38, no. 5, pp. 372–373, 2011.

[14] K. T. Bernstein, S. C. Stephens, P. M. Barry et al., "*Chlamydia trachomatis* and *Neisseria gonorrhoeae* transmission from the oropharynx to the Urethra among men who have sex with men," *Clinical Infectious Diseases*, vol. 49, no. 12, pp. 1793–1797, 2009.

[15] American Congress of Obstetricians and Gynecologists, "Gonorrhea, chlamydia, and syphilis," Tech. Rep. FAQ071, American Congress of Obstetricians and Gynecologists, Washington, DC, USA, 2016.

[16] E. Lanjouw, J. M. Ossewaarde, A. Stary, F. Boag, and W. I. van der Meijden, "2010 European guideline for the management of *Chlamydia trachomatis* infections," *International Journal of STD and AIDS*, vol. 21, no. 11, pp. 729–737, 2010.

[17] C. Bignell, M. Unemo, and European STI Guidelines Editorial Board, "2012 European guideline on the diagnosis and treatment of gonorrhoea in adults," *International Journal of STD & AIDS*, vol. 24, no. 2, pp. 85–92, 2013.

[18] British Association for Sexual Health and HIV, *Sexually Transmitted Infections: UK National Screening and Testing Guidelines*, 2006.

[19] N. H. T. M. Dukers-Muijrers, J. Schachter, G. A. F. S. van Liere, P. F. G. Wolffs, and C. J. P. A. Hoebe, "What is needed to guide testing for anorectal and pharyngeal *Chlamydia trachomatis* and *Neisseria gonorrhoeae* in women and men? Evidence and opinion," *BMC Infectious Diseases*, vol. 15, no. 1, article 533, 2015.

[20] Australian Sexual Health Alliance, *Australian STI Management Guidelines for Use in Primary Care*, Australian Government Department of Health, Darlinghurst, Australia, 2016.

[21] D. A. Lewis and E. Marumo, "Revision of the national guideline for first-line comprehensive management and control of sexually transmitted infections: what's new and why?" *Southern African Journal of Infectious Diseases*, vol. 24, no. 2, 2009, http://sajei.co.za/index.php/SAJEI/article/view/161.

[22] F. D. H. Koedijk, J. E. A. M. van Bergen, N. H. T. M. Dukers-Muijrers, A. P. van Leeuwen, C. J. P. A. Hoebe, and M. A. B. van der Sande, "The value of testing multiple anatomic sites for gonorrhoea and chlamydia in sexually transmitted infection centres in the Netherlands, 2006–2010," *International Journal of STD & AIDS*, vol. 23, no. 9, pp. 626–631, 2012.

[23] J. A. Bazan, P. Carr Reese, A. Esber et al., "High prevalence of rectal gonorrhea and chlamydia infection in women attending a sexually transmitted disease clinic," *Journal of Women's Health*, vol. 24, no. 3, pp. 182–189, 2015.

[24] P. M. Barry, C. K. Kent, S. S. Philip, and J. D. Klausner, "Results of a program to test women for rectal chlamydia and gonorrhea," *Obstetrics and Gynecology*, vol. 115, no. 4, pp. 753–759, 2010.

[25] C. S. Danby, L. A. Cosentino, L. K. Rabe et al., "Patterns of extragenital chlamydia and gonorrhea in women and men who have sex with men reporting a history of receptive anal intercourse," *Sexually Transmitted Diseases*, vol. 43, no. 2, pp. 105–109, 2016.

[26] A. Diaz, C. Garriga, J. A. Varela et al., "Gonorrhoea diagnoses in a network of STI clinics in Spain during the period 2006-2010: differences by sex and transmission route," *BMC Public Health*, vol. 13, article 1093, 2013.

[27] A. L. Garner, G. Schembri, T. Cullen, and V. Lee, "Should we screen heterosexuals for extra-genital chlamydial and gonococcal infections?" *International Journal of STD and AIDS*, vol. 26, no. 7, pp. 462–466, 2015.

[28] C. M. Giannini, H. K. Kim, J. Mortensen, J. Mortensen, K. Marsolo, and J. Huppert, "Culture of non-genital sites increases the detection of gonorrhea in women," *Journal of Pediatric and Adolescent Gynecology*, vol. 23, no. 4, pp. 246–252, 2010.

[29] J. Gratrix, A. E. Singh, J. Bergman et al., "Evidence for increased chlamydia case finding after the introduction of rectal screening among women attending 2 Canadian sexually transmitted infection clinics," *Clinical Infectious Diseases*, vol. 60, no. 3, pp. 398–404, 2015.

[30] T. Hunte, M. Alcaide, and J. Castro, "Rectal infections with chlamydia and gonorrhoea in women attending a multiethnic sexually transmitted diseases urban clinic," *International Journal of STD and AIDS*, vol. 21, no. 12, pp. 819–822, 2010.

[31] M. Javanbakht, P. Gorbach, A. Stirland, M. Chien, P. Kerndt, and S. Guerry, "Prevalence and correlates of rectal chlamydia and gonorrhea among female clients at sexually transmitted disease clinics," *Sexually Transmitted Diseases*, vol. 39, no. 12, pp. 917–922, 2012.

[32] W. D. Jenkins, L. L. Nessa, and T. Clark, "Cross-sectional study of pharyngeal and genital chlamydia and gonorrhoea infections in emergency department patients," *Sexually Transmitted Infections*, vol. 90, no. 3, pp. 246–249, 2014.

[33] R. B. Jones, R. A. Rabinovitch, B. P. Katz et al., "Chlamydia trachomatis in the pharynx and rectum of heterosexual patients at risk for genital infection," *Annals of Internal Medicine*, vol. 102, no. 6, pp. 757–762, 1985.

[34] J. Ladd, Y.-H. Hsieh, M. Barnes, N. Quinn, M. Jett-Goheen, and C. A. Gaydos, "Female users of internet-based screening for rectal STIs: descriptive statistics and correlates of positivity," *Sexually Transmitted Infections*, vol. 90, no. 6, pp. 485–490, 2014.

[35] Y. Linhart, T. Shohat, Z. Amitai et al., "Sexually transmitted infections among brothel-based sex workers in Tel-Aviv area, Israel: high prevalence of pharyngeal gonorrhoea," *International Journal of STD & AIDS*, vol. 19, no. 10, pp. 656–659, 2008.

[36] K. H. Mayer, T. Bush, K. Henry et al., "Ongoing sexually transmitted disease acquisition and risk-taking behavior among US HIV-infected patients in primary care: implications for prevention interventions," *Sexually Transmitted Diseases*, vol. 39, no. 1, pp. 1–7, 2012.

[37] K. Musil, M. Currie, M. Sherley, and S. Martin, "Rectal chlamydia infection in women at high risk of chlamydia attending Canberra Sexual Health Centre," *International Journal of STD & AIDS*, vol. 27, no. 7, pp. 526–530, 2015.

[38] L. Ostergaard, T. Agner, E. Krarup, U. B. Johansen, K. Weismann, and E. Gutschik, "PCR for detection of *Chlamydia trachomatis* in endocervical, urethral, rectal, and pharyngeal swab samples obtained from patients attending an STD clinic," *Genitourinary Medicine*, vol. 73, no. 6, pp. 493–497, 1997.

[39] R. P. H. Peters, N. Nijsten, J. Mutsaers, C. L. Jansen, S. A. Morré, and A. P. van Leeuwen, "Screening of oropharynx and anorectum increases prevalence of *Chlamydia trachomatis* and *Neisseria gonorrhoeae* infection in female STD clinic visitors," *Sexually Transmitted Diseases*, vol. 38, no. 9, pp. 783–787, 2011.

[40] R. P. H. Peters, J. H. Dubbink, L. van der Eem et al., "Cross-sectional study of genital, rectal, and pharyngeal chlamydia and gonorrhea in women in rural South Africa," *Sexually Transmitted Diseases*, vol. 41, no. 9, pp. 564–569, 2014.

[41] M. Raychaudhuri and H. D. L. Birley, "Audit of routine rectal swabs for gonorrhoea culture in women," *International Journal of STD and AIDS*, vol. 21, no. 2, pp. 143–144, 2010.

[42] M. Sethupathi, A. Blackwell, and H. Davies, "Rectal *Chlamydia trachomatis* infection in women. Is it overlooked?" *International Journal of STD and AIDS*, vol. 21, no. 2, pp. 93–95, 2010.

[43] S. G. Shaw, M. Hassan-Ibrahim, and S. Soni, "Are we missing pharyngeal and rectal infections in women by not testing those who report oral and anal sex?" *Sexually Transmitted Infections*, vol. 89, no. 5, p. 397, 2013.

[44] J. D. Trebach, C. P. Chaulk, K. R. Page, S. Tuddenham, and K. G. Ghanem, "*Neisseria gonorrhoeae* and *Chlamydia trachomatis* among women reporting extragenital exposures," *Sexually Transmitted Diseases*, vol. 42, no. 5, pp. 233–239, 2015.

[45] G. A. F. S. van Liere, C. J. P. A. Hoebe, A.-M. Niekamp, F. D. H. Koedijk, and N. H. T. M. Dukers-Muijrers, "Standard symptom- and sexual history–based testing misses anorectal *Chlamydia trachomatis* and *Neisseria gonorrhoeae* infections in swingers and men who have sex with men," *Sexually Transmitted Diseases*, vol. 40, no. 4, pp. 285–289, 2013.

[46] G. A. F. S. van Liere, C. J. P. A. Hoebe, P. F. G. Wolffs, and N. H. T. M. Dukers-Muijrers, "High co-occurrence of anorectal chlamydia with urogenital chlamydia in women visiting an STI clinic revealed by routine universal testing in an observational study: a recommendation towards a better anorectal chlamydia control in women," *BMC Infectious Diseases*, vol. 14, no. 1, article 274, 2014.

[47] G. A. F. S. van Liere, C. J. P. A. Hoebe, and N. H. T. M. Dukers-Muijrers, "Evaluation of the anatomical site distribution of chlamydia and gonorrhoea in men who have sex with men and in high-risk women by routine testing: cross-sectional study revealing missed opportunities for treatment strategies," *Sexually Transmitted Infections*, vol. 90, no. 1, pp. 58–60, 2014.

[48] G. A. van Liere, M. S. van Rooijen, C. J. Hoebe et al., "Prevalence of and Factors Associated with Rectal-Only Chlamydia and Gonorrhoea in Women and in Men Who Have Sex with Men," *PLOS ONE*, vol. 10, no. 10, p. e0140297, 2015.

[49] J. J. van der Helm, C. J. P. A. Hoebe, M. S. van Rooijen et al., "High performance and acceptability of self-collected rectal swabs for diagnosis of *Chlamydia trachomatis* and *Neisseria gonorrhoeae* in men who have sex with men and women," *Sexually Transmitted Diseases*, vol. 36, no. 8, pp. 493–497, 2009.

[50] A. Ding and R. Challenor, "Rectal chlamydia in heterosexual women: more questions than answers," *International Journal of STD & AIDS*, vol. 25, no. 8, pp. 587–592, 2014.

[51] L. A. Cosentino, T. Campbell, A. Jett et al., "Use of nucleic acid amplification testing for diagnosis of anorectal sexually transmitted infections," *Journal of Clinical Microbiology*, vol. 50, no. 6, pp. 2005–2008, 2012.

[52] L. H. Bachmann, R. E. Johnson, H. Cheng et al., "Nucleic acid amplification tests for diagnosis of *Neisseria gonorrhoeae* and *Chlamydia trachomatis* rectal infections," *Journal of Clinical Microbiology*, vol. 48, no. 5, pp. 1827–1832, 2010.

[53] P. M. Barry, C. K. Kent, S. S. Philip, and J. D. Klausner, "Results of a program to test women for rectal chlamydia and gonorrhea," *Obstetrics & Gynecology*, vol. 115, no. 4, pp. 753–759, 2010.

[54] S. Alexander, C. Ison, J. Parry et al., "Self-taken pharyngeal and rectal swabs are appropriate for the detection of *Chlamydia trachomatis* and *Neisseria gonorrhoeae* in asymptomatic men who have sex with men," *Sexually Transmitted Infections*, vol. 84, no. 6, pp. 488–492, 2008.

[55] N. T. Annan, A. K. Sullivan, A. Nori et al., "Rectal chlamydia—a reservoir of undiagnosed infection in men who have sex with men," *Sexually Transmitted Infections*, vol. 85, no. 3, pp. 176–179, 2009.

[56] J. Baker, M. Plankey, Y. Josayma et al., "The prevalence of rectal, urethral, and pharyngeal *Neisseria gonorrheae* and *Chlamydia trachomatis* among asymptomatic men who have sex with men in a prospective Cohort in Washington, D.C.," *AIDS Patient Care and STDs*, vol. 23, no. 8, pp. 585–588, 2009.

[57] L. A. Barbee, J. C. Dombrowski, R. Kerani, and M. R. Golden, "Effect of nucleic acid amplification testing on detection of extragenital gonorrhea and chlamydial infections in men who have sex with men sexually transmitted disease clinic patients," *Sexually Transmitted Diseases*, vol. 41, no. 3, pp. 168–172, 2014.

[58] P. D. Benn, G. Rooney, C. Carder et al., "*Chlamydia trachomatis* and *Neisseria gonorrhoeae* infection and the sexual behaviour of men who have sex with men," *Sexually Transmitted Infections*, vol. 83, no. 2, pp. 106–112, 2007.

[59] E. P. F. Chow, J. Tomnay, G. Fehler et al., "Substantial increases in chlamydia and gonorrhea positivity unexplained by changes in individual-level sexual behaviors among men who have sex with men in an Australian sexual health service from 2007 to 2013," *Sexually Transmitted Diseases*, vol. 42, no. 2, pp. 81–87, 2015.

[60] M. J. Currie, S. J. Martin, T. M. Soo, and F. J. Bowden, "Screening for chlamydia and gonorrhoea in men who have sex with men in clinical and non-clinical settings," *Sexual Health*, vol. 3, no. 2, pp. 123–126, 2006.

[61] T. Dang, K. Jaton-Ogay, M. Flepp et al., "High prevalence of anorectal chlamydial infection in HIV-infected men who have sex with men in Switzerland," *Clinical Infectious Diseases*, vol. 49, no. 10, pp. 1532–1535, 2009.

[62] S. Dudareva-Vizule, K. Haar, A. Sailer et al., "Prevalence of pharyngeal and rectal *Chlamydia trachomatis* and *Neisseria gonorrhoeae* infections among men who have sex with men in Germany," *Sexually Transmitted Infections*, vol. 90, no. 1, pp. 46–51, 2014.

[63] J. Gratrix, A. E. Singh, J. Bergman et al., "Prevalence and characteristics of rectal chlamydia and gonorrhea cases among men who have sex with men after the introduction of nucleic acid amplification test screening at 2 Canadian sexually transmitted infection clinics," *Sexually Transmitted Diseases*, vol. 41, no. 10, pp. 589–591, 2014.

[64] R. A. Gunn, C. J. O'Brien, M. A. Lee, and R. A. Gilchick, "Gonorrhea screening among men who have sex with men: value of multiple anatomic site testing, San Diego, California, 1997–2003," *Sexually Transmitted Diseases*, vol. 35, no. 10, pp. 845–848, 2008.

[65] J. Hocking and C. K. Fairley, "Associations between condom use and rectal or urethral chlamydia infection in men," *Sexually Transmitted Diseases*, vol. 33, no. 4, pp. 256–258, 2006.

[66] E. Jiménez, M. G. Pedrazuela, M. M. Pérez, S. F. de Mosteyrín, J. J. Arrieta, and M. L. F. Guerrero, "Prevalence of pharyngeal infection by *Neisseria gonorrhoeae* among human immunodeficiency virus-positive men who have sex with men in downtown Madrid, 2011," *International Journal of STD & AIDS*, vol. 24, no. 11, pp. 875–878, 2013.

[67] S. Keaveney, C. Sadlier, S. O'Dea, S. Delamere, and C. Bergin, "High prevalence of asymptomatic sexually transmitted infections in HIV-infected men who have sex with men: a stimulus to improve screening," *International Journal of STD and AIDS*, vol. 25, no. 10, pp. 758–761, 2014.

[68] C. K. Kent, J. K. Chaw, W. Wong et al., "Prevalence of rectal, urethral, and pharyngeal chlamydia and gonorrhea detected in 2 clinical settings among men who have sex with men: San Francisco, California, 2003," *Clinical Infectious Diseases*, vol. 41, no. 1, pp. 67–74, 2005.

[69] A. A. Kim, C. K. Kent, and J. D. Klausner, "Risk factors for rectal gonococcal infection amidst resurgence in HIV transmission," *Sexually Transmitted Diseases*, vol. 30, no. 11, pp. 813–817, 2003.

[70] J. D. Klausner, K. T. Bernstein, M. Pandori et al., "Clinic-based testing for rectal and pharyngeal *Neisseria gonorrhoeae* and *Chlamydia trachomatis* infections by community-based organizations—five cities, United States, 2007," *Morbidity and Mortality Weekly Report*, vol. 58, pp. 716–719, 2009.

[71] N. A. Lister, N. J. Chaves, C. W. Pang, A. Smith, and C. K. Fairley, "Clinical significance of questionnaire-elicited or clinically reported anorectal symptoms for rectal *Neisseria gonorrhoeae* and *Chlamydia trachomatis* amongst men who have sex with men," *Sexual Health*, vol. 5, no. 1, pp. 77–82, 2008.

[72] K. Manavi, A. McMillan, and H. Young, "The prevalence of rectal chlamydial infection amongst men who have sex with men attending the genitourinary medicine clinic in Edinburgh," *International Journal of STD and AIDS*, vol. 15, no. 3, pp. 162–164, 2004.

[73] A. McMillan, R. G. Sommerville, and P. M. K. McKie, "Chlamydial infection in homosexual men: frequency of isolation of *Chlamydia trachomatis* from the urethra, ano-rectum, and pharynx," *British Journal of Venereal Diseases*, vol. 57, no. 1, pp. 47–49, 1981.

[74] M. J. Mimiaga, K. H. Mayer, S. L. Reisner et al., "Asymptomatic gonorrhea and chlamydial infections detected by nucleic acid amplification tests among Boston area men who have sex with men," *Sexually Transmitted Diseases*, vol. 35, no. 5, pp. 495–498, 2008.

[75] M. J. Mimiaga, D. J. Helms, S. L. Reisner et al., "Gonococcal, chlamydia, and syphilis infection positivity among MSM attending a large primary care clinic, Boston, 2003 to 2004," *Sexually Transmitted Diseases*, vol. 36, no. 8, pp. 507–511, 2009.

[76] S. R. Morris, J. D. Klausner, S. P. Buchbinder et al., "Prevalence and incidence of pharyngeal gonorrhea in a longitudinal sample of men who have sex with men: the EXPLORE study," *Clinical Infectious Diseases*, vol. 43, no. 10, pp. 1284–1289, 2006.

[77] K. V. Ota, D. N. Fisman, I. E. Tamari et al., "Incidence and treatment outcomes of pharyngeal *Neisseria gonorrhoeae* and *Chlamydia trachomatis* infections in men who have sex with men: a 13-year retrospective cohort study," *Clinical Infectious Diseases*, vol. 48, no. 9, pp. 1237–1243, 2009.

[78] J. Park, J. L. Marcus, M. Pandori, A. Snell, S. S. Philip, and K. T. Bernstein, "Sentinel surveillance for pharyngeal chlamydia and gonorrhea among men who have sex with men—San Francisco, 2010," *Sexually Transmitted Diseases*, vol. 39, no. 6, pp. 482–484, 2012.

[79] M. E. Patton, S. Kidd, E. Llata et al., "Extragenital gonorrhea and chlamydia testing and infection among men who have sex with men—STD Surveillance Network, United States, 2010–2012," *Clinical Infectious Diseases*, vol. 85, no. 11, pp. 1564–1570, 2014.

[80] R. P. H. Peters, S. P. Verweij, N. Nijsten et al., "Evaluation of sexual history-based screening of anatomic sites for chlamydia trachomatis and neisseria gonorrhoeae infection in men having sex with men in routine practice," *BMC Infectious Diseases*, vol. 11, article 203, 2011.

[81] L. Pinsky, D. B. Chiarilli, J. D. Klausner et al., "Rates of asymptomatic nonurethral gonorrhea and chlamydia in a population

of university men who have sex with men," *Journal of American College Health*, vol. 60, no. 6, pp. 481–484, 2012.

[82] G. Rieg, R. J. Lewis, L. G. Miller, M. D. Witt, M. Guerrero, and E. S. Daar, "Asymptomatic sexually transmitted infections in HIV-infected men who have sex with men: prevalence, incidence, predictors, and screening strategies," *AIDS Patient Care and STDs*, vol. 22, no. 12, pp. 947–954, 2008.

[83] A. M. Rompalo, C. B. Price, P. L. Roberts, and W. E. Stamm, "Potential value of rectal-screening cultures for *Chlamydia trachomatis* in homosexual men," *Journal of Infectious Diseases*, vol. 153, no. 5, pp. 888–892, 1986.

[84] E. J. Sanders, E. Wahome, H. S. Okuku et al., "Evaluation of WHO screening algorithm for the presumptive treatment of asymptomatic rectal gonorrhoea and chlamydia infections in at-risk MSM in Kenya," *Sexually Transmitted Infections*, vol. 90, no. 2, pp. 94–99, 2014.

[85] M. E. Sexton, J. J. Baker, K. Nakagawa et al., "How reliable is self-testing for gonorrhea and chlamydia among men who have sex with men?" *Journal of Family Practice*, vol. 62, no. 2, pp. 70–78, 2013.

[86] S. Soni and J. A. White, "Self-screening for *Neisseria gonorrhoeae* and chlamydia trachomatis in the human immunodeficiency virus clinic-high yields and high acceptability," *Sexually Transmitted Diseases*, vol. 38, no. 12, pp. 1107–1109, 2011.

[87] S. R. Tabet, M. R. Krone, M. A. Paradise, L. Corey, W. E. Stamm, and C. L. Celum, "Incidence of HIV and sexually transmitted diseases (STD) in a cohort of HIV-negative men who have sex with men (MSM)," *AIDS*, vol. 12, no. 15, pp. 2041–2048, 1998.

[88] M. M. Taylor, D. R. Newman, J. Gonzalez, J. Skinner, R. Khurana, and T. Mickey, "HIV status and viral loads among men testing positive for rectal gonorrhoea and chlamydia, Maricopa County, Arizona, USA, 2011–2013," *HIV Medicine*, vol. 16, no. 4, pp. 249–254, 2015.

[89] D. J. Templeton, F. Jin, J. Imrie et al., "Prevalence, incidence and risk factors for pharyngeal chlamydia in the community based Health in Men (HIM) cohort of homosexual men in Sydney, Australia," *Sexually Transmitted Infections*, vol. 84, no. 5, pp. 361–363, 2008.

[90] D. J. Templeton, F. Jin, L. P. McNally et al., "Prevalence, incidence and risk factors for pharyngeal gonorrhoea in a community-based HIV-negative cohort of homosexual men in Sydney, Australia," *Sexually Transmitted Infections*, vol. 86, no. 2, pp. 90–96, 2010.

[91] J. Tongtoyai, C. S. Todd, W. Chonwattana et al., "Prevalence and correlates of *Chlamydia trachomatis* and *Neisseria gonorrhoeae* by anatomic site among urban Thai men who have sex with men," *Sexually Transmitted Diseases*, vol. 42, no. 8, pp. 440–449, 2015.

[92] A. N. Turner, P. C. Reese, M. Ervin, J. A. Davis, K. S. Fields, and J. A. Bazan, "HIV, rectal chlamydia, and rectal gonorrhea in men who have sex with men attending a sexually transmitted disease clinic in a midwestern US city," *Sexually Transmitted Diseases*, vol. 40, no. 6, pp. 433–438, 2013.

[93] L. A. Vodstrcil, C. K. Fairley, G. Fehler et al., "Trends in chlamydia and gonorrhea positivity among heterosexual men and men who have sex with men attending a large urban sexual health service in Australia," *BMC Infectious Diseases*, vol. 11, p. 158, 2011.

[94] N. A. Lister, A. Smith, T. Read, and C. K. Fairley, "Testing men who have sex with men for *Neisseria gonorrhoeae* and *Chlamydia trachomatis* prior to the introduction of guidelines at an STD clinic in Melbourne," *Sexual Health*, vol. 1, no. 1, pp. 47–50, 2004.

[95] W. M. Geisler, W. L. H. Whittington, R. J. Suchland, and W. E. Stamm, "Epidemiology of anorectal chlamydial and gonococcal infections among men having sex with men in Seattle: utilizing serovar and auxotype strain typing," *Sexually Transmitted Diseases*, vol. 29, pp. 189–195, 2002.

[96] A. McMillan and H. Young, "Clinical correlates of rectal gonococcal and chlamydial infections," *International Journal of STD & AIDS*, vol. 17, no. 6, pp. 387–390, 2006.

[97] J. L. Marcus, K. T. Bernstein, S. C. Stephens et al., "Sentinel surveillance of rectal chlamydia and gonorrhea among males—San Francisco, 2005–2008," *Sexually Transmitted Diseases*, vol. 37, no. 1, pp. 59–61, 2010.

[98] N. Ryder, C. Bourne, and B. Donovan, "Different trends for different sexually transmissible infections despite increased testing of men who have sex with men," *International Journal of STD and AIDS*, vol. 22, no. 6, pp. 335–337, 2011.

[99] A. McMillan, K. Manavi, and H. Young, "Concurrent gonococcal and chlamydial infections among men attending a sexually transmitted diseases clinic," *International Journal of STD and AIDS*, vol. 16, no. 5, pp. 357–361, 2005.

[100] P. A. Chan, M. Janvier, N. E. Alexander, E. M. Kojic, and K. Chapin, "Recommendations for the diagnosis of *Neisseria gonorrhoeae* and *Chlamydia trachomatis*, including extra-genital sites," *Medicine and Health, Rhode Island*, vol. 95, no. 8, pp. 252–254, 2012.

[101] C. D. den Heijer, G. A. van Liere, C. J. Hoebe et al., "Who tests whom? A comprehensive overview of Chlamydia trachomatis test practices in a Dutch region among different STI care providers for urogenital, anorectal and oropharyngeal sites in young people: a cross-sectional study," *Sexually Transmitted Infections*, vol. 92, no. 3, pp. 211–217, 2016.

[102] W. Dimech, M. S. C. Lim, C. Van Gemert et al., "Analysis of laboratory testing results collected in an enhanced chlamydia surveillance system in Australia, 2008–2010," *BMC Infectious Diseases*, vol. 14, article 325, 2014.

[103] D. Ivens, K. MacDonald, L. Bansi, and A. Nori, "Screening for rectal chlamydia infection in a genitourinary medicine clinic," *International Journal of STD and AIDS*, vol. 18, no. 6, pp. 404–406, 2007.

[104] K. Oda, H. Yano, N. Okitsu et al., "Detection of *Chlamydia trachomatis* or *Neisseria gonorrhoeae* in otorhinolaryngology patients with pharyngeal symptoms," *Sexually Transmitted Infections*, vol. 90, article 99, 2014.

[105] S. B. Patterson, D. Rivera, T. S. Sunil, and J. F. Okulicz, "Evaluation of extragenital screening for gonorrhea and chlamydia in HIV-infected active duty Air Force members," *MSMR*, vol. 21, no. 11, pp. 7–9, 2014.

[106] C. Rodriguez-Hart, R. A. Chitale, R. Rigg, B. Y. Goldstein, P. R. Kerndt, and P. Tavrow, "Sexually transmitted infection testing of adult film performers: is disease being missed?" *Sexually transmitted diseases*, vol. 39, no. 12, pp. 989–994, 2012.

[107] C. Tipple, S. C. Hill, and A. Smith, "Is screening for pharyngeal *Chlamydia trachomatis* warranted in high-risk groups?" *International Journal of STD and AIDS*, vol. 21, no. 11, pp. 770–771, 2010.

[108] R. K. Bolan and M. R. Beymer, "One size does not fit all: the public health ramifications of proposed food and drug administration premarket review for extragenital gonorrhea and chlamydia testing," *Sexually Transmitted Diseases*, vol. 42, no. 7, pp. 403–404, 2015.

[109] J. Schachter, J. Moncada, S. Liska, C. Shayevich, and J. D. Klausner, "Nucleic acid amplification tests in the diagnosis of chlamydial and gonococcal infections of the oropharynx and rectum in men who have sex with men," *Sexually Transmitted Diseases*, vol. 35, no. 7, pp. 637–642, 2008.

[110] L. H. Bachmann, R. E. Johnson, H. Cheng, L. E. Markowitz, J. R. Papp, and I. W. H. Edward, "Nucleic acid amplification tests for diagnosis of *Neisseria gonorrhoeae* oropharyngeal infections," *Journal of Clinical Microbiology*, vol. 47, no. 4, pp. 902–907, 2009.

[111] D. M. Whiley, J. W. Tapsall, and T. P. Sloots, "Nucleic acid amplification testing for *Neisseria gonorrhoeae*: an ongoing challenge," *Journal of Molecular Diagnostics*, vol. 8, no. 1, pp. 3–15, 2006.

[112] V. Schick, B. Van Der Pol, B. Dodge, A. Baldwin, and J. Dennis Fortenberry, "A mixed methods approach to assess the likelihood of testing for STI using self-collected samples among behaviourally bisexual women," *Sexually Transmitted Infections*, vol. 91, no. 5, pp. 329–333, 2015.

[113] A. M. Roth, J. G. Rosenberger, M. Reece, and B. Van Der Pol, "Expanding sexually transmitted infection screening among women and men engaging in transactional sex: the feasibility of field-based self-collection," *International Journal of STD and AIDS*, vol. 24, no. 4, pp. 323–328, 2013.

[114] B. Dodge, B. Van Der Pol, J. G. Rosenberger et al., "Field collection of rectal samples for sexually transmitted infection diagnostics among men who have sex with men," *International Journal of STD & AIDS*, vol. 21, no. 4, pp. 260–264, 2010.

[115] J. G. Rosenberger, B. Dodge, B. Van Der Pol, M. Reece, D. Herbenick, and J. D. Fortenberry, "Reactions to self-sampling for ano-rectal sexually transmitted infections among men who have sex with men: a qualitative study," *Archives of Sexual Behavior*, vol. 40, no. 2, pp. 281–288, 2011.

[116] B. Dodge, B. Van Der Pol, M. Reece et al., "Rectal self-sampling in non-clinical venues for detection of sexually transmissible infections among behaviourally bisexual men," *Sexual Health*, vol. 9, no. 2, pp. 190–191, 2012.

[117] A. H. Freeman, K. T. Bernstein, R. P. Kohn, S. Philip, L. M. Rauch, and J. D. Klausner, "Evaluation of self-collected versus clinician-collected swabs for the detection of *Chlamydia trachomatis* and *Neisseria gonorrhoeae* pharyngeal infection among men who have sex with men," *Sexually Transmitted Diseases*, vol. 38, no. 11, pp. 1036–1039, 2011.

[118] F. Nyatsanza, A. Trivedy, and G. Brook, "The effect of introducing routine self-taken extra-genital swabs in a genitourinary medicine clinic cohort. A before and after study," *International Journal of STD & AIDS*, 2015.

[119] E. Lanjouw, J. M. Ossewaarde, A. Stary, F. Boag, and W. I. van der Meijden, "2010 European guideline for the management of *Chlamydia trachomatis* infections," *International Journal of STD & AIDS*, vol. 21, no. 11, pp. 729–737, 2010.

[120] M. S. van Rooijen, M. F. S. van der Loeff, S. A. Morré, A. P. van Dam, A. G. C. L. Speksnijder, and H. J. C. de Vries, "Spontaneous pharyngeal *Chlamydia trachomatis* RNA clearance. A cross-sectional study followed by a cohort study of untreated STI clinic patients in Amsterdam, the Netherlands," *Sexually Transmitted Infections*, vol. 91, no. 3, pp. 157–164, 2015.

[121] S. K. Apewokin, W. M. Geisler, and L. H. Bachmann, "Spontaneous resolution of extragenital chlamydial and gonococcal infections prior to therapy," *Sexually Transmitted Diseases*, vol. 37, no. 5, pp. 343–344, 2010.

[122] C.-Y. Lau and A. K. Qureshi, "Azithromycin versus doxycycline for genital chlamydial infections: a meta-analysis of randomized clinical trials," *Sexually Transmitted Diseases*, vol. 29, no. 9, pp. 497–502, 2002.

[123] F. Y. S. Kong, S. N. Tabrizi, M. Law et al., "Azithromycin versus doxycycline for the treatment of genital chlamydia infection: a meta-analysis of randomized controlled trials," *Clinical Infectious Diseases*, vol. 59, no. 2, pp. 193–205, 2014.

[124] W. M. Geisler, A. Uniyal, J. Y. Lee et al., "Azithromycin versus doxycycline for urogenital *Chlamydia trachomatis* infection," *The New England Journal of Medicine*, vol. 373, pp. 2512–2521, 2015.

[125] F. Y. S. Kong, S. N. Tabrizi, C. K. Fairley et al., "The efficacy of azithromycin and doxycycline for the treatment of rectal chlamydia infection: a systematic review and meta-analysis," *Journal of Antimicrobial Chemotherapy*, vol. 70, no. 5, Article ID dku574, pp. 1290–1297, 2014.

[126] J. S. Hocking, F. Y. S. Kong, P. Timms, W. M. Huston, and S. N. Tabrizi, "Treatment of rectal chlamydia infection may be more complicated than we originally thought," *Journal of Antimicrobial Chemotherapy*, vol. 70, no. 4, pp. 961–964, 2014.

[127] S. J. Jordan and W. M. Geisler, "Azithromycin for rectal chlamydia: is it time to leave azithromycin on the shelf?...Not yet," *Sexually Transmitted Diseases*, vol. 41, no. 2, pp. 86–88, 2014.

[128] N. M. Steedman and A. McMillan, "Treatment of asymptomatic rectal *Chlamydia trachomatis*: is single-dose azithromycin effective?" *International Journal of STD & AIDS*, vol. 20, no. 1, pp. 16–18, 2009.

[129] E. Hathorn, C. Opie, and P. Goold, "What is the appropriate treatment for the management of rectal *Chlamydia trachomatis* in men and women?" *Sexually Transmitted Infections*, vol. 88, no. 5, pp. 352–354, 2012.

[130] F. Drummond, N. Ryder, H. Wand et al., "Is azithromycin adequate treatment for asymptomatic rectal chlamydia?" *International Journal of STD and AIDS*, vol. 22, no. 8, pp. 478–480, 2011.

[131] C. M. Khosropour, J. C. Dombrowski, L. A. Barbee, L. E. Manhart, and M. R. Golden, "Comparing azithromycin and doxycycline for the treatment of rectal chlamydial infection: a retrospective cohort study," *Sexually Transmitted Diseases*, vol. 41, no. 2, pp. 79–85, 2014.

[132] A. Elgalib, S. Alexander, C. Y. W. Tong, and J. A. White, "Seven days of doxycycline is an effective treatment for asymptomatic rectal *Chlamydia trachomatis* infection," *International Journal of STD and AIDS*, vol. 22, no. 8, pp. 474–477, 2011.

[133] K. Manavi, F. Zafar, and H. Shahid, "Oropharyngeal gonorrhoea: rate of co-infection with sexually transmitted infection, antibiotic susceptibility and treatment outcome," *International Journal of STD and AIDS*, vol. 21, no. 2, pp. 138–140, 2010.

[134] P. J. Horner, "Azithromycin antimicrobial resistance and genital *Chlamydia trachomatis* infection: duration of therapy may be the key to improving efficacy," *Sexually Transmitted Infections*, vol. 88, no. 3, pp. 154–156, 2012.

[135] D. J. Templeton, P. Read, R. Varma, and C. Bourne, "Australian sexually transmissible infection and HIV testing guidelines for asymptomatic men who have sex with men 2014: a review of the evidence," *Sexual Health*, vol. 11, no. 3, pp. 217–229, 2014.

[136] F. Y. S. Kong and J. S. Hocking, "Treatment challenges for urogenital and anorectal *Chlamydia trachomatis*," *BMC Infectious Diseases*, vol. 15, no. 1, article 293, 2015.

[137] M. Y Chen, K. Stevens, R. Tideman et al., "Failure of 500 mg of ceftriaxone to eradicate pharyngeal gonorrhoea, Australia,"

The Journal of Antimicrobial Chemotherapy, vol. 68, no. 6, pp. 1445–1447, 2013.

[138] J. Tapsall, P. Read, C. Carmody et al., "Two cases of failed ceftriaxone treatment in pharyngeal gonorrhoea verified by molecular microbiological methods," *Journal of Medical Microbiology*, vol. 58, no. 5, pp. 683–687, 2009.

[139] M. Ohnishi, T. Saika, S. Hoshina et al., "Ceftriaxone-resistant *Neisseria gonorrhoeae*, Japan," *Emerging Infectious Diseases*, vol. 17, no. 1, pp. 148–149, 2011.

[140] M. Unemo, D. Golparian, M. Potocnik, and S. Jeverica, "Treatment failure of pharyngeal gonorrhoea with internationally recommended first-line ceftriaxone verified in Slovenia, September 2011," *Euro Surveillance: Bulletin Européens sur les Maladies Transmissibles*, vol. 17, no. 25, 2012.

[141] M. Unemo, D. Golparian, and A. Hestner, "Ceftriaxone treatment failure of pharyngeal gonorrhoea verified by international recommendations, Sweden, July 2010," *Eurosurveillance*, vol. 16, no. 6, Article ID 19792, 2011.

[142] Y. H. Grad, R. D. Kirkcaldy, D. Trees et al., "Genomic epidemiology of *Neisseria gonorrhoeae* with reduced susceptibility to cefixime in the USA: a retrospective observational study," *The Lancet Infectious Diseases*, vol. 14, no. 3, pp. 220–226, 2014.

[143] D. Golparian, A. Ohlsson, H. Janson et al., "Four treatment failures of pharyngeal gonorrhoea with ceftriaxone (500 mg) or cefotaxime (500 mg), Sweden, 2013 and 2014," *Euro Surveillance: European communicable disease bulletin*, vol. 19, no. 30, Article ID 20862, 2013.

[144] Centers for Disease Control and Prevention (CDC), "Update to CDC's sexually transmitted diseases treatment guidelines, 2010: oral cephalosporins no longer a recommended treatment for gonococcal infections," *Morbidity and Mortality Weekly Report*, vol. 61, no. 31, pp. 590–594, 2012.

[145] P. J. Read, E. A. Limnios, A. McNulty, D. Whiley, and M. M. Lahra, "One confirmed and one suspected case of pharyngeal gonorrhoea treatment failure following 500 mg ceftriaxone in Sydney, Australia," *Sexual Health*, vol. 10, no. 5, pp. 460–462, 2013.

[146] J. Gratrix, J. Bergman, C. Egan, S. J. Drews, R. Read, and A. E. Singh, "Retrospective review of pharyngeal gonorrhea treatment failures in Alberta, Canada," *Sexually Transmitted Diseases*, vol. 40, no. 11, pp. 877–879, 2013.

[147] A. Hustig, C. Bell, and R. Waddell, "An audit of pharyngeal gonorrhoea treatment in a public sexual health clinic in Adelaide, South Australia," *International Journal of STD and AIDS*, vol. 24, no. 5, pp. 399–400, 2013.

[148] T. Matsumoto, T. Muratani, K. Takahashi et al., "Multiple doses of cefodizime are necessary for the treatment of *Neisseria gonorrhoeae* pharyngeal infection," *Journal of Infection and Chemotherapy*, vol. 12, no. 3, pp. 145–147, 2006.

[149] J. S. Moran and W. C. Levine, "Drugs of choice for the treatment of uncomplicated gonococcal infections," *Clinical Infectious Diseases*, vol. 20, supplement 1, pp. S47–S65, 1995.

[150] L. M. Newman, J. S. Moran, and K. A. Workowski, "Update on the management of gonorrhea in adults in the United States," *Clinical Infectious Diseases*, vol. 44, supplement 3, pp. S84–S101, 2007.

[151] M. Y. Chen, K. Stevens, R. Tideman et al., "Failure of 500 mg of ceftriaxone to eradicate pharyngeal gonorrhoea, Australia," *The Journal of Antimicrobial Chemotherapy*, vol. 68, no. 6, pp. 1445–1447, 2013.

[152] K. Manavi, H. Young, and A. McMillan, "The outcome of oropharyngeal gonorrhoea treatment with different regimens,"

[153] M. Bissessor, D. M. Whiley, C. K. Fairley et al., "Persistence of *Neisseria gonorrhoeae* DNA following treatment for pharyngeal and rectal gonorrhea is influenced by antibiotic susceptibility and reinfection," *Clinical Infectious Diseases*, vol. 60, no. 4, pp. 557–563, 2015.

International Journal of STD & AIDS, vol. 16, no. 1, pp. 68–70, 2005.

[154] L. Sathia, B. Ellis, S. Phillip, A. Winston, and A. Smith, "Pharyngeal gonorrhoea—is dual therapy the way forward?" *International Journal of STD and AIDS*, vol. 18, no. 9, pp. 647–648, 2007.

[155] L. A. Barbee, R. P. Kerani, J. C. Dombrowski, O. O. Soge, and M. R. Golden, "A retrospective comparative study of 2-drug oral and intramuscular cephalosporin treatment regimens for pharyngeal gonorrhea," *Clinical Infectious Diseases*, vol. 56, no. 11, pp. 1539–1545, 2013.

[156] C. A. Renault, D. M. Israelski, V. Levy, B. K. Fujikawa, T. A. Kellogg, and J. D. Klausner, "Time to clearance of *Chlamydia trachomatis* ribosomal RNA in women treated for chlamydial infection," *Sexual Health*, vol. 8, no. 1, pp. 69–73, 2011.

[157] Centers for Disease Control and Prevention, "Recommendations for the laboratory-based detection of Chlamydia trachomatis and Neisseria gonorrhoeae—2014," *Morbidity and Mortality Weekly Report (MMWR)*, vol. 63, pp. 1–19, 2014.

[158] M. R. Beymer, E. Llata, A. M. Stirland et al., "Evaluation of gonorrhea test of cure at 1 week in a Los Angeles community-based clinic serving men who have sex with men," *Sexually Transmitted Diseases*, vol. 41, no. 10, pp. 595–600, 2014.

[159] P. Pathela, S. L. Braunstein, S. Blank, and J. A. Schillinger, "HIV incidence among men with and those without sexually transmitted rectal infections: estimates from matching against an HIV case registry," *Clinical Infectious Diseases*, vol. 57, no. 8, pp. 1203–1209, 2013.

[160] K. T. Bernstein, J. L. Marcus, G. Nieri, S. S. Philip, and J. D. Klausner, "Rectal gonorrhea and chlamydia reinfection is associated with increased risk of HIV seroconversion," *Journal of Acquired Immune Deficiency Syndromes*, vol. 53, no. 4, pp. 537–543, 2010.

[161] K. J. P. Craib, D. R. Meddings, S. A. Strathdee et al., "Rectal gonorrhea as an independent risk factor for HIV infection in a cohort of homosexual men," *Genitourinary Medicine*, vol. 71, no. 3, pp. 150–154, 1995.

[162] N. M. Zetola, K. T. Bernstein, E. Wong, B. Louie, and J. D. Klausner, "Exploring the relationship between sexually transmitted diseases and HIV acquisition by using different study designs," *Journal of Acquired Immune Deficiency Syndromes*, vol. 50, no. 5, pp. 546–551, 2009.

[163] A. P. Craig, F. Kong, L. Yeruva et al., "Is it time to switch to doxycycline from azithromycin for treating genital chlamydial infections in women? Modelling the impact of autoinoculation from the gastrointestinal tract to the genital tract," *BMC Infectious Diseases*, vol. 15, article 200, 2015.

[164] W. E. Lafferty, J. P. Hughes, and H. H. Handsfield, "Sexually transmitted diseases in men who have sex with men: acquisition of gonorrhea and nongonococcal urethritis by fellatio and implications for STD/HIV prevention," *Sexually Transmitted Diseases*, vol. 24, no. 5, pp. 272–278, 1997.

[165] A. McMillan, H. Young, and A. Moyes, "Rectal gonorrhoea in homosexual men: source of infection," *International Journal of STD and AIDS*, vol. 11, no. 5, pp. 284–287, 2000.

[166] M. Bissessor, S. N. Tabrizi, C. K. Fairley et al., "Differing Neisseria gonorrhoeae bacterial loads in the pharynx and

rectum in men who have sex with men: implications for gonococcal detection, transmission, and control," *Journal of Clinical Microbiology*, vol. 49, no. 12, pp. 4304–4306, 2011.

[167] G. A. F. S. Van Liere, J. A. M. C. Dirks, C. J. P. A. Hoebe, P. F. Wolffs, and N. H. T. M. Dukers-Muijrers, "Anorectal *Chlamydia trachomatis* load is similar in men who have sex with men and women reporting anal sex," *PLoS ONE*, vol. 10, no. 8, Article ID e0134991, 2015.

[168] H. W. Chesson, K. T. Bernstein, T. L. Gift, J. L. Marcus, S. Pipkin, and C. K. Kent, "The cost-effectiveness of screening men who have sex with men for rectal chlamydial and gonococcal infection to prevent HIV infection," *Sexually Transmitted Diseases*, vol. 40, no. 5, pp. 366–371, 2013.

[169] J. C. Dombrowski, "Do women need screening for extragenital gonococcal and chlamydial infections?" *Sexually Transmitted Diseases*, vol. 42, no. 5, pp. 240–242, 2015.

[170] U. Marcus, J. Ort, M. Grenz, K. Eckstein, K. Wirtz, and A. Wille, "Risk factors for HIV and STI diagnosis in a community-based HIV/STI testing and counselling site for men having sex with men (MSM) in a large german city in 2011-2012," *BMC Infectious Diseases*, vol. 15, article 14, 2015.

[171] E. R. Cachay, A. Sitapati, J. Caperna et al., "Denial of risk behavior does not exclude asymptomatic anorectal sexually transmitted infection in HIV-infected men," *PLoS ONE*, vol. 4, no. 12, Article ID e8504, 2009.

[172] J. L. Marcus, K. T. Bernstein, R. P. Kohn, S. Liska, and S. S. Philip, "Infections missed by urethral-only screening for chlamydia or gonorrhea detection among men who have sex with men," *Sexually Transmitted Diseases*, vol. 38, no. 10, pp. 922–924, 2011.

[173] K. Wada, S. Uehara, R. Mitsuhata et al., "Prevalence of pharyngeal Chlamydia trachomatis and Neisseria gonorrhoeae among heterosexual men in Japan," *Journal of Infection and Chemotherapy*, vol. 18, no. 5, pp. 729–733, 2012.

13

Influenza Vaccination among Pregnant Women: Patient Beliefs and Medical Provider Practices

Lauren M. Stark,[1] Michael L. Power,[1] Mark Turrentine,[2] Renee Samelson,[3] Maryam M. Siddiqui,[4] Michael J. Paglia,[5] Emmie R. Strassberg,[5] Elizabeth Kelly,[6] Katie L. Murtough,[7] and Jay Schulkin[7]

[1]Research Department, American College of Obstetricians and Gynecologists, 409 12th Street SW, Washington, DC 20024, USA
[2]Department of Obstetrics & Gynecology, Kelsey-Seybold Clinic, 1111 Augusta Drive, Houston, TX 77057, USA
[3]Division of Maternal Fetal Medicine, Department of Obstetrics & Gynecology, Albany Medical Center, 391 Myrtle Avenue, Suite 2, Albany, NY 12208, USA
[4]The University of Chicago Medicine, 5841 S. Maryland Avenue, MC 2050, Chicago, IL 60637, USA
[5]Department of Maternal-Fetal Medicine, Geisinger Health System, 100 N Academy Avenue, Danville, PA 17822, USA
[6]Department of Obstetrics & Gynecology, Albany Medical Center, 391 Myrtle Avenue, 2nd floor, MC 74, Albany, NY 12208, USA
[7]American College of Obstetricians and Gynecologists, 409 12th Street SW, Washington, DC 20024, USA

Correspondence should be addressed to Lauren M. Stark; lstark@acog.org

Academic Editor: Bryan Larsen

ACOG's research department recruited four medical centers to participate in a study on the attitudes and practices of medical providers and pregnant patients regarding influenza vaccination. Medical providers and patients were given voluntary surveys and medical record data was collected over two flu seasons, from 2013 to 2015. Discrepancies between self-reports of medical providers and patients and medical records were observed. Nearly 80% of patients self-reported accepting the influenza vaccine, but medical record data only reported 36% of patients accepting the vaccine. Similarly, all medical providers reported giving recommendations for the vaccine, but only 85% of patients reported receiving a recommendation. Age, education, a medical provider's recommendation, and educational materials were found to positively influence patient beliefs about the influenza vaccine. Accepting the vaccine was influenced by a patient's previous actions, beliefs, and a medical provider's recommendation. Patients who reported previously not accepting the vaccine and had negative feelings towards the vaccine but accepted it while pregnant reported concern for the health and safety of their baby. Future research should focus on groups that may be less likely to accept the vaccine and ways to dispel negative myths. Medical provider should continue to strongly recommend the vaccine and provide educational materials.

1. Introduction

Influenza vaccination is recommended during pregnancy to prevent harm to both mothers and fetuses. Pregnant women are at an increased risk of developing serious illness from the flu due to changes within their immune system; as well they are at risk for complications such as premature birth if they develop the flu [1]. While many anti-immunization groups have raised concerns over ill effects of vaccinations, no scientific evidence has supported their claims [2, 3]. Additionally, accepting the vaccination is associated with lower rates of influenza diagnosis, which, if contracted, is associated with higher rates of fetal mortality [4]. In 2014, the American College of Obstetricians and Gynecologists (ACOG) reaffirmed their committee opinion recommending that all pregnant women should accept the influenza vaccination, unless there are valid medical reasons such as allergic reactions. Despite the preventive benefits from the influenza vaccine, during the 2014-2015 flu season, only 50% of pregnant women accepted the influenza vaccine [2]. This is well below the 80% goal set by Healthy People 2020, a national government program that has established benchmarks to improve health outcomes of Americans [5]. Studies suggest that pregnant women are concerned about contracting influenza from the vaccine and about harming their baby, which decreases their likelihood of accepting the vaccine while pregnant [6, 7]. In a review of barriers associated with immunization in pregnancy, however, Shavell et al. noted multiple studies which found that concern for their baby can increase vaccination rates among pregnant women and that a physician's recommendation has a strong impact on vaccination rates [7]. In 2013, ACOG launched a study on influenza vaccination among pregnant women through the Expanded Collaborative Ambulatory Research Network (ECARN). The purpose of this study was to understand the attitudes and practices of patients and medical providers regarding the influenza vaccination, as well as identifying potential barriers that exist in vaccine acceptance among pregnant women.

2. Materials and Methods

Since 1995, the Collaborative Ambulatory Research Network (CARN) conducted by ACOG has surveyed obstetricians and gynecologists (OB/GYNs) on their knowledge, attitudes, and beliefs regarding a number of obstetric and gynecological issues to provide up-to-date information for improving educational materials and ACOG guidelines. One of the main goals of CARN is to improve patient health by understanding the resources and guidelines OB/GYNs need, as well as the barriers they perceive to providing quality healthcare. ECARN expands on this effort by providing access to patients and their medical records. In this way, provider perspectives can be assessed in conjunction with patient perceptions and medical record data.

ECARN was created to help bridge the data gap between providers, patients, and records. Medical centers and private OB/GYN offices are enlisted to take part in studies that collect data from medical providers and patient self-reports, as well as medical record data. Communication between medical providers and patients is imperfect, and both medical provider and patients surveys are subject to biased responses based on social desirability and recall error. By comparing the two perspectives and including medical record data, discrepancies can give insight into where additional resources or education is needed.

Four sites were recruited for the ECARN study, which varied in location, size, and demographics (see Table 1): Kelsey-Seybold Clinic (Texas), the Women's Health Center of Albany Medicine (New York), the University of Chicago Medicine (Illinois), and Geisinger Health System (Pennsylvania). As an expansion of CARN, ECARN sites were recruited from the CARN member database from those who had expressed interest in conducting patient-centered research. Data collection was overseen by a lead medical provider at each site, who was responsible for collecting materials, shipping them to ACOG, and serving as a lead for answering any questions by medical staff or patients. Individual sites received approval from a local IRB, and ACOG research staff created and provided all sites with the appropriate materials for data collection, including patient and medical provider surveys, patient information sheets, data collection procedures for staff, site surveys, and return mailing materials. Data was collected

during the 2013-2014 flu season, September 2013 to April 2014, and during the 2014-2015 flu season, September 2014 to April 2015.

Patients were recruited by medical staff who were knowledgeable of the study and provided with an information sheet describing voluntary consent to participate. All pregnant patients were provided a questionnaire regarding their opinions and practices of the influenza vaccination and medical providers filled out a data sheet at the time of their visit. Each patient's medical record was marked to show they received the survey, but no identifiable information was collected with the survey or data sheet. All medical providers were similarly given a questionnaire to fill out at the beginning of data collection. In addition to OB/GYNs, one site also included non-MD obstetric providers (e.g., nurse midwives); however, given the small number (6), all medical providers were combined together for analysis. Two sites collected prospective medical record data on forms provided by ACOG which recorded basic information such as status of receiving the influenza vaccine and delivery outcomes. The two other sites conducted a retrospective data pull from their electronic medical records (EMR) after their survey collection period had ended. These results are discussed individually and combined as "medical record data" below.

All surveys were sealed in envelopes and collected by individual sites. Surveys and data sheets were sent to ACOG for analysis after the end of data collection. No identifying information was collected. Results were analyzed aggregately, by site, and combined. The majority of data was entered by hand by ACOG staff into Microsoft Excel 2013©, with the exception of two sites who provided an electronic format of their medical records. Data was analyzed using IBM SPSS Statistics 20.0, IBM Corp.©, Armonk, NY.

All responses indicating the patient had already accepted or had the intention to accept the influenza vaccine during pregnancy were grouped together and are referred to as accepted in this paper. These groups were combined due to variance in survey participation dates. Some patients received the survey at the beginning of the flu season; thus it was unlikely that they had accepted the vaccine already, and others received the survey at the end of the flu season. This is further discussed as a limitation below. A binary logistic regression was used to determine the significance of factors for accepting the influenza vaccination (no or yes). Independent variables included previous influenza vaccination practices, site, age, education, race, receiving a medical provider's recommendation, receiving educational materials, and patient belief scores. Similarly, a multinomial logistic regression was used to analyze factors influencing patient beliefs. Patient beliefs score ranged from 4 to 20, adding the score of 4 different questions pertaining to patient attitudes on their own and their baby's health and safety regarding the influenza vaccine. Each question asked patients to rate their beliefs on a 5-point scale, from "strongly disagree" (1) to "strongly agree" (5). Patient belief scores were grouped into 3 categories (4–9, 10–15, and 16–20) for the multinomial analysis. Similar to the binary logistic model, independent variables included previous influenza vaccination practices,

TABLE 1: Demographic information.

Data collection, flu season	Site 1 2013-2014	Site 2 2013-2014	Site 3 2014-2015	Site 4 2014-2015**	Total —
Medical provider demographics					
Sample size	11	33	8	24	76
Gender					
Female	54.5%	72.7%	62.5%	79.2%	71.1%
Male	45.5%	27.3%	37.5%	20.8%	28.9%
Mean year of birth*					
Female	1971	1978	1966	1977	1976
Male	1965	1960	1961	1966	1962
Total	1968	1973	1965	1975	1972
Years in practice					
Female	13.7	5.25	14.2	9.6	8.5
Male	17.2	23.6	20	15	19.7
Total	15.27	10.24	16.38	10.78	11.8
Patient demographics					
Sample size	280	365	66	273	984
Race					
Hispanic, Latino, or Spanish	34.9%	11.2%	6.9%	1.5%	13.1%
White	46%	66.8%	40.3%	96.7%	59%
Black or African American	25.2%	17.3%	41.7%	1.5%	14.8%
American Indian or Alaska Native	1.4%	0.3%	—	0.4%	.05%
Asian, Native Hawaiian, or other Pacific Islander	12.9%	7.4%	9.7%	1.8%	7.7%
Other	12.9%	6.6%	1.4%	1.8%	5.9%
Age					
Mean	30.86	28.97	30.98	28.69	29.6
18–27	23.1%	41.2%	19.7%	42.4%	35%
28–34	55.2%	41.8%	54.5%	45%	47.3%
35–47	21.7%	17%	25.8%	12.5%	17.7%
Education					
Less than high school diploma	2.5%	9.6%	—	5.2%	5.7%
High school diploma, GED, or equivalent	12.2%	28.7%	13.6%	27.4%	22.5%
More than high school diploma	85.3%	61.7%	86.4%	67.4%	71.5%

*Statistically significant at the 95% level.
**Medical record data also collected for the 2013-2014 flu season.

site, age, education, race, receiving a medical provider's recommendation, and receiving educational materials.

Patients were compared based on their previous influenza vaccination practices. Four groups were created to compare patient belief scores. Group A was comprised of patients who previously did not and continued not to get the vaccine. Group B was comprised of patients who previously accepted the vaccine but did not while pregnant. Group C was comprised of patients who previously did not but decided to get the vaccine while pregnant. Finally, Group D was comprised of patients who previously accepted the vaccine and continued to accept the vaccine when pregnant. An exploratory analysis of differences between the groups was conducted using Pearson chi-square tests.

3. Results

A total of 76 providers and 984 patients responded to the surveys (see Table 1). Providers were asked about

their attitudes and practices towards administration of the influenza vaccine, and patients were asked about their beliefs and practices towards getting the influenza vaccine. Medical records data served as a backup to the recall issues that come from surveys to show how many patients actually accepted the vaccination. Provider and patient perspectives, along with medical record data, are analyzed and compared below.

3.1. Medical Providers Self-Reports. The 76 medical providers included obstetrician-gynecologists attending physicians and residents, nurse practitioners, physician assistants, and nurse midwives and varied demographically across the four sites (Table 1). The only statistically significant difference was that male providers were more likely to be older, and, similarly, in clinical practice for more years than female providers ($p < .01$). Nearly all providers responded that primary or preventive care was an important part of their practice;

Table 2: Physician beliefs.

	Site 1 (%)	Site 2 (%)	Site 3 (%)	Site 4 (%)	Total (%)		
					F	M	T
Safety of administration in 1st trimester							
Not concerned	63.6	57.6	87.5	29.2	48.1	63.6	52.6
Slightly concerned	—	12.1	—	33.3	16.7	13.6	15.8
Concerned	18.2	9.1	—	16.7	14.8	4.5	11.8
Very concerned	18.2	21.2	12.5	20.8	20.4	18.2	19.7
Health of mother and fetus if flu is contracted							
Not concerned	—	—	—	—	—	—	—
Slightly concerned	—	3	—	—	1.9	—	1.3
Concerned	18.2	6.1	12.5	29.2	18.5	9.1	15.8
Very concerned	81.8	90.9	87.5	70.8	79.6	90.9	82.9

48.7% answered "very important," and 48.7% answered "important."

Providers were asked about their attitudes regarding safety of the influenza vaccine (Table 2). Neither site nor age was a significant factor in determining beliefs. Nearly one-third of medical providers (31.5%) were concerned or very concerned about safety of administration of influenza vaccine in the 1st trimester. Only in site 4 did a demographic variable prove statistically significant; female providers were more concerned than male providers ($p < .01$). All providers were concerned with the health of the mother and fetus if the mother contracted the flu during pregnancy (82.9% very concerned, 15.8% concerned, and 1.3% slightly concerned).

All providers recommended the influenza vaccine to their pregnant patients (Table 3). The majority (90.7%) recommended it during any trimester, and the remaining 9.3% recommended it any time after the 1st trimester. Sites varied in their responses; all of Site 1 providers recommended the vaccination during any trimester, whereas the remaining sites differed. However, this discrepancy was not statistically significant. Similarly, practice site was not statistically significant for providing educational materials, despite variation among responses (Table 3). Overall, 53.9% of providers reported they always provided educational materials, 27.6% sometimes provided educational materials, and 15.8% never provided educational materials. Within sites, gender was a significant factor for Sites 2 and 3. In Site 2, women were more likely to never or only sometimes provide educational materials than men (50% versus 22.2%; $p = .047$); however the opposite was found in Site 3 (100% of men never provided educational materials versus only 20% of women; $p < .01$).

3.2. Patient Self-Reports.

Overall, 77.9% of patients stated that they had already (71.1%) or were planning on (6.8%) accepting the influenza vaccine while pregnant. Individual sites ranged from 69.7% to 87.1% acceptance rates. The majority of patients who listed where they accepted the vaccination received it from their respective hospital group. Binary logistic regression was used to determine the significance of factors for accepting the influenza vaccination within individual sites and aggregated (see Supplementary Table 6 in Supplementary Material available online

at http://dx.doi.org/10.1155/2016/3281975). Within individual sites, the only significant variable was accepting the influenza vaccine in previous years. At Site 1, sometimes accepting the influenza vaccination increased the odds ratio by 3.804 ($p = .012$) and usually or always by an odds ratio of 27.296 ($p < .01$). At Site 2, sometimes accepting the influenza vaccination increased the odds ratio by 3.288 ($p < .01$) and usually or always by an odds ratio of 24.809 ($p < .01$). At Site 3, usually or always accepting the influenza vaccination increased the odds ratio by 18.308 ($p < .01$). At Site 4, sometimes accepting the influenza vaccination increased the odds ratio by 3.667 ($p < .01$) and usually or always by an odds ratio of 35.648 ($p < .01$).

Aggregated, the patient's individual beliefs and practices made a difference in vaccination acceptance. The binary logistic regression produced a Nagelkerke R square of .653 and the Hosmer and Lemeshow test produced a significance level of .683, indicating that the model is good fit. Among the covariates, for every 1-point increase in a patient's influenza vaccine belief score, the odds ratio of accepting the vaccine was increased by 1.708 ($p < .01$). Additionally, accepting the influenza vaccine usually or always in previous years increased the probability of accepting the influenza vaccine while pregnant, by an odds ratio of 4.867 ($p < .01$). Finally, a medical provider's recommendation also increased the odds ratio of accepting the vaccine by 2.603 ($p < .01$). Medical center site, education level, age, receiving educational materials, and race were not statistically significant.

Overall, patients had positive beliefs about the vaccination, which, as stated above, was a significant factor in accepting the influenza vaccination. Nearly half (49.5%) scored between 16 and 20, and another 40.8% scored between 10 and 15. Only 9.7% of patients scored between 4 and 9. Nearly all patients who scored above 16 accepted the influenza vaccination (98.3%), and most patients with a score of 4–9 declined the vaccine (84%). Patients who scored in the middle (10–15) produced the highest variation; 68.4% accepted the vaccination, and 31.6% did not accept the vaccination.

A multinomial logistic regression determined a number of factors which were statistically significant in the patient reporting positive beliefs about the influenza vaccine (see Supplementary Table 7). The likelihood ratio chi-square was

TABLE 3: Physician results.

	Provide educational materials			Recommend vaccine	
	Never	*Sometimes*	*Always*	*Any trimester*	*Any time after 1st trimester*
Site					
Site 1	—	9.1%	90.9%	100%	—
Site 2	21.2%	21.2%	51.5%	87.9%	12.1%
Site 3	25%	25%	50%	87.5%	12.5%
Site 4	12.5%	45.8%	41.7%	91.3%	8.7%
Total	*15.8%*	*27.6%*	*53.9%*	*90.7%*	*9.3%*

TABLE 4: Group characteristics.

	Group A $N = 168$	Group B $N = 18$	Group C $N = 167$	Group D $N = 489$	Pearson Chi-square p value
Influenza vaccine practices					
Accepted vaccine in previous years	No	Yes	No	Yes	
Accepted vaccine while pregnant	No	No	Yes	Yes	
Race					
Hispanic, Latino, or Spanish	18.6%	5.6%	7.8%	16.8%	
White	61.7%	66.7%	70.1%	69.7%	
Black or African American	19.8%	11.1%	19.8%	15%	.001
American Indian or Alaska Native	2.4%	—	0.6%	—	
Asian, Native Hawaiian, or other Pacific Islander	9%	22.2%	3.6%	6.8%	
Other	6.6%	—	6%	6.8%	
Age					
18–27	49.7%	35.3%	32.9%	30.7%	
28–34	36.5%	64.7%	52.7%	48.7%	.000
35–47	13.8%	—	14.4%	20.6%	
Education					
Less than high school diploma	3.6%	—	6%	4.8%	
High school diploma, GED, or equivalent	37.5%	33.3%	23.4%	17.4%	.000
More than high school diploma	58.9%	66.7%	70.7%	77.9%	
Received educational materials	50.9%	44.4%	70.7%	71.8%	.000
Received medical provider's recommendation	73.5%	61.1%	91.6%	89%	.000

106.752 ($p < .01$) and the Nagelkerke R square was .125. Only three independent variables were found to be statistically significant. Patient age was statistically significant to score 10–15 in comparison to the scoring in the lowest group, increasing the odds ratio by 1.056 ($p = .027$) for every 1-year increase. Patient age was also statistically significant in scoring 16–20; for every 1-year increase, the odds ratio increased by 1.095 ($p < .01$). In addition, having a high school degree decreased the probability of scoring 16–20 by 92.1% (odds ratio of .079; $p = .015$). Finally, receiving educational materials increased the odds ratio of scoring 16–20 by 2.287 ($p < .01$).

As stated above, the patient belief score had a strong effect on the likelihood of accepting the influenza vaccine while pregnant. To further explore this, we compared four groups of patients based on their past immunization history and acceptance of vaccination while pregnant (e.g., previously did not accept the vaccine but accepted the vaccine while pregnant; see Tables 4 and 5). Most interesting are groups B and C, patients who changed from their previous practice patterns. The majority of Group C answered "don't know" for believing people should get the influenza vaccine, and the rest disagreed more than agreed, however, for the remainder of the questions that indicated the importance of vaccine while pregnant and for the safety of their baby. This is stark contrast to those in Group A who had similar previous practices and continued to not accept the vaccine. The same pattern is true for Group B patients in comparison to Group D. Group B patients were overwhelmingly strong believers in flu shots (83.8%); however, they showed variance in the other answers. Most prominent was the fact that 44.5% of patients answered agree or strongly agree with concern about the flu shot harming the baby than concern for getting the flu, in comparison to Group D where only 17.3% agreed.

TABLE 5: Patient flu vaccine practices and beliefs.

	Opinion (%)				
	Strongly disagree	*Disagree*	*Don't know*	*Agree*	*Strongly agree*
I am a strong believer that people should get flu shots					
Group A	24.6	26.4	46.1	2.4	0.6
Group B	5.6	—	27.8	44.4	22.2
Group C	6.7	20.6	50.3	18.2	4.2
Group D	—	0.4	15.8	40.5	43.3
It is important for my health and safety to get a flu shot while I am pregnant					
Group A	25.1	34.7	34.1	6	—
Group B	5.6	—	27.8	44.4	22.2
Group C	1.8	4.8	24.8	40.6	27.9
Group D	—	0.2	6.3	33.9	59.5
It is important for the health and safety of my baby that I get a flu shot while I am pregnant					
Group A	4.8	16.4	26.1	28.5	24.2
Group B	5.6	5.6	33.3	33.3	22.2
Group C	0.6	4.9	22	42.1	30.5
Group D	—	0.4	8	31.8	59.8
I am more worried about the flu shot harming my baby than I am about what would happen if I get the flu					
Group A	4.8	16.4	26.1	28.5	24.2
Group B	—	27.8	27.8	5.6	38.9
Group C	12.3	38.9	27.2	15.4	6.2
Group D	27.3	40.9	14.6	7.6	9.7
Mean score					
Group A	9.24				
Group B	13.61				
Group C	14.11				
Group D	16.99				

These four groups were demographically different based on an exploratory analysis (see Table 5). Group A was more likely to be non-White, particularly Hispanic/Latino and Black/African American, younger, and less educated. Group C had the highest percentage of White patients, was older, and had a higher education. Group B was more likely to be Asian, Native Hawaiian, or Pacific Islander and also had a high school degree or higher. Group D also had higher percentages of Hispanic/Latino patients, were older, and had higher education. Most significantly, and similar to our statistical analysis findings, Groups C and D who accepted the vaccine had much higher rates of receiving the educational materials and medical providers' recommendations compared to Groups A and B (Table 5).

3.3. Discrepancies between Patients and Medical Providers. There were some discrepancies between patient and medical provider self-reports of practices and opinions. Medical providers were asked why they believe patients do not accept the influenza vaccination. Nearly all (85.5%) chose "(patients) are afraid it is not safe," and 65.8% chose "(patients) do not think they need vaccines." Another third wrote in additional

reasons, the majority of which were fear of needles and fear of getting sick. Medical providers' beliefs were fairly consistent with their patients'; however the majority of patients who gave answers for not accepting the vaccination were afraid of getting sick. A large amount of patients also stated that they do not think they need vaccines, they do not believe in the vaccine, or they are concerned it is not safe for their babies.

81.5% of medical providers stated they provided educational materials to their patients (53.9% always and 27.6% sometimes), but only 66.4% of patients reported receiving educational materials. There were significant differences among sites regarding educational materials. A larger number of patients at Sites 1 and 4 reported receiving educational materials, 74.3% and 68.4%, respectively, versus 60.2% in Site 2, and 60.6% at Site 3 ($p < .01$). Providers also differed within sites; 10 of the 11 providers in Site 1 reported providing educational materials always. The other 3 sites were fairly similar; more than 75% reported always or sometimes providing educational materials. Gender was also significant within sites; at Site 2 men were more likely to offer educational materials, but, at Site 3, women were more likely to offer educational materials. Similarly, 85.6% of patients reported receiving a recommendation from their medical provider while 100% of medical providers stated they recommend the vaccination. While the sites did not vary dramatically, Site 1 again was consistent in having 100% of providers recommend the vaccine at any trimester, compared to the other three sites, in which about 90% of providers recommended the vaccine at any trimester.

3.4. Discrepancies between Self-Reported Data and Medical Record Data. Overall, medical record data showed that only 36.1% of patients accepted the influenza vaccine. Averaging by site, 48.1% of patients accepted the influenza vaccine (Site 1: 53.6%; Site 2: 67.6%; Site 3: 38.9%; and Site 4: 32.1%). This was significantly lower than patient self-reports (77.9%). However, if sites are split between those who used prospective data (1 and 2) and those who conducted a retrospective data pull (3 and 4), medical records show that prospective data observed that 58% of patients accept the vaccine versus 80.6% of self-reports; and retrospective data observed that only 32.9% of patients accept the vaccine versus 72.8% of self-reports.

Of the patients who accepted the influenza vaccine, 74.5% accepted the influenza vaccination within their respective site's office/hospital which was similar to self-reported data. Other locations included the patients' place of employment, a referring doctor, or a commercial pharmacy. The percentage of patients who accepted the vaccine was pretty evenly split among trimesters: 30.1% during the 1st, 31.9% during the 2nd, and 38% during the 3rd. This split however may be accounted for by the patient's pregnancy dates and correspondence with flu season. We did not ask patients when they became pregnant; thus we cannot compare if the trimester of vaccination was correlated with how far long they were in their pregnancy. However, the majority of patients who were still pregnant at the end of the study accepted the influenza vaccine during the first trimester (47.4%) and 16.4% in the 2nd and 36.2% in the 3rd trimester. Patients who delivered full term accepted the influenza vaccine mainly in the 2nd trimester (43.3%) or 3rd trimester (41.9%). Similarly, 45.6% of patients who delivered prematurely accepted the vaccine in the 2nd trimester and 27.5% in the 3rd and 26.9% in the 1st trimester. The majority of patients who accepted the influenza vaccine delivered full term (47.3%) or were still pregnant (41.4%); 5.8% had a preterm delivery, and 1.4% miscarried or had a stillborn delivery.

4. Discussion

77.9% of patients self-reported accepting the influenza vaccination, and medical record data observed 36.1% of patients accepting the vaccination. There are a number of possibilities for the gap that exists between self-reported and medical record data, including overreporting by patients. Given that patients filled out the survey in their doctor's office, where influenza vaccines are socially desirable, patients may have overreported their willingness to accept the vaccine, when, in reality, they did not. Similarly, because the survey was voluntary, it is possible that those who filled out the questionnaire were more inclined than other patients who did not respond to the survey in favor of influenza vaccinations. The demographics of the sites which were primarily persons being White and highly educated may also skew the results and be missing a population of women who have lower rates of vaccination. Additionally, patient responses are limited by the date they filled out the survey (beginning and end of the flu season) and when their pregnancy began. It is possible, for example, that a woman received the influenza vaccine in October prior to becoming pregnant in January, and she still reported receiving the influenza vaccination. However, the majority of patients had already accepted the vaccine; only 6.8% reported a future intention.

An alternative is that medical record data was inaccurate. Two sites used data sheets over the course of the data collection period to record rates, and two sites conducted a data pull from their EMR which may be a limitation given medical provider recall error or show limitations with EMR data. Additionally, the stage of pregnancy each patient was in was difficult to compare. In one piece of EMR data, patients who delivered at the beginning of collection (e.g., September) and who had just begun their pregnancy at the end (e.g., April) were excluded given the likelihood that they would accept the vaccine during a different influenza season; however, we were not able to exclude these patients from the remaining sites. The difference between the prospective and retrospective data also suggests that EMR data may not be as accurate as intended. Retrospective studies utilizing medical records will search for items (i.e., the flu immunization) by codes primarily used for billing and are subject to errors of omission and commission by medical coders. A potential for underascertainment and misclassification bias exist. It is likely that a combination of EMR and self-reported limitation created the large gap. An additional sampling bias among patients, medical providers, and sites is also a limitation. The number of medical providers and patients varied by site which may suggest differences in practices depending on size or type of medical site.

Not surprisingly, a patient's beliefs had a strong impact on accepting the influenza vaccination while pregnant, and the greatest impact on vaccination was a patient's past immunization record (accepting the vaccine or not the same as previous years). In line with previous research, fear of contracting influenza, fear that the vaccine was unsafe, and belief of not needing the vaccine were all reasons women did not accept the vaccine, and belief of the positive benefits of vaccine was reason to accept the vaccine [8]. Our results also showed that receiving a recommendation from a doctor and receiving educational materials were significant factors in increasing the acceptance of the vaccination or impacting their beliefs, which are also in line with previous studies [8]. However, it is also important to note that only 18 patients changed their previous practices of vaccine acceptance to nonacceptance while pregnant. While the small number is better in terms of vaccine uptake, it also limits our ability to conduct further statistical analysis on why these patients changed.

The large number of patients who changed behaviors from nonacceptance to acceptance of vaccine indicates a success in increasing immunization among pregnant women.

The largest contrast within these patients compared to those who did not change their behavior was concern for the baby. Future research should consider ways to more effectively communicate to patients the safety and importance of the vaccine for the health of the baby, as well as research the difference between educational levels. Patients with a high school degree, but not more than a high school degree, were more likely to get the influenza vaccine and have positive beliefs about the vaccine, which could suggest targeting educational materials towards patients with lower and higher educational levels. While it seems contradictory that more education would reduce influenza vaccinations, one hypothesis could be that more educated women research a variety of media sources, including antivaccine reports and blogs. While not statistically significant in our logistic regression analyses, our exploratory analysis of patients who changed behaviors suggests that non-White women are less likely to accept the vaccine. These results are similar to other studies, which have shown that non-White and lower educated women are less likely to accept the flu vaccine as well [8]. However, our sample was primarily White and highly educated and therefore these results cannot be generalized to the larger US population without additional research and analysis.

5. Conclusion

In summary, our findings showed the importance of providing educational materials and a recommendation from a medical provider in acceptance of influenza vaccination. In addition, our findings suggested that non-White and less educated women may be less likely to accept the vaccine while pregnant. Future research should explore reasons pregnant patients would be inclined to change previous immunization behavior more thoroughly. In addition, our findings showed discrepancies between patients and medical providers self-reports and medical record data. Improving medical record tools, communication between medical providers and patients, and determining more accurate ways of measuring self-reported vaccination rates should also be considered for future research.

Disclosure

The funding agreement ensured the authors' independence in designing the study, interpreting the data, and writing and publishing the report.

Competing Interests

The authors declare that there are no competing interests regarding the publication of this paper.

Acknowledgments

Financial support for this study was provided in part by Grant UA6MC19010 from the Maternal and Child Health Bureau (Title V, Social Security Act, Health Resources and Services Administration, and Department of Health and Human Services).

References

[1] ACOG, "Influenza vaccination during pregnancy. Committee Opinion No. 608. American College of Obstetricians and Gynecologists," *Obstetrics & Gynecology*, vol. 124, pp. 648–651, 2014.

[2] Center for Disease Control, Science Summary: CDC Studies on Thimerosal in Vaccines, http://www.cdc.gov/vaccinesafety/pdf/cdcstudiesonvaccinesandautism.pdf.

[3] Institute of Medicine of the National Academies Press, Immunization Safety Review: Vaccines and Autism Immunization Safety Review Committee, 2004.

[4] S. E. Håberg, L. Trogstad, N. Gunnes et al., "Risk of fetal death after pandemic influenza virus infection or vaccination," *New England Journal of Medicine*, vol. 368, no. 4, pp. 333–340, 2013.

[5] Department of Health and Human Services, Healthy People 2020 topics and objectives: immunization and infectious diseases, http://www.healthypeople.gov/2020/topics-objectives/topic/immunization-and-infectious-diseases/objectives.

[6] J. R. Gorman, N. T. Brewer, J. B. Wang, and C. D. Chambers, "Theory-based predictors of influenza vaccination among pregnant women," *Vaccine*, vol. 31, no. 1, pp. 213–218, 2012.

[7] V. I. Shavell, M. H. Moniz, B. Gonik, and R. H. Beigi, "Influenza immunization in pregnancy: overcoming patient and health care provider barriers," *American Journal of Obstetrics and Gynecology*, vol. 207, no. 3, pp. S67–S74, 2012.

[8] C. Y. S. Yuen and M. Tarrant, "Determinants of uptake of influenza vaccination among pregnant women—a systematic review," *Vaccine*, vol. 32, no. 36, pp. 4602–4613, 2014.

14

Pelvic Surgical Site Infections in Gynecologic Surgery

Mark P. Lachiewicz,[1] Laura J. Moulton,[2] and Oluwatosin Jaiyeoba[2]

[1]Department of Gynecology and Obstetrics, Emory University School of Medicine, 1639 Pierce Drive, 4th Floor WMB, Atlanta, GA 30322, USA
[2]Cleveland Clinic Foundation, Women's Health Institute, Cleveland, OH, USA

Correspondence should be addressed to Mark P. Lachiewicz; mlachiewicz@gmail.com

Academic Editor: Per Anders Mardh

The development of surgical site infection (SSI) remains the most common complication of gynecologic surgical procedures and results in significant patient morbidity. Gynecologic procedures pose a unique challenge in that potential pathogenic microorganisms from the skin or vagina and endocervix may migrate to operative sites and can result in vaginal cuff cellulitis, pelvic cellulitis, and pelvic abscesses. Multiple host and surgical risk factors have been identified as risks that increase infectious sequelae after pelvic surgery. This paper will review these risk factors as many are modifiable and care should be taken to address such factors in order to decrease the chance of infection. We will also review the definitions, microbiology, pathogenesis, diagnosis, and management of pelvic SSIs after gynecologic surgery.

1. Introduction

The development of surgical site infection (SSI) results in significant patient morbidity. Postoperative infection remains the most common complication of surgical procedures in gynecology [1]. Prior to the advent of routine antimicrobial prophylaxis, pelvic infection rates after vaginal hysterectomy were as high as 33%, with pelvic cellulitis seen most frequently [2]. The widespread implementation of antibiotic prophylaxis prior to surgery, as well as recognition of modifiable risk factors for postoperative infection, has led to a significant reduction in postoperative infection rates. In a recent cross-sectional analysis of the 2005–2009 American College of Surgeon's National Surgical Quality Improvement Program participant data files, there was a 2.7% occurrence for superficial, deep, and organ space infections after hysterectomy [3]. This paper will review the definitions, microbiology, pathogenesis, and risk factors of pelvic SSIs after gynecologic surgery with a focus on vaginal cuff cellulitis, pelvic cellulitis, and pelvic abscesses. We will also review the diagnosis and management of these conditions.

2. Definition of Pelvic Infections after Gynecologic Surgery

The Centers for Disease Control and Prevention (CDC) defines a SSI as an infection occurring within 30 days of an operation occurring in one of 3 locations: superficial at the incision site, deep at the incision site, or in other organs or spaces opened or manipulated during an operation [4].

2.1. Superficial Incisional SSI Includes Vaginal Cuff Cellulitis. Infection involves only the skin and subcutaneous tissue of the incision and at least one of the following:

(1) purulent drainage with or without laboratory confirmation, from the superficial incision;

(2) organisms isolated from an aseptically obtained culture of fluid or tissue from the superficial incision;

(3) at least one of the following signs or symptoms of infection: pain or tenderness, localized swelling, redness, or heat and superficial incision being deliberately opened by surgeon, unless incision is culture-negative.

2.2. Deep Incisional SSI Includes Pelvic Cellulitis. The infection involves deep soft tissue (e.g., fascia, muscle) of the incision and at least one of the following:

(1) purulent drainage from the deep incision but not from the organ/space component of the surgical site;

(2) a deep incision which spontaneously dehisces or is deliberately opened by a surgeon when the patient has at least one of the following signs or symptoms: fever (>38°C), localized pain, or tenderness, unless incision is culture-negative;

(3) an abscess or other evidence of infection involving the deep incision being found on direct examination, during reoperation, or by histopathologic or radiologic examination.

2.3. Organ/Space SSIs Include Adnexal Infections and Pelvic Abscesses. Infection involves any part of the anatomy (e.g., organs and spaces) other than the incision that was opened or manipulated during an operation and at least one of the following:

(1) purulent drainage from a drain that is placed through a stab wound into the organ/space;

(2) organisms isolated from an aseptically obtained culture of fluid or tissue in the organ/space;

(3) an abscess or other evidence of infection involving the organ/space that is found on direct examination, during reoperation, or by histopathologic or radiologic examination [4].

3. Microbiology and Pathogenesis

Microbial contamination of the surgical site by endogenous skin or vaginal flora is a fundamental precursor to postoperative SSI. The risk of infection is significantly elevated when there is an increased concentration and virulence of contaminating bacteria. Quantitatively, it has been shown that the risk for developing an infection increases markedly if the operating site is contaminated with $>10^5$ microorganisms per gram of tissue. However, in the presence of foreign bodies, such as suture material, this required inoculum decreases to 10^3 microorganisms per gram of tissue [5–9]. Conversely, both systemic and local host immune defense mechanisms function to contain inoculated bacteria and prevent infection. Prophylactic antibiotics in the tissue augment the natural host immunity.

For most SSIs, the source of pathogens is the endogenous flora of the patient's skin, which consists of predominantly aerobic gram-positive cocci [7, 10]. However, gynecologic procedures pose a unique challenge in that potential pathogenic microorganisms may come from the skin or ascend from the vagina and endocervix to the operative sites, including the abdominal incision and vaginal cuff. The endogenous vaginal flora is a complex and dynamic mix of pathogenic and nonpathogenic bacteria composed of facultative and obligate anaerobic gram-positive and gram-negative species. Therefore, gynecologic SSIs are more likely to be polymicrobial and may include gram-negative bacilli, enterococci, group B streptococci, and anaerobes as a result of incisions involving the vagina and perineum. If the balance of pathogenic to nonpathogenic bacteria is disrupted, these bacteria can gain access to the sterile tissue of the pelvis and can lead to infection. Bacterial vaginosis (BV) is a well-documented risk factor for SSI after pelvic surgery, specifically vaginal cuff cellulitis. BV is a complex alteration in the vaginal flora resulting in an increased concentration of potentially pathogenic anaerobic bacteria at levels reported at 1000–10000-fold greater than normal [8, 10, 11].

The development of infection results from ineffective host defense mechanisms and insufficient antibiotic prophylaxis in the setting of a high bacterial inoculum in virulent species [9]. Microorganisms produce toxins and other virulence factors that increase their ability to invade, cause damage to, and survive within or on host tissue. In the case of postoperative pelvic abscess, it is hypothesized that blood, lymphatic and serous fluid, necrotic debris, and fibrillar hemostats can accumulate in the lower pelvis and around the vaginal vault and produce a simple fluid collection. This fluid collection can subsequently become infected through contamination from the skin, through the vaginal opening, or after bowel resections and may result in formation of pelvic abscess. The incidence of pelvic abscess in gynecologic surgery is estimated at 1% [8, 11–14].

4. Risk Factors

Multiple host and surgical factors have been identified that increase the risk of infectious sequelae after pelvic surgery. Many of these risk factors are modifiable and care should be taken to address such factors in order to decrease the chance of infection.

5. Host Risk Factors

The preoperative evaluation of a patient provides an excellent opportunity to evaluate for the presence of modifiable and nonmodifiable host risk factors for SSIs. A cross-sectional analysis of the 2005–2009 American College of Surgeon's National Surgical Quality Improvement Program patient files identified many risk factors for SSI [3]. Obesity significantly influences risk for gynecologic and obstetrical SSI, specifically in patients with a BMI of greater than 30 or with depth of subcutaneous tissue greater than 2 cm. Diabetes mellitus is associated with elevated risk of infection postoperatively, particularly in patients with perioperative serum glucose levels greater than 150 mg/dL and preoperative hemoglobin HbA_{1c} greater than 6.5%. Patients with preexisting medical illness such as diabetes should be medically optimized prior to surgery. Preoperative anemia and history of cerebrovascular accidents were also associated with deep and organ space SSI [3]. There are several other well-documented risk factors for SSI within the surgical literature including tobacco use, corticosteroid use, malnutrition, and increased age [15–19]. History of radiation to the surgical site also elevates risk of infection [7]. Bacterial vaginosis is associated with a significantly elevated risk of postoperative infections, specifically

TABLE 1: Antimicrobial prophylaxis in gynecologic surgery.

Type of procedure	Recommended agents	Alternative agents in pts with β-lactam allergy
Hysterectomy	Cefazolin, cefotetan, cefoxitin, or ampicillin-sulbactam[a]	Clindamycin or vancomycin + aminoglycoside[b]; or aztreonam alone; or fluoroquinolone alone[a,c]; or metronidazole + aminoglycoside or fluoroquinolone
Laparoscopic procedure, low-risk	None	None
Laparoscopic procedure, high-risk[d]	Cefazolin, cefoxitin, cefotetan, ampicillin-sulbactam[a]	Clindamycin or vancomycin + aminoglycoside[b]; or aztreonam alone; or fluoroquinolone alone[a,c]; or metronidazole + aminoglycoside or fluoroquinolone
Clean-contaminated cancer surgery	Cefazolin + metronidazole, cefuroxime + metronidazole, ampicillin-sulbactam[a]	Clindamycin

Adapted from [25].

[a] Due to increasing resistance of *Escherichia coli* to fluoroquinolones and ampicillin-sulbactam, local population susceptibility profiles should be reviewed prior to use.

[b] Gentamicin.

[c] Ciprofloxacin or levofloxacin; fluoroquinolones are associated with an increased risk of tendonitis and tendon rupture in all ages. However, this risk would be expected to be quite small with single-dose antibiotic prophylaxis. Although the use of fluoroquinolones may be necessary for surgical antibiotic prophylaxis in some children, they are not drugs of first choice in the pediatric population due to an increased incidence of adverse events as compared with controls in some clinical trials.

[d] Factors that indicate a high risk of infectious complications include emergency procedures, diabetes, long procedure duration, age of >70 years, American Society of Anesthesiologists classification of 3 or greater, pregnancy, immunosuppression, and insertion of prosthetic device.

vaginal cuff cellulitis. Therefore preoperative screening and treatment is an important deterrent to postoperative infection [11, 20]. Colonization or infection with other organisms at the time of operation including Group B streptococci, *Trichomonas*, *S. aureus* nasal carriage, and history of MRSA have been demonstrated to elevate risk [21–23]. Prolonged preoperative hospitalization should be avoided to decrease the risk of patients becoming colonized with nosocomial bacteria, as these microorganisms tend to be more resistant to antibiotics compared to endogenous bacteria [24].

6. Surgical Risk Factors

6.1. Preoperative Risk Factors. Prophylactic antibiotics decrease the bacterial inoculum burden on the skin and make the operative site less hospitable to the growth of bacteria. Furthermore, antibiotics concentrate in white blood cells resulting in enhanced phagocytosis of pathogenic bacteria [2]. The antibiotic of choice for prophylaxis should have broad coverage, be inexpensive, and be easy to administer. Cefazolin meets this criterion. Antibiotics should be administered within an hour of incision. Current recommendations for pre-op antibiotics were recently revised. Patients undergoing an extended procedure (≥ 3 hours) or with a total blood loss ≥ 1500 mL should receive a second dose of antibiotic. Obese women with a weight of ≥ 120 kg should receive an increased dose of antibiotics. For example, cefazolin should be increased to 3 grams in these patients, as opposed to the standard 2 grams in women with a weight of less than 120 kg. Recommended antimicrobial prophylaxis regimens, doses, and redosing intervals for gynecologic surgery are listed in Tables 1 and 2 [25].

Preoperative preparation of the skin and vagina with Povidone-Iodine or chlorhexidine gluconate is universally recommended to reduce risk of postoperative cuff cellulitis and abscess. Despite concerns about using chlorhexidine gluconate to prep the vagina, the American Congress of Obstetricians and Gynecologists (ACOG) recently supported the use of chlorhexidine gluconate to prep the vagina [26]. A recent analysis demonstrated an elevation in superficial SSI with route of hysterectomy, with the abdominal method associated with higher rate of infection compared to the vaginal approach. Comparatively, the rates of deep superficial and organ space infections were similar regardless of surgical approach [3].

6.2. Intraoperative Risk Factors. Intraoperative events including increased blood loss greater than 500 mL, prolonged surgical procedure greater than 140 minutes, and blood transfusion are associated with development of deep and organ space SSI [3, 13, 23]. Staple closure was associated with significantly increased wound infectious morbidity compared to closure with sutures in a randomized control trial by Figueroa et al. [27]. Fibrillar oxidized regenerated cellulose may contribute to pelvic abscess formation. The hemostatic agent can trap tissue debris, protect bacteria from host-defense mechanisms, and with unopposed bacterial proliferation lead to abscess formation [8].

For operations performed laparoscopically, direct trocar insertion and open technique may confer a lower postinfection rate than entry with the Veress needle [28]. Single-port laparoscopic hysterectomy appears to have a lower infection rate than traditional four-port laparoscopic hysterectomy [29]. Removal of fallopian tubes at the time of hysterectomy may also significantly decrease the risk of infectious complications [30]. Robotic-assisted procedures do not appear to confer any advantage versus convention laparoscopy from an infectious standpoint [31].

TABLE 2: Recommended doses and redosing intervals for commonly used antimicrobials for surgical prophylaxis for gynecological procedures[a].

Antimicrobial	Recommended dose	Half-life (hours)	Recommended redosing interval (hours)[b]
Ampicillin-sulbactam	3 g (ampicillin 2 g/sulbactam 1 g)	0.8–1.3	2
Aztreonam	2 g	1.3–2.4	4
Cefazolin	2 g, 3 g for pts weighing ≥120 kg	1.2–2.2	4
Cefuroxime	1.5 g	1-2	4
Cefoxitin	2 g	0.7–1.1	2
Cefotetan	2 g	2.8–4.6	6
Ciprofloxacin	400 mg	3-7	NA
Clindamycin	900 mg	2-4	6
Gentamicin	5 mg/kg based on dosing weight (single dose)[c]	2-3	NA
Levofloxacin	500 mg	6–8	NA
Metronidazole	500 mg	6–8	NA

Adapted from [25].

[a] Dosing and redosing interval for adult patients with normal renal function.

[b] Redosing in the operating room is recommended at an interval of approximately two times the half-life of the agent in patients with normal renal function. Recommended redosing intervals marked as "not applicable" (NA) are based on typical case length; for unusually long procedures, redosing may be needed.

[c] In general, gentamicin for surgical antibiotic prophylaxis should be limited to a single dose given preoperatively. Dosing is based on the patient's actual body weight. If the patient's actual weight is more than 20% above ideal body weight (IBW), the dosing weight (DW) can be determined as follows: DW = IBW + 0.4(actual weight − IBW).

Patients undergoing pelvic lymphadenectomy, para-aortic lymphadenectomy, splenectomy, bowel resection, or pelvic exenteration for surgical treatment of gynecologic malignancies are associated with increased risk of deep superficial and organ space SSIs [8, 23].

6.3. *Postoperative Risk Factors.* Postoperative anemia has been defined as a significant risk factor for all classifications of SSI in obstetrical and gynecologic surgery [32]. Poor glucose control, defined as levels greater than 200 mg/dL within the first 48 hours postoperatively, increased the likelihood of pelvic infections [33]. Increased length of duration of hospital stay perioperatively has also been correlated with increased incidence of SSIs [7].

7. Clinical Features and Management of SSI

Typically, postoperative pelvic infections, including vaginal cuff cellulitis and pelvic abscess, present with complaint of pelvic pain with fever with associated tachycardia and leukocytosis. The approach to management depends on the clinical status of the patient and characteristics of the pelvic infection. Appropriate antimicrobial therapy of pelvic abscesses includes coverage against aerobic and anaerobic bacteria with an ability to penetrate abscess cavities while remaining stable in an acidic, hypoxic environment, typical of an abscess [34].

8. Vaginal Cuff Cellulitis

Vaginal cuff cellulitis is an infection of the superficial tissues at the vaginal surgical margin after vaginal hysterectomy. Patients typically present after hospital discharge with moderate, but increasing, lower abdominal pain with purulent yellow vaginal discharge. Physical examination will reveal the vaginal surgical margin to be tenderness out of proportion to what is expected with hyperemia and edema. The adnexa and parametria are nontender. Treatment is outpatient oral antibiotic therapy with a single broad-spectrum agent with close follow-up to assure treatment efficacy [7, 9, 35].

Recommended regimens for treatment of vaginal cuff cellulitis include

(i) amoxicillin/clavulanate 875/125 mg PO bid,

(ii) ciprofloxacin 500 mg po bid with metronidazole 500 mg po bid,

(iii) TMP-SMX DS po bid with metronidazole 500 mg po bid [7].

9. Pelvic Cellulitis

Patient with pelvic cellulitis typically presents 5 to 10 days after surgery with fever, vague abdominal pain, or the sensation of pelvic fullness. Associated symptoms may include anorexia, but they typically do not have gastrointestinal or urinary complaints. Physical examination will reveal regional tenderness to palpation, with edema in the absence of masses or peritoneal signs. Ultrasound will demonstrate no masses. Hospitalization is indicated and patients should be treated with an intravenous broad-spectrum antibiotic regimen until they have been afebrile for 24–48 hours and may be discharged on an oral antibiotic regimen with coverage for gram-positive, gram-negative, and anaerobic bacteria [7, 36]. Antibiotics regimens are the same as for pelvic abscesses and are discussed below.

10. Pelvic Abscess

Pelvic abscesses are a rare but serious complication of pelvic surgery occurring when pelvic cellulitis or pelvic hematoma spread into the parametrial soft tissue [9]. Pelvic abscess symptoms mirror that of pelvic cellulitis, with the addition of a palpable mass corresponding to the collection of infected fluid or visualization of the fluid collection by ultrasonography, computed tomography (CT), or magnetic resonance image (MRI). As soon as the diagnosis is reached, broad-spectrum antibiotics should be administered intravenously until patient is afebrile for 48–72 hours. Drainage via ultrasound or CT guidance, laparoscopy, or laparotomy may be required [7, 36].

11. Antibiotic Therapy

Candidates for antibiotic therapy alone may be recommended for the following women:

(i) hemodynamically stable,

(ii) no signs of sepsis or rupture of the abscess,

(iii) adequate response to antibiotic therapy,

(iv) pelvic abscess ≤8 cm in diameter [37].

Patients are empirically started on antibiotics and one intravenous antibiotic regimen that has been studied extensively is the combination of clindamycin (900 mg every 8 hours) or metronidazole (500 mg every 12 hours) plus penicillin (5 million units every 6 hours) or ampicillin (2 g every 6 hours) plus gentamicin (5 mg/kg ideal body weight every 24 hours). Aztreonam (2 g every 8 hours) is substituted for gentamicin in patients who have renal impairment [38, 39].

Additional agents with therapeutic utility include single agent treatment with an extended-spectrum cephalosporin (e.g., cefoxitin, cefotetan, cefotaxime, and ceftizoxime), an extended-spectrum penicillin (e.g., piperacillin-tazobactam), beta-lactamase inhibitors plus a beta-lactam (e.g., ticarcillin-clavulanate), and carbapenems (ertapenem or meropenem) [38, 39].

While treatment regimens containing aminoglycosides have been used effectively in the treatment of pelvic abscesses, this class of antibiotics has their activity reduced at low pH, at low oxygen tension, and in the presence of drug-binding purulent debris [40]. Ceftriaxone is a third-generation cephalosporin that has a much higher serum level to minimum inhibitory concentration ratio when compared with aminoglycosides. It has high antibacterial potency, broad spectrum of activity, low potential for toxicity, and favorable pharmacokinetics. Furthermore, ceftriaxone is highly protein bound causing it to have the longest half-life of amongst the drugs in its class which translates to convenient once daily dosing [41].

Clindamycin is actively transported into polymorphonuclear leukocytes and macrophages and has been demonstrated in relatively high concentrations, compared with peak serum levels, in experimental abscesses [42]. An important use of clindamycin is in treatment of infections likely to involve B. fragilis or other penicillin-resistant anaerobic bacteria. It is beneficial where there is spillage of fecal flora, associated with tissue damage. Studies suggest that clindamycin decreases the likelihood of abscess formation involving fecal organisms like B. fragilis but must be coadministered

with an aminoglycoside, a third-generation cephalosporin like ceftriaxone or aztreonam, because additional activity is required against Enterobacteriaceae. Given reports of increasing resistance of Bacteroides species to clindamycin, use of clindamycin may be entirely replaced in the future with other agents, such as metronidazole, where resistant strains are rare [34, 43].

Based on the available literature, we recommend metronidazole (500 mg every 12 hours) plus ceftriaxone (2 g every 24 hours) as our first line treatment for pelvic abscesses.

Parenteral antibiotics should be continued until the patient is afebrile for 24–48 hours. Patient should subsequently receive oral antibiotics to complete a 14-day course of therapy. Patients should be switched to antibiotics based on culture and sensitivities when available. Combination of oral metronidazole (500 mg every 12 hours) and trimethoprim/sulfamethoxazole (160/800 mg every 12 hours) or amoxicillin/clavulanate (875/125 mg every 12 hours) monotherapy can be used due to excellent polymicrobial coverage [39].

12. Drainage or Surgical Therapy

Traditionally, the treatment algorithm was to start antibiotics and monitor a patient for improvement. Recent evidence suggests it is acceptable or may be of benefit to choose primary drainage with concomitant antibiotic therapy or after initiation of antibiotic therapy. Routine drainage of pelvic abscesses can decrease prolonged hospitalizations and improve reproductive outcomes [37, 44]. This strategy has been recommended as a first-line procedure especially in women of reproductive age. Drainage at an early time-point after admission to hospital is also more efficient than medical treatment alone with regard to treatment success in addition to decreasing mean hospital stay [45, 46].

Regardless, drainage should be performed if an adequate response to antibiotic therapy is not registered within 2-3 days or if the pelvic abscess is >8 cm [37, 47].

Criteria for failure may include the following:

(i) Patients with no radiological reduction in abscess size. Greater than a 50% reduction should be seen.

(ii) Patients whose abscess progressively increased in size.

(iii) New onset fever or persistent fevers.

(iv) Clinical deterioration with persistent or worsening abdominal/pelvic tenderness despite appropriate antibiotic therapy.

(v) Patients meeting criteria for sepsis. Septic patients should be continued on antibiotics and taken to the operating room for emergent operative treatment.

(vi) Ruptured or suspected intra-abdominal rupture of abscess. Abscess rupture is life-threatening emergency that can result in sepsis and septic shock. Ruptured abscess should be treated immediately. Surgical intervention is advocated in these patients to improve their outcome. These patients should also be continued on antibiotics and taken to the operating room for emergent operative treatment.

Drainage can be performed by laparoscopy and has several advantages compared to laparotomy [44]. However, CT- or ultrasound-guided drainage in combination with antibiotics has emerged as a preferred alternative approach in hemodynamically stable patients with excellent results, even with large abscesses [48, 49]. This approach has several advantages compared to antibiotic therapy alone as well as laparoscopy and antibiotics, including no required anesthesia, immediate pain relief, and reduced duration of hospital stay [46, 48]. Therefore, our preferred method of drainage is percutaneous drainage guided by CT or ultrasound. Pelvic cuff abscesses can also be drained by ultrasound guided transvaginal aspiration with excellent outcomes [50, 51]. If the abscess is accessible via the vaginal apex or cul-de-sac, a transvaginal aspiration may be a more appropriate option. While colpotomy or placement of a transvaginal drain (i.e., Foley or Malecot) has been used successfully in the past, the complication rate may be higher than aspiration alone without additional benefit [52–55]. Exudate should be sent for gram stain, culture, and sensitivity. Antibiotics should be adjusted based on culture and sensitivities.

Based on the above studies, our recommendations regarding drainage are the following: pelvic abscess >8 cm should be drained in addition to the administration of empiric parenteral antibiotics; cultures and sensitivities should be obtained; early drainage of a pelvic abscess is safe, improves outcomes, reduces hospitalization, and is appropriate for the clinician to consider as primary therapy; and the preferred method for drainage is percutaneous by the interventional radiologist or transvaginally if the patient is hemodynamically stable.

13. Summary and Recommendations

(i) Postoperative cuff and pelvic abscesses are among the most common complications of gynecologic surgeries.

(ii) Evaluation for preoperative and postoperative risk factors and managing modifiable risk factors can decrease infection rates.

(iii) Pelvic abscesses are usually polymicrobial and contain both aerobic and anaerobic bacteria.

(iv) Pelvic cellulitis typically presents 5 to 10 days after surgery with fever, vague abdominal pain, or the sensation of pelvic fullness. Pelvic abscess symptoms mirror that of pelvic cellulitis with the addition of a palpable mass corresponding to the collection of infected fluid or radiographic evidence of abscess.

(v) Approach to management depends on the clinical status of the patient and characteristics of the pelvic abscess. Treatment with antibiotics alone is appropriate for women who meet the following criteria: being hemodynamically stable, having pelvic abscess <8 cm in diameter, and having adequate response to antibiotic therapy.

(vi) Our recommended antibiotic regimen for pelvic abscesses is metronidazole (500 mg every 12 hours) plus ceftriaxone (2 g every 24 hours) (Table 3).

TABLE 3: Recommended antibiotic regimen for pelvic infections after gynecologic surgery.

Infection type	Antimicrobials	Duration of treatment
Vaginal cuff cellulitis	Oral regimen Amoxicillin/clavulanate 875/125 mg q 12 h OR Ciprofloxacin 500 mg q 12 h PLUS Metronidazole 500 mg q 12 h OR Trimethoprim/sulfamethoxazole 160/800 mg q 12 h PLUS Metronidazole 500 mg q 12 h	7–14 days
Pelvic cellulitis and pelvic abscesses[a]	Parenteral regimens Clindamycin 900 mg q 8 h or Metronidazole 500 mg q 12 h PLUS Ceftriaxone 2 g q 24 h OR Clindamycin 900 mg q 8 h or Metronidazole 500 mg q 12 h PLUS Penicillin 5 million u q 6 h or Ampicillin 2 g q 6 h PLUS Gentamicin 5 mg/kg IBW q 24 h OR Aztreonam 2 g q 8 h[b] Oral regimen Metronidazole 500 mg q 12 h PLUS Trimethoprim/sulfamethoxazole 160/800 mg q 12 h OR Amoxicillin/clavulanate (875/125 mg q 12)	14 days

[a] Parenteral antibiotics should be continued until the patient is afebrile for 24–48 hours. Patient should subsequently receive oral antibiotics to complete 14-day course of antibiotics.

[b] Aztreonam 2 g q 8 h may be substituted for gentamicin in patients who have renal impairment.

(vii) Minimally invasive drainage, laparoscopy, or exploratory laparotomy may be required in women with abscesses >8 cm or who show no signs of improvement but are not worsening clinically.

(viii) Clinically worsening patients, suspected rupture, and septic patients require immediate laparotomy which may be life-saving.

(ix) Duration of therapy is for at least 14 days or more depending on resolution of the pelvic abscess.

Conflict of Interests

The authors declare that there is no conflict of interests regarding the publication of this paper.

References

[1] Antibiotic Prophylaxis for Gynecologic Procedures, "Practice bulletin No. 104. American College of Obstetricians and Gynecologists," *Obstetrics & Gynecology*, vol. 113, no. 5, pp. 1180–1189, 2009.

[2] W. Jamie and P. Duff, "Preventing infections during elective C/S and abdominal hysterectomy," *Contemporary Obstetrics and Gynecology*, vol. 48, no. 1, pp. 60–69, 2003.

[3] A. G. Lake, A. M. McPencow, M. A. Dick-Biascoechea, D. K. Martin, and E. A. Erekson, "Surgical site infection after hysterectomy," *The American Journal of Obstetrics and Gynecology*, vol. 209, no. 5, pp. 490.e1–490.e9, 2013.

[4] T. C. Horan, R. P. Gaynes, W. J. Martone, W. R. Jarvis, and T. G. Emori, "CDC definitions of nosocomial surgical site infections, 1992: a modification of CDC definitions of surgical wound infections," *Infection Control and Hospital Epidemiology*, vol. 13, no. 10, pp. 606–608, 1992.

[5] R. C. James and C. J. MacLeod, "Induction of staphylococcal infections in mice with small inocula introduced on sutures," *British Journal of Experimental Pathology*, vol. 42, pp. 266–277, 1961.

[6] W. A. Altemeier, W. R. Culbertson, and R. P. Hummel, "Surgical considerations of endogenous infections—sources, types, and methods of control," *Surgical Clinics of North America*, vol. 48, no. 1, pp. 227–240, 1968.

[7] G. B. Lazenby and D. E. Soper, "Prevention, diagnosis, and treatment of gynecologic surgical site infections," *Obstetrics and Gynecology Clinics of North America*, vol. 37, no. 3, pp. 379–386, 2010.

[8] A. Fagotti, B. Costantini, F. Fanfani et al., "Risk of postoperative pelvic abscess in major gynecologic oncology surgery: one-year single-institution experience," *Annals of Surgical Oncology*, vol. 17, no. 9, pp. 2452–2458, 2010.

[9] C. Faro and S. Faro, "Postoperative pelvic infections," *Infectious Disease Clinics of North America*, vol. 22, no. 4, pp. 653–663, 2008.

[10] P. Duff and R. C. Park, "Antibiotic prophylaxis in vaginal hysterectomy: a review," *Obstetrics and Gynecology*, vol. 55, no. 5, pp. 193–202, 1980.

[11] D. E. Soper, "Bacterial vaginosis and postoperative infections," *The American Journal of Obstetrics and Gynecology*, vol. 169, no. 2, pp. 467–469, 1993.

[12] P. Duff, "Infections in pregnancy," in *Obstetrics and Gynecology: Principles for Practice*, F. W. Ling and P. Duff, Eds., pp. 125–127, McGraw-Hill, New York, NY, USA, 1st edition, 2001.

[13] W. M. Weinstein, A. B. Onderdonk, J. G. Bartlett, and S. L. Gorbach, "Experimental intra abdominal abscesses in rats: development of an experimental model," *Infection and Immunity*, vol. 10, no. 6, pp. 1250–1255, 1974.

[14] R. L. Sweet and R. S. Gibbs, "Mixed anaerobic-aerobic pelvic infection and pelvic abscess," in *Infectious Diseases of the Female Genital Tract*, R. L. Sweet and R. S. Gibbs, Eds., pp. 75–108, Williams & Wilkins, Baltimore, Md, USA, 1990.

[15] D. W. Spelman, P. Russo, G. Harrington et al., "Risk factors for surgical wound infection and bacteraemia following coronary artery bypass surgery," *Australian and New Zealand Journal of Surgery*, vol. 70, no. 1, pp. 47–51, 2000.

[16] H. Karim, K. Chafik, K. Karim et al., "Risk factors for surgical wound infection in digestive surgery. Retrospective study of 3,000 surgical wounds," *Tunisie Medicale*, vol. 78, no. 11, pp. 634–640, 2000.

[17] J. Gerberding, R. Gaynes, T. Horan et al., "National Nosocomial Infections Surveillance (NNIS) system report, data summary from January 1990–May 1999, issued June 1999," *The American Journal of Infection Control*, vol. 27, no. 6, pp. 520–532, 1999.

[18] R. Anielski and M. Barczyński, "Postoperative wound infections. III. Patient related risk factors," *Przegląd lekarski*, vol. 55, no. 11, pp. 565–571, 1998.

[19] E. C. Vamvakas and J. H. Carven, "Transfusion of white-cell-containing allogeneic blood components and postoperative wound infection: Effect of confounding factors," *Transfusion Medicine*, vol. 8, no. 1, pp. 29–36, 1998.

[20] P.-G. Larsson and B. Carlsson, "Does pre- and postoperative metronidazole treatment lower vaginal cuff infection rate after abdominal hysterectomy among women with bacterial vaginosis?" *Infectious Disease in Obstetrics and Gynecology*, vol. 10, no. 3, pp. 133–140, 2002.

[21] P. Litta, P. Vita, J. Konishi de Toffoli, and G. L. Onnis, "Risk factors for complicating infections after cesarian sections," *Clinical and Experimental Obstetrics and Gynecology*, vol. 22, no. 1, pp. 71–75, 1995.

[22] D. E. Soper, R. C. Bump, and W. G. Hurt, "Bacterial vaginosis and trichomoniasis vaginitis are risk factors for cuff cellulitis after abdominal hysterectomy," *The American Journal of Obstetrics and Gynecology*, vol. 163, no. 3, pp. 1016–1023, 1990.

[23] J. N. Bakkum-Gamez, S. C. Dowdy, B. J. Borah et al., "Predictors and costs of surgical site infections in patients with endometrial cancer," *Gynecologic Oncology*, vol. 130, no. 1, pp. 100–106, 2013.

[24] A. B. Cavanillas, R. Rodriguez-Contreras, M. D. Rodriguez et al., "Preoperative stay as a risk factor for nosocomial infection," *European Journal of Epidemiology*, vol. 7, no. 6, pp. 670–676, 1991.

[25] D. W. Bratzler, E. P. Dellinger, K. M. Olsen et al., "Clinical practice guidelines for antimicrobial prophylaxis in surgery," *The American Journal of Health-System Pharmacy*, vol. 70, no. 3, pp. 195–283, 2013.

[26] American College of Obstetricians and Gynecologists Women's Health Care Physicians; Committee on Gynecologic Practice, "Committee Opinion No. 571: solutions for surgical preparation of the vagina," *Obstetrics & Gynecology*, vol. 122, no. 3, pp. 718–720, 2013.

[27] D. Figueroa, V. C. Jauk, J. M. Szychowski, R. Garner, J. R. Biggio, and W. W. Andrews, "Surgical staples compared with subcuticular suture for skin closure after cesarean delivery: A randomized controlled trial," *Obstetrics and Gynecology*, vol. 121, no. 1, 2013.

[28] R. Angioli, C. Terranova, C. de Cicco Nardone et al., "A comparison of three different entry techniques in gynecological laparoscopic surgery: a randomized prospective trial," *European Journal of Obstetrics Gynecology and Reproductive Biology*, vol. 171, no. 2, pp. 339–342, 2013.

[29] M. Li, Y. Han, and Y. C. Feng, "Single-port laparoscopic hysterectomy versus conventional laparoscopic hysterectomy: a prospective randomized trial," *Journal of International Medical Research*, vol. 40, no. 2, pp. 701–708, 2012.

[30] F. Ghezzi, A. Cromi, G. Siesto, V. Bergamini, F. Zefiro, and P. Bolis, "Infectious morbidity after total laparoscopic hysterectomy: does concomitant salpingectomy make a difference?" *BJOG: An International Journal of Obstetrics & Gynaecology*, vol. 116, no. 4, pp. 589–593, 2009.

[31] E. B. Rosero, K. A. Kho, G. P. Joshi, M. Giesecke, and J. I. Schaffer, "Comparison of robotic and laparoscopic hysterectomy for benign gynecologic disease," *Obstetrics and Gynecology*, vol. 122, no. 4, pp. 778–786, 2013.

[32] T. A. Jido and I. D. Garba, "Surgical-site infection following Cesarean section in Kano, Nigeria," *Annals of Medical and Health Sciences Research*, vol. 2, no. 1, pp. 33–36, 2012.

[33] A. J. Mangram, T. C. Horan, M. Pearson et al., "Guideline for prevention of surgical site infection," *Infection Control and Hospital Epidemiology*, vol. 20, no. 4, pp. 247–264, 1999.

[34] J. Oteo, B. Aracil, J. I. Alós, and J. L. Gómez-Garcés, "High prevalence of resistance to clindamycin in *Bacteroides fragilis* group isolates," *Journal of Antimicrobial Chemotherapy*, vol. 45, no. 5, pp. 691–693, 2000.

[35] D. L. Stevens, A. L. Bisno, H. F. Chambers et al., "Practice guidelines for the diagnosis and management of skin and soft tissue infections," *Clinical Infectious Diseases*, vol. 41, no. 10, pp. 1373–1406, 2005.

[36] J. W. Larsen, W. D. Hager, C. H. Livengood, and U. Hoyme, "Guidelines for the diagnosis, treatment and prevention of postoperative infections," *Infectious Disease in Obstetrics and Gynecology*, vol. 11, no. 1, pp. 65–70, 2003.

[37] J. DeWitt, A. Reining, J. E. Allsworth, and J. F. Peipert, "Tuboovarian abscesses: is size associated with duration of hospitalization & complications?" *Obstetrics and Gynecology International*, vol. 2010, Article ID 847041, 5 pages, 2010.

[38] P. Duff, "Antibiotic selection in obstetric patients," *Infectious Disease Clinics of North America*, vol. 11, no. 1, pp. 1–12, 1997.

[39] P. Duff, "Antibiotic selection in obstetrics: making cost-effective choices," *Clinical Obstetrics & Gynecology*, vol. 45, no. 1, pp. 59–72, 2002.

[40] D. N. Gilbert and J. E. Leggett, "Aminoglycosides," in *Principles and Practice of Infectious Disease*, G. L. Mandel, J. E. Bennett, and R. Dolin, Eds., p. 367, Churchill-Livingstone Elsevier, Philadelphia, Pa, USA, 7th edition, 2010.

[41] D. R. Andes and W. A. Craig, "Cephalosporins," in *Principles and Practice of Infectious Disease*, G. L. Mandel, J. E. Bennett, and R. Dolin, Eds., pp. 334–335, Churchill Livingstone, Philadelphia, Pa, USA, 7th edition, 2010.

[42] S. Sivapalasingam and N. H. Steigbigel, "Macrolides, clindamycin, and ketolides," in *Principles and Practice of Infectious Disease*, G. L. Mandel, J. E. Bennett, and R. Dolin, Eds., pp. 442–443, Churchill Livingstone Elsevier, Philadelphia, Pa, USA, 7th edition, 2010.

[43] R. Schaumann, M. Funke, E. Janssen, and A. C. Rodloff, "*In Vitro* activities of clindamycin, imipenem, metronidazole, and piperacillin-tazobactam against susceptible and resistant isolates of *Bacteroides fragilis* evaluated by kill kinetics," *Antimicrobial Agents and Chemotherapy*, vol. 56, no. 6, pp. 3413–3416, 2012.

[44] M. Rosen, D. Breitkopf, and K. Waud, "Tubo-ovarian abscess management options for women who desire fertility," *Obstetrical and Gynecological Survey*, vol. 64, no. 10, pp. 681–689, 2009.

[45] M. A. Aboulghar, R. T. Mansour, and G. I. Serour, "Ultrasonographically guided transvaginal aspiration of tuboovarian abscesses and pyosalpinges: an optional treatment for acute pelvic inflammatory disease," *The American Journal of Obstetrics and Gynecology*, vol. 172, no. 5, pp. 1501–1503, 1995.

[46] T. Perez-Medina, M. A. Huertas, and J. M. Bajo, "Early ultrasound-guided transvaginal drainage of tubo-ovarian abscesses: a randomized study," *Ultrasound in Obstetrics and Gynecology*, vol. 7, no. 6, pp. 435–438, 1996.

[47] S. D. Reed, D. V. Landers, and R. L. Sweet, "Antibiotic treatment of tuboovarian abscess: comparison of broad-spectrum β-lactam agents versus clindamycin-containing regimens," *The American Journal of Obstetrics and Gynecology*, vol. 164, no. 6, pp. 1556–1562, 1991.

[48] K. Gjelland, E. Ekerhovd, and S. Granberg, "Transvaginal ultrasound-guided aspiration for treatment of tubo-ovarian abscess: a study of 302 cases," *The American Journal of Obstetrics and Gynecology*, vol. 193, no. 4, pp. 1323–1330, 2005.

[49] N. Goharkhay, U. Verma, and F. Maggiorotto, "Comparison of CT- or ultrasound-guided drainage with concomitant intravenous antibiotics vs. intravenous antibiotics alone in the management of tubo-ovarian abscesses," *Ultrasound in Obstetrics & Gynecology*, vol. 29, no. 1, pp. 65–69, 2007.

[50] P. J. Corsi, S. C. Johnson, B. Gonik, S. L. Hendrix, S. G. McNeeley Jr., and M. P. Diamond, "Transvaginal ultrasound-guided aspiration of pelvic abscesses," *Infectious Diseases in Obstetrics and Gynecology*, vol. 7, no. 5, pp. 216–221, 1999.

[51] A. L. Nelson, R. M. Sinow, R. Renslo, M. J. Renslo, and F. Atamdede, "Endovaginal ultrasonographically guided transvaginal drainage for treatment of pelvic abscesses," *The American Journal of Obstetrics and Gynecology*, vol. 172, no. 6, pp. 1926–1935, 1995.

[52] M. E. Rivlin, "Clinical outcome following vaginal drainage of pelvic abscess," *Obstetrics and Gynecology*, vol. 61, no. 2, pp. 169–173, 1983.

[53] M. R. N. Darling, A. Golan, and A. Rubin, "Colpotomy drainage of pelvic abscesses," *Acta Obstetricia et Gynecologica Scandinavica*, vol. 62, no. 3, pp. 257–259, 1983.

[54] M. E. Rivlin, A. Golan, and M. R. Darling, "Diffuse peritoneal sepsis associated with colpotomy drainage of pelvic abscess," *Journal of Reproductive Medicine for the Obstetrician and Gynecologist*, vol. 27, no. 7, pp. 406–410, 1982.

[55] P. R. Rubenstein, D. R. Mishell Jr., and W. J. Ledger, "Colpotomy drainage of pelvic abscess," *Obstetrics and Gynecology*, vol. 48, no. 2, pp. 142–145, 1976.

15

Antiretroviral Resistance and Pregnancy Characteristics of Women with Perinatal and Nonperinatal HIV Infection

Gweneth B. Lazenby,[1] Okeoma Mmeje,[2] Barbra M. Fisher,[3]
Adriana Weinberg,[3] Erika K. Aaron,[4] Maria Keating,[4] Amneris E. Luque,[5]
Denise Willers,[6] Deborah Cohan,[7] and Deborah Money[8]

[1]Department of Obstetrics and Gynecology, Medical University of South Carolina, 96 Jonathan Lucas Street, Suite 624,
 Charleston, SC 29425, USA
[2]Department of Obstetrics and Gynecology, University of Michigan, L4100 Women's Hospital, 1500 East Medical Center Drive,
 Ann Arbor, MI 48109, USA
[3]Department of Pediatrics, University of Colorado Anschutz Medical Campus, 12700 E. 19th Box B168, Aurora, CO 80045, USA
[4]Department of Medicine, Drexel University, 1427 Vine Street, 2nd Floor, Philadelphia, PA 19102, USA
[5]Department of Medicine, University of Rochester, 601 Elmwood Avenue, Box 689, Rochester, NY 14642, USA
[6]Department of Obstetrics and Gynecology, Washington University, 4921 Parkview Place, St. Louis, MO 63110, USA
[7]Department of Obstetrics and Gynecology, University of California, 350 Parnassus Avenue No. 908, San Francisco, CA 94117, USA
[8]Department of Obstetrics and Gynecology, University of British Columbia, 1190 Hornby Street, 4th Floor, Vancouver,
 BC, Canada V6Z 2K5

Correspondence should be addressed to Gweneth B. Lazenby; lazenbgb@musc.edu

Academic Editor: Bryan Larsen

Objective. To compare HIV drug resistance in pregnant women with perinatal HIV (PHIV) and those with nonperinatal HIV (NPHIV) infection. *Methods.* We conducted a multisite cohort study of PHIV and NPHIV women from 2000 to 2014. Sample size was calculated to identify a fourfold increase in antiretroviral (ARV) drug resistance in PHIV women. Continuous variables were compared using Student's t-test and Wilcoxon rank-sum tests. Categorical variables were compared using χ^2 and Fisher's exact tests. Univariate analysis was used to determine factors associated with antiretroviral drug resistance. *Results.* Forty-one PHIV and 41 NPHIV participants were included. Women with PHIV were more likely to have drug resistance than those with NPHIV ((55% versus 17%, $p = 0.03$), OR 6.0 (95% CI 1.0–34.8), $p = 0.05$), including multiclass resistance (15% versus 0, $p = 0.03$), and they were more likely to receive nonstandard ARVs during pregnancy (27% versus 5%, $p = 0.01$). PHIV and NPHIV women had similar rates of preterm birth (11% versus 28%, $p = 0.08$) and cesarean delivery (47% versus 46%, $p = 0.9$). Two infants born to a single NPHIV woman acquired HIV infection. *Conclusions.* PHIV women have a high frequency of HIV drug resistance mutations, leading to nonstandard ARVs use during pregnancy. Despite nonstandard ARV use during pregnancy, PHIV women did not experience increased rates of adverse pregnancy outcomes.

1. Introduction

Less than one percent of women living with HIV have perinatally acquired HIV infection (PHIV). According to recent Centers for Disease Control and Prevention (CDC) HIV surveillance data, approximately 2,388 PHIV women are living in the United States [1]. Due to lifelong HIV infection, many women with PHIV have been exposed to multiple antiretroviral (ARV) therapy regimens. These exposures may include inadequate therapy during periods when there were limited ARV therapy options, such as mono and dual therapy. As a consequence of suboptimal therapy, inconsistent drug adherence, and/or prolonged intermittent exposure to multiple ARV classes, PHIV women may have HIV that has developed significant drug resistance [2–5].

Antiretroviral drug resistance can limit options for therapy during pregnancy and potentially complicate obstetrical care for HIV-infected women. PHIV women who have developed ARV drug resistance may require ARV therapies which are less well studied in pregnancy and may have unknown toxicities [6, 7]. Potentially secondary to noncompliance or a suboptimal ARV regimen, PHIV patients may have poor viral suppression during pregnancy resulting in cesarean delivery and a higher risk of perinatal transmission [3, 4, 8, 9]. Examples of other risks specific to PHIV pregnant women include complex psychosocial issues, unplanned pregnancies, and transmission of HIV to susceptible partners [3, 6, 10, 11].

ARV resistance rates have been reported as high as 30–50% in PHIV pregnant women [4, 9, 12]. ARV resistance mutations and drug classes affected are not well described in previous studies of PHIV pregnant women [4, 9, 12]. The primary objective of this study was to determine if PHIV pregnant women are more likely than pregnant women with nonperinatal HIV infection (NPHIV) to have ARV drug resistance. We describe the ARV classes affected by HIV genotypic mutations in both PHIV and NPHIV women. Our secondary objective is to describe and compare potential adverse maternal and neonatal outcomes among PHIV and NPHIV pregnant women.

2. Materials and Methods

The primary objective of this study was to determine how much more likely PHIV women are to have HIV genotypic mutations that confer clinically significant ARV resistance during pregnancy compared to NPHIV women. Prior data indicated the probability of genotypic resistance to ARVs, specifically nonnucleoside reverse transcriptase inhibitors (NNRTIs), in drug naïve NPHIV pregnant women to be 13–17% [13]. Based on previous reports, PHIV women may have ARV resistance rates as high as 50%. We anticipated a noncollinear relationship between ARV resistance and timing of HIV infection. In order to demonstrate odds ratio of at least 4.0 (13% × 4 = 52%) for ARV resistance in PHIV pregnant women relative to NPHIV women, 41 cases (PHIV) and 41 controls (NPHIV) were required to reject the null hypothesis that this odds ratio equals one with a probability of 0.8. The Type I error probability associated with this test of the null hypothesis was 0.05. The study was not powered to determine differences in pregnancy outcomes between PHIV and NPHIV.

Because PHIV is a rare condition in pregnancy, a multisite, retrospective cohort study was conducted to enroll the necessary sample size of PHIV participants. To identify potential study sites, an email was sent to all providers participating in the Reproductive Infectious Diseases listserv (ReproIDHIV Listserv) [14]. Collaborators from twenty-two sites responded with interest and were provided a copy of the protocol. Seven sites at academic medical centers in British Columbia, California, Colorado, Missouri, New York,

Pennsylvania, and South Carolina elected to participate and the study protocol was approved by the institutional review boards at each site (IRB #13184). The study was supported by the departmental resources of the investigators.

Pregnant women with PHIV who received prenatal care at any of the study sites from 2000 to 2014 were eligible for participation. A woman was considered to have PHIV if her HIV serostatus was confirmed and determined to be acquired from her biological, serostatus-confirmed HIV-infected mother in the absence of any other risk factors (i.e., blood transfusion). Investigators at all 7 sites were responsible for identifying PHIV women for the study. Control participants were identified as pregnant women with NPHIV receiving prenatal care during the study period at any study site. A woman was considered to have NPHIV if she was diagnosed with HIV at ≥ 11 years of age in the absence of questionable perinatal infection (HIV-infected mother) or other risk factors for childhood infection (breastfeeding from an HIV-infected mother or blood transfusion). NPHIV participants were selected based on a similar age to study participants (± 1 year of age). Participants were age-matched in order to reduce an uneven distribution of age-related medical comorbidities, such as preexisting hypertension and diabetes, which may potentially impact pregnancy outcomes. The majority of NPHIV were identified by the Principal Investigator from one academic institution.

The medical records of participants were reviewed by site specific investigators to obtain data from maternal antepartum, intrapartum, and postpartum care. Variables of interest were collected for all participants when available. Maternal variables included age, race, ethnicity, marital status, insurer, current partner's HIV status, history of opportunistic infections, existing medical and psychiatric diagnoses, gestational age at entry into prenatal care and at delivery, HIV RNA viral load (copies/mL) and CD4 cell count (cells/mm^3) at entry into prenatal care and at delivery, ARV regimens before, during, and after pregnancy, HIV genotypic mutations associated with clinical drug resistance, evidence of sexually transmitted infections ((STIs): *Neisseria gonorrhea*, *Chlamydia trachomatis*, *Trichomonas vaginalis*, *Treponema pallidum*, human papilloma virus, hepatitis B and C, and herpes simplex virus), number of prenatal visits, antepartum complications, intrapartum prophylaxis IV zidovudine (AZT) when indicated, mode of delivery, postpartum infections including chorioamnionitis, and birth outcomes (e.g., live birth, intrauterine fetal demise, and spontaneous or elective abortion). Maternal antepartum complications of interest were hypertensive disorders of pregnancy, diabetes, maternal infection(s), preterm labor, anemia, and fetal anomaly and/or aneuploidy. In participants who gave birth to a live infant, data were collected from neonatal records up to 18 months of age. Variables of interest included birth weight, Apgar scores, level of nursery admit, neonatal postexposure ARV prophylaxis, duration of ARV prophylaxis, and HIV status. Neonates were considered HIV-infected if at least two positive HIV DNA PCR tests were confirmed before 18 months of age [15]. To protect confidentiality, all participants' data were deidentified.

TABLE 1: Maternal characteristics of pregnant women with perinatal and nonperinatal HIV infection.

	Perinatal HIV ($n = 41$)	Nonperinatal HIV ($n = 41$)	p value
Mean age, (years)	20.9 (±3.2)	21.7 (±3.1)	0.2
Black/African American	21 (51%)	29 (71%)	0.07
Hispanic/Latino	5 (12%)	4 (10%)	1.0
Mean years living with HIV infection	20.5 (±3.5)	2.4 (±2.8)	<0.0001
Current HIV-infected sexual partner	1/24 (4%)	7/22 (32%)	0.02
Parity	0 (0-1)	1 (0–2)	0.0004
History of sexually transmitted infection(s) (STI)	22 (51%)	25 (61%)	0.5
History of abnormal pap smear	17/37 (46%)	8/38 (21%)	0.02
Hepatitis B and/or C coinfection	2 (5%)	3 (8%)	0.7
History of opportunistic infection(s)	7/40 (18%)	0	
History of a psychiatric illness, including depression	20/40 (50%)	11 (27%)	0.03
Medical comorbidity[a]	12 (29%)	19 (46%)	0.11
STI diagnosis during pregnancy	5 (13%)	11 (27%)	0.11

All denominators are $n = 41$ unless otherwise stated. Continuous variables are represented as means (±standard deviation) and medians (interquartile range). Continuous variables are compared using Student's t-test for means, pooled for equal variances and Wilcoxon rank-sum tests are used to compare medians. Medical comorbidities excluding HIV, hepatitis, and psychiatric illness, including hypertensive disorders, asthma, anemia, cholelithiasis, transaminitis, obesity, and neuropathy[a].

Study site investigators collected and managed data using REDCap™ (Research Electronic Data Capture), a secure, web-based application designed to support data capture [16]. Statistical analysis was performed using SAS® 9.4 software (Cary, N.C.). Continuous variables were compared using Student's t-test (means) and Wilcoxon rank-sum tests (medians). Continuous variables were tested for normality, and medians were compared when data were not normally distributed. Categorical variables were compared using χ^2 and Fischer's exact tests. Univariate logistic regression was used to determine factors associated with the presence of ARV drug resistance.

3. Results

As determined by the sample size calculation, 41 PHIV and 41 NPHIV women were included in the analysis (Figure 1). The mean age of participants at the time of pregnancy was 21 years (standard deviation (SD) ± 3) with a range of 14–30 years. The median parity of women was one (interquartile range (IQR), 0-1). The median gestational age at which women presented for prenatal care was 11 weeks (IQR, 7–14 weeks), and the mean number of prenatal visits prior to delivery was 10 (SD ± 5). The HIV status of the participants' male partner was recorded in approximately half of the women. NPHIV women were more likely to report an HIV-infected partner(s) than PHIV women (32% versus 4%, $p = 0.02$). When comparing PHIV and NPHIV women, there were no differences in race, ethnicity, age, and prenatal care initiation or duration. NPHIV women were more likely to be parous than PHIV women (1 (IQR 0–4) versus 0 (IQR 0–2), $p = 0.0004$), and PHIV women were more likely to have a history of abnormal cervical cytology (50% versus 27%, $p = 0.03$). All pregnancies were singleton gestations (Tables 1 and 2).

The mean duration of known HIV infection for PHIV women was 21 (SD ± 4) years and it was 2 (SD ± 3) years

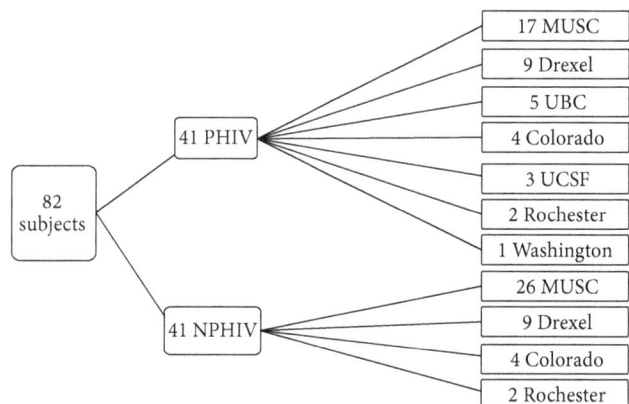

FIGURE 1: Site recruitment of pregnant women with perinatal and nonperinatal HIV infection. Site key: MUSC, Medical University of South Carolina, Charleston, SC; Drexel, Drexel University, Philadelphia, PA; UBC, University of British Columbia, Vancouver, BC; Colorado, University of Colorado, Aurora, CO; UCSF, University of California San Francisco, San Francisco, CA; Rochester, University of Rochester, Rochester, NY; Washington, Washington University, Saint Louis, MO.

for NPHIV women ($p < 0.0001$). Of the participants with NPHIV infection, 21 were diagnosed with HIV within one year of pregnancy and 20 were known to have HIV of duration of more than one year. Forty-three percent of all participants (36/82) reported current ARV use at initial presentation for prenatal care. PHIV women were more likely to report taking ARVs at presentation (68% versus 23%, $p = 0.006$). Although only 27 PHIV women were on ARVs at conception, all PHIV women in this study were exposed to ARVs during their lifetime prior to enrollment. The specific ARV regimens prescribed to individual subjects throughout their lives prior to enrollment in this study are not available for inclusion in

Table 2: Antepartum, intrapartum, and neonatal findings among pregnant women with perinatal HIV and nonperinatal HIV infection.

	Perinatal HIV ($n = 41$)	Nonperinatal HIV ($n = 41$)	p value
Antepartum			
Gestational age in weeks at initial obstetric visit[a]	11 (6–14)	11 (8–18)	0.2
ARV use at time of conception	27 (68%)	9 (23%)	<0.0001
Initial HIV RNA viral load (copies/mL) in pregnancy	19,945 (99–20,915)	4,800 (41–19,047)	0.8
Initial CD4 cell count (cells/mm³) in pregnancy	426 (±271)	516 (±212)	0.1
Number of obstetric visits prior to delivery	10.4 (±5.2)	9.9 (±5.3)	0.7
Pregnancy complications[b]	17/38 (45%)	24 (59%)	0.2
ARV use during pregnancy prior to delivery	41 (100%)	38 (93%)	0.2
Intrapartum and postpartum			
Gestational age at delivery	38 (38–39)	38 (34–39)	0.4
Preterm delivery (<37 weeks)	4/37 (11%)	11/39 (28%)	0.08
HIV RNA viral load (copies/mL) at delivery	40 (0–2,500)	0 (0–1,680)	0.3
HIV RNA viral load > 1,000 copies/mL at delivery	10 (26%)	11 (28%)	0.9
HIV RNA viral load < 40 copies/mL at delivery	23 (56%)	26 (63%)	0.5
CD4 cell count (cells/mm³) at delivery[a]	484 (265–612)	514 (373–646)	0.2
CD4 cell count (cells/mm³) below 200 at delivery	11 (27%)	4 (10%)	0.08
IV AZT administered at least 3 hours prior to delivery when indicated	28/35 (80%)	31/37 (84%)	0.7
Cesarean delivery	18/38 (47%)	18/39 (46%)	0.9
Any maternal intrapartum or postpartum infection	5/37 (14%)	7/38 (18%)	0.6
Neonatal			
Live birth	37/38 (97%)	39/40 (98%)	1.0
Birth weight (gm)[a]	3,065 (2,659–3,370)	2,742 (2,435–3,200)	0.02
Low birth weight (<2,500 gm)	8/37 (22%)	13/38 (34%)	0.2
NICU admission	5/35 (14%)	10/35 (29%)	0.2
Duration of postexposure prophylaxis with oral AZT (weeks)	6 (6)	6 (6)	0.6
Perinatal HIV infection	0/30	2/32 (6%)	0.5

All denominators are $n = 41$ unless otherwise stated. Continuous variables are represented as means (±standard deviation) and medians (interquartile range). Continuous variables are compared using Wilcoxon rank-sum tests to compare medians (Monte Carlo estimates were used to compare some medians[a]) and pooled Student's t-test is used for means. Pregnancy complications included hyperemesis gravidarum, urinary tract infection/pyelonephritis, hypertensive disorders of pregnancy, cervical incompetence, threatened preterm labor, abruption, preterm birth (<37 weeks), preterm rupture of membranes, and anemia[b].

this study. Of the NPHIV participants with HIV diagnosis greater than one year, only 30% reported current ARV use at initial presentation for prenatal care. The median HIV RNA viral load (copies/mL) and mean CD4 cell count (cells/mm³) collected within three months of the initial prenatal visit were not significantly different between PHIV and NPHIV women. Of the women reporting ARV use at their initial pregnancy visit, PHIV women were more likely than NPHIV women to have HIV RNA viral load $\geq 1,000$ copies/mL (46% versus 0, $p = 0.01$) (Tables 1 and 2).

Over half of participants (24 PHIV and 25 NPHIV) had an HIV RNA viral load $\geq 1,000$ copies/mL at their initial prenatal evaluation. When using an HIV RNA viral load $\geq 1,000$ copies/mL as criteria for collecting a genotype (HIV-1 genotype, ViroSeq®, ARUP laboratories, Salt Lake City, UT), 60% of participants would have been eligible for genotypic testing for HIV drug resistance. Not all participants who were eligible for resistance testing had a genotype collected within three months of their initial pregnancy visit. Collection of an HIV genotype during this time period was reported in 34 (42%) participants. Although similar numbers of PHIV

and NPHIV women met criteria for resistance evaluation by genotype (24 PHIV and 25 NPHIV), PHIV participants were more likely to have genotypic testing collected within three months of their initial pregnancy visit compared to NPHIV counterparts (22 PHIV (54%) and 12 NPHIV (29%), $p = 0.03$). When accounting for genotype collection within three months of presentation for prenatal care, 55% PHIV versus 17% NPHIV had drug resistance ($p = 0.03$) (Figure 2).

In addition to genotype resistance noted in 12 PHIV and two NPHIV women within three months of initial prenatal care, ARV drug resistance was documented for seven additional participants either before pregnancy or during pregnancy. ARV drug resistance was documented in 21 participants (17 PHIV and four NPHIV), but 18 resistance patterns were available for analysis (15 PHIV and 3 NPHIV participants). Drug resistance to the NNRTI class was the most common mutation for both groups. Multiclass ARV drug resistance, resistance to more than one ARV class, occurred exclusively in PHIV women (16% versus 0, $p = 0.03$). Genotypic resistance to multiple ARV drug classes was documented in 6 PHIV women (NRTIs $n = 6$, NNRTIs $n = 11$, and protease

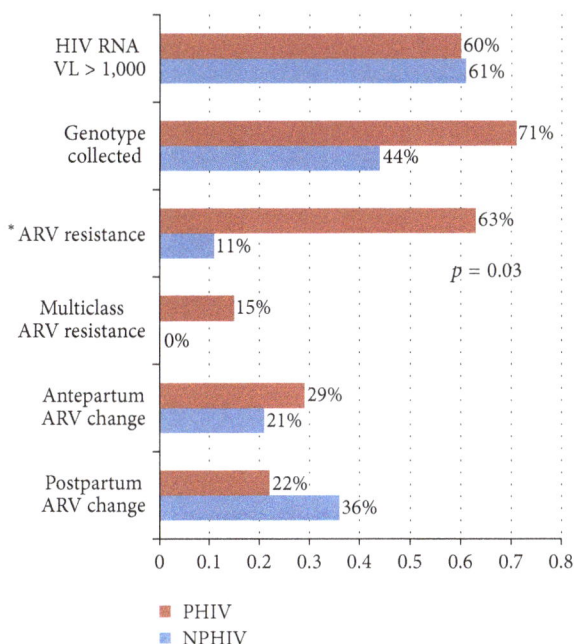

FIGURE 2: Antiretroviral drug resistance testing and therapy changes in women with perinatal and nonperinatal HIV infection. The proportion of women with a genotype collected and ARV resistance accounts for the number of participants eligible to have a genotype evaluated (HIV RNA viral load > 1,000 copies/mL). *ARV resistance and multidrug resistance rates were significantly different between groups.

inhibitors (PIs) n = 6). NPHIV women had resistance to NRTI (n = 1) and NNRTIs (n = 2), but no PIs resistance was noted. ARV regimens were adjusted during pregnancy in seven women (five PHIV and two NPHIV) secondary to drug resistance (Table 3).

Univariate analysis was performed to identify which maternal factors were associated with the ARV resistance mutations. Among women who had an HIV genotype collected, PHIV infection was associated with an increased risk of drug resistance (OR 6.0 (95% CI, 1.03–34.8), p = 0.05). PHIV infection was the only variable with a statistically significant association to ARV drug resistance. Other variables analyzed were the duration of HIV infection prior to pregnancy, elevated HIV viral load at presentation for pregnancy, medical comorbidities, race/ethnicity, history of psychiatric illness, and maternal age.

The majority of participants had documented ARV use during pregnancy (100% PHIV and 93% NPHIV, p = 0.24) (Table 2). PHIV women were more likely to take integrase inhibitors (20% versus 2%, p = 0.03). Fusion inhibitors (n = 3) and CCR5 antagonists (n = 1) were used exclusively in PHIV women. Resistance testing and results for these alternative drug classes were not available for analysis. At the time of delivery, there was no significant difference in the number of women from either group taking NRTIs, NNRTIs, and PIs (Table 3). An appendix in Supplementary Material available online at http://dx.doi.org/10.1155/2016/4897501 which provides a detailed description of the types of ARVs prescribed

before, during, and after pregnancy for all study participants is available upon request.

Medical and psychiatric illnesses were common among study participants. Psychiatric illness was more common in women with PHIV (50% PHIV versus 27% NPHIV, p = 0.03). Depression was the most common psychiatric diagnosis, affecting 43% of PHIV and 22% of NPHIV women. NPHIV and PHIV women had similarly high rates of medical comorbidities in pregnancy (46% NPHIV versus 29% PHIV, p = 0.1). The most common medical comorbidities reported were asthma, obesity, chronic hypertension, and anemia. Only PHIV women had prior history of opportunistic infection(s). Rates of STIs were similar between PHIV and NPHIV women (p = 0.1). The following STIs were common among participants in both groups: genital herpes (68%), *T. vaginalis* (22%), *C. trachomatis* (14%), and *N. gonorrhoeae* (3%). Chronic hepatitis was infrequent among participants (6%); three women had hepatitis B and two had hepatitis C. Both groups had similar rates of pregnancy-related complications (45% versus 59%, p = 0.2). The most common complications of pregnancy were hypertensive disorders of pregnancy (12%), preterm labor/shortened cervical length/preterm delivery (20%), and premature rupture of membranes (2%) (Tables 1 and 2).

Live birth rates and cesarean delivery rates were similar among PHIV and NPHIV women ((97% PHIV versus 98% NPHIV, p = 1.0) and (47% PHIV versus 46% NPHIV, p = 0.9), resp.). At the time of delivery, the proportions of participants with HIV RNA viral load ≥ 1,000 copies/mL and HIV RNA viral loads below the level of detection (<40 copies/mL) were similar between groups ((26% PHIV versus 28% NPHIV, p = 0.9) and (56% PHIV versus 63% NPHIV, p = 0.5), resp.). The difference in the proportion of participants with HIV RNA viral loads between 40 and 999 copies/mL near delivery was not statistically significant (18% PHIV and 9% NPHIV, p = 0.18). Similar proportions of participants received at least three hours of intrapartum IV AZT when indicated (80% versus 84%, = 0.7) (Table 2).

The median gestational age at the time of delivery was 38 weeks in both groups. Preterm birth (<37 weeks gestation) rates were not significantly different between groups (11% PHIV versus 28% NPHIV, p = 0.08). Median birth weights were lower in the NPHIV women (2,742 (IQR 2,435–3,200) versus 3,065 (IQR 2,659–3,370), p = 0.02), but the proportion of low birth weight (<2,500 gm) infants was similar (34% NPHIV versus 22% PHIV, p = 0.2). Neonatal intensive care unit admissions were not significantly different between groups (29% NPHIV versus 14% PHIV, p = 0.2). The median duration of neonatal postexposure AZT prophylaxis was six weeks for both groups. HIV perinatal transmission was documented among two infants (2/32, 6%) born to a single NPHIV mother one year apart. The mother did not have prenatal care and did not take ARVs during either pregnancy. Both infants were born preterm, one by spontaneous vaginal delivery complicated by previable premature rupture of membranes and chorioamnionitis and the other by emergent cesarean delivery in the setting of abruption and preeclampsia. There were no documented cases of HIV perinatal transmission among women with PHIV (Table 2).

TABLE 3: Antiretroviral drug resistance patterns in HIV-infected pregnant women.

Subject number	NRTI resistance	NNRTI resistance	PI resistance	ARV regimen change during pregnancy	ART prior to delivery
PHIV n = 15	N = 6	N = 11	N = 6	N = 5	
1		✓		✓	AZT/3TC, DDI, NVP, NFV
3			✓		FTC/TDF, DRV, RIT
5	✓			✓	FTC/TDF, LPV/RIT
10			✓		ABC/AZT/3TC
12		✓	✓	✓	FTC/TDF, DRV, RIT, T-20
16			✓		FTC/TDF, LPV/RIT
28	✓	✓		✓	ABC/3TC, EFV, DRV, RIT
29		✓			ABC, TDF, LPV/RIT
46		✓			FTC/TDF, RAL
50		✓	✓		ATZ/3TC, LOP/RIT
58	✓	✓			ETV, DRV, RIT, RAL
60	✓	✓	✓	✓	TPV, RIT, MVC, T-20, DTG
77	✓	✓			FTC/TDF, EVG, COB
78	✓	✓			DRV, RIT, RAL, ETV
79		✓			DRV, RIT, FTC/TDF, ABC/3TC
NPHIV n = 3	N = 1	N = 2	N = 0	N = 2	
18		✓			AZT/3TC, LPV/RIT
25		✓		✓	AZT/3TC, RAL
56	✓				AZT/3TC, NFV

The genotypic mutation types were not recorded for 3 subjects: 2 PHIV (#80 and 81) and 1 NPHIV (#76). The ART regimens at delivery for these subjects were #80, FTC/TDF/RPV; #81, FTC/ETC/EVG/COB; and #76, ABC/3TC, ETV. #76 required a change in ART during pregnancy. ART, antiretroviral therapy; NRTI, nucleoside reverse transcriptase inhibitor; NNRTI, nonnucleoside reverse transcriptase inhibitor; PI, protease inhibitor; 3TC, lamivudine; ABC, abacavir; ATV, atazanavir; COB, cobicistat; DRV, darunavir; DTG, dolutegravir; EFV, efavirenz; ETV, etravirine; EVG, elvitegravir; FTC, emtricitabine; LPV, lopinavir; MVC, maraviroc; NFV, nelfinavir; NVP, nevirapine; TDF, tenofovir; RAL, raltegravir; RIT, ritonavir; RPV, rilpivirine; T-20, enfuvirtide.

4. Conclusions

HIV genotypic patterns suggestive of clinically relevant ARV drug resistance were documented in PHIV pregnant women three times more frequently than NPHIV pregnant women. Previous studies have documented clinically relevant genotypic mutations in 30–50% of PHIV pregnant women and in 13–17% of NPHIV pregnant women [4, 9, 12]. We anticipated and found comparatively higher rates of ARV drug resistance among PHIV women likely due to their lifelong HIV infection and potential intermittent exposure to multiple ARV classes and suboptimal ARV regimens. Providers caring for HIV-infected pregnant women should be aware of the potential for high rates of ARV resistance among all pregnant women in this age group but especially among women born with HIV infection.

Compared to previous studies, we were able to document the patterns of HIV drug resistance in PHIV pregnant women. The genotypic resistance in NPHIV women was limited to the NRTI and NNRTI classes compared to multiple ARV classes in PHIV women. Six PHIV women had multidrug resistant HIV infection, and one PHIV women had resistance mutations to all three major ARV classes (NRTI, NNRTIs, and PIs). Due to multidrug resistance, PHIV women were more likely to be prescribed ARV combinations that are nonstandard regimens for the prevention of perinatal transmission [15]. During the study period, nonstandard ARV therapies prescribed for PHIV pregnant women included integrase inhibitors, fusion inhibitors, and CCR5 antagonists. Given the importance of HIV viral suppression during pregnancy, providers caring for pregnant women with PHIV should be familiar with the potential use and limitations of these alternative ARVs during pregnancy.

Our findings of high rates of ARV drug resistance support the recommendation for HIV genotype analysis in early pregnancy. Genotypic testing should be collected and assessed as early as possible in all HIV-infected women [15]. These tests should be repeated during later pregnancy in women with poorly suppressed HIV RNA viral loads. When resistance to standard ARV classes used for prevention of perinatal transmission is suspected, providers should consider alternative drug classes and order additional resistance testing for integrase inhibitors, fusion inhibitors, or CCR5 antagonists.

PHIV women were more likely to report ARV use at the time of pregnancy diagnosis, but overall use of ARVs prior to conception was low. Only 68% of PHIV women and even fewer NPHIV women (23%) were on ARV therapy at initial presentation for pregnancy care. Only 30% of NPHIV women diagnosed with HIV at least one year prior to pregnancy reported ARV use at presentation for care. In previous studies, PHIV women were more likely to have poor viral suppression during pregnancy, likely due to inconsistent drug adherence [3–5, 8]. In contrast to these reports, PHIV women in our study had similar rates of virological suppression and comparable CD4 cell counts to NPHIV women during pregnancy. Providers caring for reproductive age women with HIV infection should be aware of their pregnancy intentions in order to reduce the risk of perinatal HIV transmission from delayed exposure to effective ARV therapy before and during pregnancy. Women currently not seeking pregnancy should be offered effective contraception [17].

Although the reduction of perinatal transmission is a primary objective of prenatal care for HIV-infected women, pregnancy is also a time when HIV-infected women are examined frequently and can be screened for other significant medical comorbidities. Current or past psychiatric illness, especially depression, was more common among PHIV women (50%). Given the potential effects of depression on pregnancy, HIV-infected women should receive a multidisciplinary approach including psychiatric evaluation and support services [10, 18]. Additionally, PHIV women were more likely to have a history of abnormal pap smears. Frequent visits during pregnancy can provide adequate time for evaluation for cervical cancer risks among HIV-infected women.

Our study revealed that HIV-serodiscordance was very common among pregnant women and their partners. PHIV women were more likely to have HIV susceptible partners (96%) compared to NPHIV women (68%). This difference is likely explained by NPHIV women potentially having acquired HIV from their current partners, as compared to PHIV counterparts, who acquired HIV at birth. Prenatal providers should be aware of the potential risk of HIV transmission to HIV susceptible partners during pregnancy. In an effort to reduce the transmission of HIV to susceptible partners, providers should provide risk reduction counseling to all serodiscordant couples and frequent HIV testing of susceptible partners and evaluate partners for HIV preexposure prophylaxis [19].

The limitations of this study are related to the retrospective cohort design. This study design was necessary given the relative rarity of the exposure of PHIV in pregnancy. Data were not available for every variable for every participant. Genotypic testing was not available for all 82 participants. This can partially be explained by 33 (40%) women having HIV RNA viral loads < 1,000 copies/mL at the time of initial pregnancy care. It is unclear to the investigators why genotypes were not collected in all 49 women who were eligible for HIV drug resistance evaluation (HIV RNA viral load ≥ 1,000 copies/mL). Three genotype resistance patterns were not available for detailed review. Another limitation of our study is that we neglected planning for and carrying out collection of information regarding substance use, including tobacco, alcohol, and prescription and/or street drugs. A prospective study design and inclusion of all PHIV and NPHIV women presenting to any site during the study period would be the most effective means for evaluating the primary outcome and potential differences in pregnancy outcomes. However, given the rarity of PHIV during pregnancy, a prospective, multisite study would exceed the resources available.

The results of this study may not be applicable to all populations. The majority of study participants were identified at an academic center in the Southeast, where the Principal Investigator practices. According to the CDC, the Southeast has the 2nd highest prevalence of HIV infection in the United States. As of 2011, the Southeast had the highest number of new HIV infections and the largest proportion of individuals living with stage 3 HIV/AIDS [1]. Perinatal transmission rates are also high in this region [1]. Due to the increased rate of perinatal HIV transmissions, it is reasonable that the majority of cases and controls are clustered in this region due to prevalence of infection. However, the entirety of PHIV cases were distributed from multiple locations in North America suggesting this data has generalizability for many centers caring for PHIV women during pregnancy.

This is the largest single group of PHIV women studied in comparison to age-matched NPHIV controls. This study adds to the medical literature by describing the types of HIV ARV mutations that affect the care of HIV-infected women during pregnancy. Based upon the data presented here, obstetric providers of PHIV and NPHIV women should have a high suspicion for clinically relevant HIV drug resistance early in pregnancy in order to best select effective therapies for the prevention of perinatal HIV transmission. Lastly, PHIV women did not experience higher rates of perinatal complications and there were no perinatal HIV transmissions to PHIV-exposed infants. Although not powered to identify any significant differences in pregnancy outcomes, our findings suggest that PHIV women may have similar pregnancy outcomes compared to NPHIV. Further investigation is needed, but providers can offer some reassurance to women living with PHIV infection that they are likely to have pregnancy outcomes comparable to other HIV-infected pregnant women.

Disclosure

Since the completion of this study, Dr. Luque has relocated to University of Texas Southwestern, 5323 Harry Hines Boulevard, Dallas, TX 75390-9173. Some of these data were presented at the 2013 Infectious Diseases Society of Obstetrics and Gynecology Annual Meeting, Albuquerque, NM.

Competing Interests

Dr. Mmeje has served as a paid consultant at World Health Organization.

Acknowledgments

The authors would like to thank the HIV-infected women and clinic staff at their study sites for participation. No financial compensation was provided.

References

[1] Centers for Disease Control and Prevention, *HIV Surveillance Report*, vol. 25, CDC, 2013.

[2] S. Crane, M. Sullivan, M. Feingold, and G. E. Kaufman, "Successful pregnancy in an adolescent with perinatally acquired human immunodeficiency virus," *Obstetrics and Gynecology*, vol. 92, no. 4, p. 711, 1998.

[3] U. K. Phillips, M. G. Rosenberg, J. Dobroszycki et al., "Pregnancy in women with perinatally acquired HIV-infection: outcomes and challenges," *AIDS Care*, vol. 23, no. 9, pp. 1076–1082, 2011.

[4] M. L. Badell, A. Kachikis, L. B. Haddad, M. L. Nguyen, and M. Lindsay, "Comparison of pregnancies between perinatally and sexually HIV-infected women: an observational study at an urban hospital," *Infectious Diseases in Obstetrics and Gynecology*, vol. 2013, Article ID 301763, 6 pages, 2013.

[5] C. Calitri, C. Gabiano, L. Galli et al., "The second generation of HIV-1 vertically exposed infants: a case series from the Italian Register for paediatric HIV infection," *BMC Infectious Diseases*, vol. 14, article 277, 2014.

[6] I. Munjal, J. Dobroszycki, E. Fakioglu et al., "Impact of HIV-1 infection and pregnancy on maternal health: comparison between perinatally and behaviorally infected young women," *Adolescent Health, Medicine and Therapeutics*, vol. 4, pp. 51–58, 2013.

[7] J. Jao, K. M. Sigel, K. T. Chen et al., "Small for gestational age birth outcomes in pregnant women with perinatally acquired HIV," *AIDS*, vol. 26, no. 7, pp. 855–859, 2012.

[8] M. L. S. Cruz, C. A. Cardoso, E. C. João et al., "Pregnancy in HIV vertically infected adolescents and young women: a new generation of HIV-exposed infants," *AIDS*, vol. 24, no. 17, pp. 2727–2731, 2010.

[9] S. F. Williams, M. H. Keane-Tarchichi, L. Bettica, A. Dieudonne, and A. D. Bardeguez, "Pregnancy outcomes in young women with perinatally acquired human immunodeficiency virus-1," *American Journal of Obstetrics and Gynecology*, vol. 200, no. 2, pp. 149.e1–149.e5, 2009.

[10] M. Millery, S. Vazquez, V. Walther, N. Humphrey, J. Schlecht, and N. Van Devanter, "Pregnancies in perinatally HIV-infected young women and implications for care and service programs," *The Journal of the Association of Nurses in AIDS Care*, vol. 23, no. 1, pp. 41–51, 2012.

[11] R. Chibber and A. Khurranna, "Birth outcomes in perinatally HIV-infected adolescents and young adults in Manipur, India: a new frontier," *Archives of Gynecology and Obstetrics*, vol. 271, no. 2, pp. 127–131, 2005.

[12] J. Kenny, B. Williams, K. Prime, P. Tookey, and C. Foster, "Pregnancy outcomes in adolescents in the UK and Ireland growing up with HIV," *HIV Medicine*, vol. 13, no. 5, pp. 304–308, 2012.

[13] F. M. Hecht and R. M. Grant, "Resistance testing in drug-naive HIV-infected patients: is it time?" *Clinical Infectious Diseases*, vol. 41, no. 9, pp. 1324–1325, 2005.

[14] S. Weber, The National Perinatal HIV Clinicians' Network: Best Practices for Linking HIV-positive Women with Care. AETC National Resource Center Website, 2013, http://aidsetc.org/blog/national-perinatal-hiv-clinicians%E2%80%99-network-best-practices-linking-hiv-positive-women-care.

[15] Panel on Treatment of HIV-Infected Pregnant Women and Prevention of Perinatal Transmission. Recommendations for Use of Antiretroviral Drugs in Pregnant HIV-1-Infected Women for Maternal Health and Interventions to Reduce Perinatal HIV Transmission in the United States, "Antiretroviral drug resistance and resistance testing in pregnancy", 2014, http://aidsinfo.nih.gov/contentfiles/lvguidelines/PerinatalGL.pdf.

[16] P. A. Harris, R. Taylor, R. Thielke, J. Payne, N. Gonzalez, and J. G. Conde, "Research electronic data capture (REDCap)—a metadata-driven methodology and workflow process for providing translational research informatics support," *Journal of Biomedical Informatics*, vol. 42, no. 2, pp. 377–381, 2009.

[17] L. Rahangdale, A. Stewart, R. D. Stewart et al., "Pregnancy intentions among women living with HIV in the United States," *Journal of Acquired Immune Deficiency Syndromes*, vol. 65, no. 3, pp. 306–311, 2014.

[18] E. Aaron, A. Bonacquisti, P. A. Geller, and M. Polansky, "Perinatal depression and anxiety in women with and without human immunodeficiency virus infection," *Women's Health Issues*, vol. 25, no. 5, pp. 579–585, 2015.

[19] US Public Health Service, Pre-exposure prophylaxis for the prevention of HIV infection in the United States: a clinical practice guideline, 2014, http://www.cdc.gov/hiv/risk/prep/index.html.

16

Influenza and Pregnancy: A Review of the Literature

Ashwini Bhalerao-Gandhi,[1] **Pankdeep Chhabra,**[2]
Saurabh Arya,[2] **and James Mark Simmerman**[3]

[1]*P. D. Hinduja Hospital and Medical Research Centre, Veer Savarkar Marg, Mahim, Mumbai 400016, India*
[2]*Sanofi Pasteur India Pvt. Ltd., 54/A, Mathuradas Vasanji Road, Andheri East, Mumbai 400093, India*
[3]*Sanofi Pasteur Thailand, 87/2 CRC Tower, 23rd Floor, Wireless Road, Bangkok 10330, Thailand*

Correspondence should be addressed to Ashwini Bhalerao-Gandhi; ashwinibgandhi@rediffmail.com

Academic Editor: Flor Munoz

Maternal influenza infection is known to cause substantial morbidity and mortality among pregnant women and young children. Many professional healthcare bodies including the World Health Organization (WHO) have identified pregnant women as a priority risk group for receipt of inactivated seasonal influenza vaccination. However influenza prevention in this group is not yet a public health priority in India. This literature review was undertaken to examine the Indian studies of influenza among pregnant women. Eight Indian studies describing influenza burden and/or outcomes among pregnant women with influenza were identified. In most studies, influenza A (pH1N1) was associated with increased maternal mortality (25–75%), greater disease severity, and adverse fetal outcomes as compared to nonpregnant women. Surveillance for seasonal influenza infections along with higher quality prospective studies among pregnant women is needed to quantify disease burden, improve awareness among antenatal care providers, and formulate antenatal influenza vaccine policies.

1. Introduction

Influenza is an acute, viral respiratory infection that causes significant morbidity and mortality among high-risk groups like pregnant women and infants. Physiological and immunological changes during pregnancy including decreased tidal volume and lung capacity, increased oxygen consumption and cardiac output, and selective suppression of T-helper-type 1 cell-mediated immunity that impairs maternal response to infection place pregnant women at high risk of complications and hospitalizations [1–3]. During the influenza pandemics of 1918, 1957, and 2009, pregnant women were at high risk of complications such as primary viral influenza pneumonia and mortality [4–6]. Even during the interpandemic period, pregnant women have been observed to be at a 18-fold higher risk of hospitalization as compared to healthy nonpregnant women and the risk is greatest among women in later stages of pregnancy [7–9]. Pregnant women with coexisting medical conditions such as asthma or diabetes are at 3-4 times greater risk of morbidity as compared to nonpregnant control subjects with similar high-risk conditions [7, 10].

Influenza infection among pregnancy is also linked to adverse pregnancy and birth outcomes. Newsome and colleagues reported that among severely ill pregnant women hospitalized for pandemic influenza A (pH1N1), 63.6% delivered preterm and 43.8% delivered low birth weight infants, compared with US averages of 12.3% for preterm birth and 8.2% for low birth weight [11]. Pregnant women hospitalized for respiratory illness during influenza season had higher odds of preterm delivery (adjusted OR 3.82, 95% CI 3.53–4.14), cesarean delivery (adjusted OR 3.47, 95% CI 3.22–3.74), and fetal distress (adjusted OR 2.33, 95% CI 2.15–2.52) and their infants were more likely to be small-for-gestational age (adjusted relative risk of 1.66; 95% CI 1.11–2.49) and have lower mean birth weight (3448.5 ± 498.2 versus 3531.3 ± 504.1 g; $P < 0.009$) as compared to pregnant women not hospitalized for respiratory illness [12, 13].

Among young infants, influenza infection may present with fever and other nonspecific symptoms such as irritability, reduced oral intake, dyspnea, vomiting, and diarrhea. In a prospective study in Bangladesh where influenza virus circulates throughout the year, about one-third of infants <6 months had serological confirmation of influenza infection [14]. In an urban setting in Dhaka, Bangladesh, 28% of influenza-positive children had pneumonia, whereas influenza virus was associated with 10% of all childhood pneumonia [15]. In a community-based study in Bangladesh among infants <6 months old, the incidence of acute respiratory infection and pneumonia due to influenza virus was 6/100 child-years (95% CI: 3–12) and 3/100 child-years (95% CI: 1–8), respectively [16]. The interaction between influenza virus and pneumococcus can increase the burden and severity of pneumonia in children, especially in the tropical countries where pneumonia is highly prevalent [17, 18].

Trivalent influenza vaccines (TIV) contain antigens from two influenza A strains (H1N1 and H3N2), and one of the two influenza B strains (Yamagata or Victoria), as recommended by WHO [19]. Immunologic responses generated by influenza immunization in pregnant women are comparable to nonpregnant women and can provide protection to the fetus and infant by efficiently transferring influenza-specific antibodies across the placenta [20–23]. In the Mother Gift's randomized blinded trial conducted in Bangladesh among 340 pregnant women in the third trimester, maternal influenza vaccination led to a 63% reduction of laboratory-confirmed influenza, 29% reduction in febrile respiratory illness among infants, and a 36% reduction in febrile respiratory illness among mothers [24]. During the period of influenza virus circulation, maternal influenza vaccination was associated with statistically significant reductions in febrile respiratory illness among mothers and infants ($P = 0.0003$), higher mean birth weight in infants ($P = 0.02$), and lower proportion of infants who were small-for-gestation age ($P = 0.03$) [25]. No differences were observed between the intervention (influenza vaccine) and control (pneumococcal polysaccharide vaccine) groups for adverse fetal, perinatal, or infant outcomes, and none of the adverse events reported were found to be related to the influenza vaccine [24]. Published reviews of observational studies and clinical trials from the past few decades provide reassuring results on the safety of seasonal influenza vaccines among pregnant women and infants [26–28].

The WHO Strategic Advisory Group of Experts (SAGE) on immunization has given highest priority to pregnant women for receiving inactivated influenza immunization [29]. In India, influenza vaccine uptake among pregnant women is extremely poor (12.8% for pandemic influenza vaccine and none for seasonal influenza) [30, 31]. The lack of disease burden data among pregnant Indian women may have contributed to the perception that prevention of influenza in pregnant women and young children may not be a public health priority. The objective of this review is to examine the published Indian studies to better understand the burden of influenza among pregnant women.

2. Review of Indian Studies

2.1. Methods. A literature search was conducted in PubMed, EMBASE, SCOPUS, and Medind databases and the website of Indian journals (http://www.indianjournals.com) to identify Indian studies that were published till 31 December 2013 and described burden of influenza and/or outcomes among pregnant women with seasonal or pandemic influenza. The search terms used included "influenza," "India," and "pregnancy." Wherever appropriate, the search also included the term "pregnan*" to capture any forms of the word "pregnant" or "pregnancy." After eliminating duplicates, titles and abstracts of citations were screened for relevance and were excluded if they did not focus on influenza epidemiology in India. On excluding review articles, editorials, case reports, and letters, potentially relevant citations included research studies that described influenza infection among pregnant women. Full texts of the potentially relevant citations and of the citations in which information was unclear in the abstract were retrieved. Finally, references of all selected articles were examined to identify additional articles.

Studies were included in the final review if they provided the number of pregnant women with influenza infection along with the data on comorbidities, maternal/fetal outcomes, trimester distribution, and severity of infection.

2.2. Results

2.2.1. Study Characteristics. Of 272 citations identified in our search, eight studies were included in the final review [32–39]. All studies were initiated during the pandemic of 2009-2010 in various regions of India (five studies were conducted in southern India, two studies in western India, and one study in northern India). Pregnant women were described as part of the overall population tested for influenza. In all studies, suspected influenza like illness (ILI)/severe acute respiratory illness (SARI) cases were confirmed for influenza by reverse transcriptase polymerase chain reaction (RT-PCR) test. All studies primarily focused on diagnosis of pandemic influenza A (pH1N1) and only two studies described prevalence of other seasonal influenza viruses [32, 33]. Three studies described the prevalence of influenza among both outpatients and inpatients [34, 35, 37], while five others focused only on severely ill patients requiring hospitalization [32, 33, 38, 39] or intensive care [36]. Only two studies provided information on influenza positivity among nonpregnant females [33, 34]. Gunasekaran observed important differences between seasonal and pandemic influenza positivity among pregnant and nonpregnant women [33]. Overall, a higher proportion of pregnant women were positive for both seasonal influenza (11.1% pregnant versus 1.4% nonpregnant) and influenza A (pH1N1) (21.4% pregnant women versus 2.7% nonpregnant). Pramanick et al. reported that, among all women presenting with ILI/SARI, influenza A (pH1N1) was positive in 25.3% of pregnant/puerperal women and 29.6% of nonpregnant women [34]. Most pregnant women with influenza A (pH1N1) infection presented to the hospital during second or third trimester. The study characteristics are described briefly in Table 1.

2.2.2. Outcomes

Maternal Mortality. Overall, the studies included in this review showed that pandemic influenza was associated with high mortality among Indian pregnant women. Across five

TABLE 1: Characteristics of included studies.

Sr. number	Author (year)	Objective	Region	Setting	Period	Sample	Outcomes	Results
1	Mathur et al. (2013) [37]	To assess the clinical profile, factors determining the response, prognosis of the disease, and outcome in H1N1 positive patients during 2009-2010 H1N1 pandemic	Jodhpur (West India)	Hospital-based, ICU/isolation patients	2009-2010	Overall population: 221 Pregnant women: 37	Clinical and epidemiological characteristics	**Prevalence of Influenza virus:** (i) Influenza A (pH1N1): 37 (23.4%) **Length of pregnancy at presentation:** (i) First trimester: 4 (11%) (ii) Second trimester: 18 (49%) (iii) Third trimester: 15 (40%) **Maternal mortality:** (i) 26 (70%) pregnant women died (ii) Mortality in third trimester: 80% **Treatment:** (i) All patients received Oseltamivir, Zanamivir, oxygen and ventilatory therapy, intravenous antibiotics and fluids, low dose steroids, and symptomatic therapy according to WHO guidelines
2	Mehta et al. (2013) [38]	To observe clinical profile of admitted patients with confirmed H1N1 swine flu infection and risk factors associated with the need of mechanical ventilation and/or death	Kochi, Kerala (South India)	Hospital-based inpatient	August 2009 to December 2011 (28 months)	Overall population: 115 Pregnant women: 6	Clinical and epidemiological characteristic Risk factors associated with mechanical ventilation/death	**Influenza virus prevalence:** (i) Influenza A (H1N1): 5.2% **Maternal mortality:** 2 women (33%) **Loss of fetus:** 2 women (33%) **Preterm delivery:** 2 women (33%) **Treatment:** All patients received Oseltamivir 75 mg twice daily for 5-10 days as per CDC guidelines
3	Ramakrishna et al. (2012) [36]	To detail the profile and outcomes of patients admitted to the intensive care unit (ICU) with pandemic Influenza A (H1N1) 2009 virus [P(H1N1)2009v] infection	Bangalore, Vellore, Manipal (South India)	Hospital-based, ICU patients	September 2009–December 2009 (4 months)	Overall population: 1902 Pregnant women: 19	(i) Hospital mortality (ii) Need for any duration of ventilation, tracheostomy, and skeletal muscle relaxants (iii) Need for renal replacement therapy (iv) Duration of ICU (v) Hospital stay	**Onset of infection:** (i) Antepartum: 14 women (ii) Postpartum: 5 women **Maternal mortality:** (i) 10 pregnant/postpartum women (52.6%) died (ii) Other outcomes were not described separately for pregnant women **Treatment:** All patients received Oseltamivir; no separate mention of timing of initiation of Oseltamivir in pregnant women

TABLE 1: Continued.

Sr. number	Author (year)	Objective	Region	Setting	Sample	Period	Outcomes	Results
4	Gunasekaran (2012) [33]	To determine the cumulative prevalence of H1N1 2009 influenza among pregnant and postpartum women in Tamil Nadu	Chennai (South India)	Hospital-based, inpatient and outpatient	Overall population: 7638 Pregnant women: 126	September 2009–May 2011 (21 months)	Clinical and epidemiological characteristics	**Prevalence of influenza virus:** (i) Influenza (pH1N1): 27 women (21.4%) (ii) Influenza A/H3: 12 women (9.5%) (iii) Influenza B: 2 women (1.6%) **Onset of infection:** (i) Antepartum: 12 women (ii) Postpartum: 15 women **ICU admission and complication:** (i) Admitted in ICU and treated for severe outcomes: 3 (11.1%) (ii) Admitted in obstetric ward and treated for moderate outcomes: 5 (18.5%) women **Maternal mortality:** (i) One woman died during postpartum period **Treatment:** Oseltamivir was initiated in patients considering their high-risk status
5	Pramanick et al. (2011) [34]	To assess the clinical profile of pregnant/puerperal women infected with pandemic H1N1 influenza A and to evaluate their outcome	Vellore (South India)	Hospital-based	Overall population: 566 Pregnant women: 20	August 2009–January 2010 (6 months)	Primary outcome (i) Maternal mortality Secondary outcomes (ii) Need for ICU admission (iii) Need for mechanical ventilation (iv) Renal failure	(i) Out of 79 pregnant women, 20 (29%) women presenting with ILI/SARI were pregnant **Onset of infection:** (i) Antepartum: 16 women (80%) (ii) Postpartum: 4 women (20%) **Length of pregnancy at presentation:** (i) Second trimester: 4 women (20%) (ii) Third trimester: 11 women (55%) (iii) 1 woman had molar pregnancy at 18 weeks of pregnancy **ICU admission:** (i) Required by 8 pregnant/postpartum (40%) **Maternal mortality:** 5 women (25%) died **Fetal mortality:** 1 **Complications:** (i) Renal failure: 4 women (20%) (ii) Mechanical ventilation: 7 women (35%) (iii) Seizures: 1 woman (5%) **Treatment:** Oseltamivir received by 18 women (90%); no mention of timing of initiation of Oseltamivir

TABLE 1: Continued.

Sr. number	Author (year)	Objective	Region	Setting	Sample	Period	Outcomes	Results
6	Puvanalingam et al. (2011) [35]	To study clinical profile of H1N1 influenza cases and to study the impact of H1N1 infection on pregnancy outcome	Chennai (South India)	Hospital-based inpatient and outpatient	Overall population: 442 Pregnant women: 12	August 2009–January 2010 (6 months)	Clinical characteristics and outcome of pregnant women	**Length of pregnancy at presentation:** (i) First trimester: 2 (16.7%) women (ii) Second trimester: none (iii) Third trimester: 10 (83.3%) women **Maternal mortality:** 3 women (25%) died **Complication:** (i) 9 women (75%) presented with pneumonia **Fetal death:** (i) 2 women (16.7%) had spontaneous abortion following intrauterine death in the third trimester Treatment: not mentioned
7	Chudasama et al. (2010) [32]	To investigated the clinicoepidemiological characteristics of patients who were hospitalized with 2009 pandemic H1N1 influenza virus infection and seasonal influenza in the Saurashtra region of India	Rajkot (West India)	Hospital-based inpatient	Overall population: 773 Pregnant women: 15	September 2009–February 2010 (6 months)	Clinical and epidemiological characteristics	**Length of pregnancy at presentation:** (i) All women presented in either 2nd or 3rd trimester **ICU admission:** (i) 11 women (73.3%) required intensive care **Treatment:** All patients received Oseltamivir, no separate mention of number of pregnant women that received the drug within 2 days of illness onset
8	Sharma et al. (2010) [39]	To describe the mortality data of severe influenza cases admitted in a tertiary care center in New Delhi	New Delhi (North India)	Hospital-based inpatient	Total: 8 women Pregnant women: 2	September 2009 to January 2010 (5 months)	Mortality	Out of 8 deaths due to influenza A (pH1N1), 2 women were pregnant **Length of pregnancy at presentation:** (i) First trimester: one woman (ii) Postpartum period: one woman, child delivered by caesarean section

studies, influenza-related maternal mortality ranged from 25% to 70% among pregnant women [34–38], whereas Gunasekaran reported mortality of 3.7% [33]. In the descriptive study by Sharma and colleagues, 2 out of eight women who died due to influenza A (pH1N1) were pregnant [39]. Pramanick and colleagues reported that mortality among pregnant women with influenza was associated with a significant delay in presentation to hospital (median time: 6 days for those who died versus 1.5 days for survivors), dyspnea, need for ICU admission, need for mechanical ventilation, and renal failure [34]. Mathur et al. observed a higher maternal mortality rate among women in third trimester (80%) as compared to women presenting in early pregnancy (63%) [37]. Mehta et al. reported a 2.9-fold higher mortality among pregnant women that was not statistically significant (OR = 2.90 (95% CI: 0.48–17.72)) [38]. Similarly, Ramakrishna et al. did not find a statistically significant difference in mortality among pregnant and nonpregnant women [36]. However, high mortality due to influenza A (pH1N1) among pregnant women was observed by Puvanalingam (25% pregnant women versus 2.7% nonpregnant), Pramanick (25% pregnant women versus 8.3% nonpregnant women, $P = 0.04$), and Mathur (70% pregnant women versus 26% nonpregnant).

Fetal and Perinatal Outcomes. Three studies reported the effect of maternal influenza infection on fetal and perinatal outcomes. These studies reported fetal mortality ranging from 5.5% to 33% and prematurity rates were from 20% to 33% [34, 35, 38].

Severity of Disease, Comorbidities, and Complications. Four studies provided data on severity, comorbidities, and complications due to influenza infection among pregnant women [32–35]. Out of 20 pregnant and postpartum women with influenza A (pH1N1) infection, Pramanick reported that 8 (40%) required ICU admission, 4 (20%) developed renal failure, and 1 (5%) developed seizures. Chudasama and colleagues reported ICU admission among 73% of pregnant and postpartum women. Palani et al. reported that 11% of pregnant women with influenza A (pH1N1) were admitted to the ICU for the management of severe outcomes. A higher proportion of pregnant women with seasonal influenza (21.4%) had asthma in comparison to pregnant women with influenza A (pH1N1) (3.7%). Puvanalingam observed that 75% of pregnant women with influenza had pneumonia in comparison to 24% nonpregnant women. Additional risk factors such as diabetes mellitus and obesity which are known to complicate pregnancy along with influenza A (pH1N1) were not described specifically among pregnant women in all studies.

3. Discussion

The eight studies that assessed the effect of influenza among pregnant Indian women were conducted in response to the 2009 influenza pandemic and only one assessed seasonal influenza infections in the postpandemic phase.

The maternal mortality rate observed in most Indian studies was higher than that reported in other countries [6, 40–42]. The mortality estimates in the Indian studies varied widely (3.7% to 70%) which could be due to the diverse study populations and differing sampling methods used.

Delay in the initiation of antiviral treatment and the presence of underlying comorbidities are associated with severe H1N1 disease [43], but not all studies provided information on these factors. Receipt of Oseltamivir to influenza-positive patients was reported in six studies, but whether it was given within the recommended duration from onset of symptoms was not mentioned in all studies. Similarly, information on comorbidities specifically among pregnant women subgroup was mentioned in only two studies [34, 35]. Other factors prevalent in developing countries that may contribute to severe disease are lack of awareness and misconceptions regarding influenza, poor diagnostic and intensive care management, and use of over-the-counter medications [44].

The finding that pregnant women with influenza (pH1N1) infection present with severe disease later in pregnancy is consistent with other studies. In a Singaporean study, women presenting in the second trimester had a 1.2-fold increase and women in the third trimester had 2.3-fold higher odds of hospitalization [45]. A similar finding was observed in a review by Liu et al. in which the results from seven studies from different geographic areas revealed that 9.1% of the cases with influenza A (pH1N1) infection occurred in the first trimester, 29.8% in the second trimester, and 47.0% in the third trimester [46].

This literature review has some limitations. We excluded studies that provided only the number of pregnant women without any other information for this group and studies that were presented only in conferences or meetings as abstracts. Among two studies that attempted to describe prevalence of seasonal influenza among pregnant women, one overestimated the burden of seasonal influenza by misclassifying patients that were negative for pandemic influenza A (pH1N1) as patients with seasonal influenza without actually testing them for influenza A (H3N2) or influenza B [32]. The other study did not describe characteristics or outcomes among women positive for influenza A/H3N2 or influenza B viruses [33].

There were methodological limitations in the included studies. Pregnant women were described as a subgroup of a population with ILI/SARI that was referred to tertiary-level hospitals, thus capturing more severe cases, while milder influenza infections might not have been captured. Some of these studies lacked power to assess the association between influenza and adverse maternal and/or fetal outcomes. Studies were also limited by retrospective study designs, short follow-up periods, small sample sizes, inadequate assessment of maternal and neonatal outcomes, and inadequate description of comorbidities or treatment. Some studies described combined outcomes among pregnant and postpartum women preventing comparisons between these two groups.

4. Conclusions

Though limited data are available from India, this review highlighted the high burden of maternal and fetal complications during pregnancy, especially due to pandemic Influenza

A (pH1N1). However, six years after the pandemic, influenza A (pH1N1) strain continues to circulate as a seasonal virus and continues to cause outbreaks, severe illness, and some deaths [47, 48]. Since most studies did not test for seasonal influenza virus (A/H3N2 or type B virus) among pregnant women, this review identified an important data gap that can be addressed by surveillance of all influenza virus serotypes circulating in India. Additionally, better quality prospective studies to assess influenza burden among pregnant women are needed to help improve awareness among antenatal care providers and better inform antenatal influenza vaccine policy in India.

Conflict of Interests

Ashwini Bhalerao-Gandhi has a speaker contract with Sanofi Pasteur, manufacturer of an influenza vaccine. Pankdeep Chhabra, Saurabh Arya, and James Mark Simmerman are employed by Sanofi Pasteur, manufacturer of an influenza vaccine.

Authors' Contribution

Pankdeep Chhabra and Saurabh Arya conducted the literature search and identified the articles to be included; Ashwini Bhalerao-Gandhi, Pankdeep Chhabra, Saurabh Arya, and James Mark Simmerman have contributed to the conception and writing of this paper, providing comments and approving the final version.

References

[1] D. J. Jamieson, R. N. Theiler, and S. A. Rasmussen, "Emerging infections and pregnancy," *Emerging Infectious Diseases*, vol. 12, no. 11, pp. 1638–1643, 2006.

[2] G. Gaunt and K. Ramin, "Immunological tolerance of the human fetus," *The American Journal of Perinatology*, vol. 18, no. 6, pp. 299–312, 2001.

[3] V. R. Laibl and J. S. Sheffield, "Influenza and pneumonia in pregnancy," *Clinics in Perinatology*, vol. 32, no. 3, pp. 727–738, 2005.

[4] J. M. Hardy, E. N. Azarowicz, A. Mannini, D. N. Medearis Jr., and R. E. Cooke, "The effect of Asian influenza on the outcome of pregnancy, Baltimore, 1957–1958," *American Journal of Public Health and the Nation's Health*, vol. 51, no. 8, pp. 1182–1188, 1961.

[5] J. Harris, "Influenza occurring in pregnant women: a statistical study of thirteen hundred and fifty cases," *The Journal of American Medical Association*, vol. 72, no. 14, pp. 978–980, 1919.

[6] D. J. Jamieson, M. A. Honein, S. A. Rasmussen et al., "H1N1 2009 influenza virus infection during pregnancy in the USA," *The Lancet*, vol. 374, no. 9688, pp. 451–458, 2009.

[7] K. M. Neuzil, G. W. Reed, E. F. Mitchel, L. Simonsen, and M. R. Griffin, "Impact of influenza on acute cardiopulmonary hospitalizations in pregnant women," *American Journal of Epidemiology*, vol. 148, no. 11, pp. 1094–1102, 1998.

[8] V. L. Rogers, J. S. Sheffield, S. W. Roberts et al., "Presentation of seasonal influenza A in pregnancy: 2003-2004 influenza season," *Obstetrics and Gynecology*, vol. 115, no. 5, pp. 924–929, 2010.

[9] D. L. Schanzer, T. W. S. Tam, J. M. Langley, and B. T. Winchester, "Influenza-attributable deaths, Canada 1990–1999," *Epidemiology and Infection*, vol. 135, no. 7, pp. 1109–1116, 2007.

[10] T. V. Hartert, K. M. Neuzil, A. K. Shintani et al., "Maternal morbidity and perinatal outcomes among pregnant women with respiratory hospitalizations during influenza season," *The American Journal of Obstetrics and Gynecology*, vol. 189, no. 6, pp. 1705–1712, 2003.

[11] K. Newsome, J. Williams, S. Way et al., "Maternal and infant outcomes among severely ill pregnant and postpartum women with 2009 pandemic influenza A (H1N1)—United States, April 2009-August 2010," *Morbidity and Mortality Weekly Report*, vol. 60, no. 35, pp. 1193–1196, 2011.

[12] A. Martin, S. Cox, D. J. Jamieson, M. K. Whiteman, A. Kulkarni, and N. K. Tepper, "Respiratory illness hospitalizations among pregnant women during influenza season, 1998–2008," *Maternal and Child Health Journal*, vol. 17, no. 7, pp. 1325–1331, 2013.

[13] S. A. McNeil, L. A. Dodds, D. B. Fell et al., "Effect of respiratory hospitalization during pregnancy on infant outcomes," *The American Journal of Obstetrics and Gynecology*, vol. 204, no. 6, pp. S54–S57, 2011.

[14] E. Henkle, M. C. Steinhoff, S. B. Omer et al., "Incidence of influenza virus infection in early infancy: a prospective study in South Asia," *Pediatric Infectious Disease Journal*, vol. 30, no. 2, pp. 170–173, 2011.

[15] W. A. Brooks, D. Goswami, M. Rahman et al., "Influenza is a major contributor to childhood pneumonia in a tropical developing country," *Pediatric Infectious Disease Journal*, vol. 29, no. 3, pp. 216–221, 2010.

[16] N. Homaira, S. P. Luby, W. A. Petri et al., "Incidence of respiratory virus-associated pneumonia in urban poor young children of dhaka, bangladesh, 2009—2011," *PLoS ONE*, vol. 7, no. 2, Article ID e32056, 2012.

[17] B. Greenwood, "The epidemiology of pneumococcal infection in children in the developing world," *Philosophical Transactions of the Royal Society B: Biological Sciences*, vol. 354, no. 1384, pp. 777–785, 1999.

[18] K. L. O'Brien, M. I. Walters, J. Sellman et al., "Severe pneumococcal pneumonia in previously healthy children: the role of preceding influenza infection," *Clinical Infectious Diseases*, vol. 30, no. 5, pp. 784–789, 2000.

[19] "Vaccines against influenza WHO position paper—November 2012," *The Weekly Epidemiological Record*, vol. 87, no. 47, pp. 461–476, 2012.

[20] J. A. Englund, I. N. Mbawuike, H. Hammill, M. C. Holleman, B. D. Baxter, and W. P. Glezen, "Maternal immunization with influenza or tetanus toxoid vaccine for passive antibody protection in young infants," *Journal of Infectious Diseases*, vol. 168, no. 3, pp. 647–656, 1993.

[21] L. A. Jackson, S. M. Patel, G. K. Swamy et al., "Immunogenicity of an inactivated monovalent 2009 H1N1 influenza vaccine in pregnant women," *Journal of Infectious Diseases*, vol. 204, no. 6, pp. 854–863, 2011.

[22] S. Y. Lin, E. T. Wu, C. H. Lin, M. K. Shyu, and C. N. Lee, "The safety and immunogenicity of trivalent inactivated influenza vaccination: a study of maternal-cord blood pairs in taiwan," *PLoS ONE*, vol. 8, no. 6, Article ID e62983, 2013.

[23] J. M. Puck, W. P. Glezen, A. L. Frank, and H. R. Six, "Protection of infants from infection with influenza A virus by transplacentally acquired antibody," *Journal of Infectious Diseases*, vol. 142, no. 6, pp. 844–849, 1980.

[24] K. Zaman, E. Roy, S. E. Arifeen et al., "Effectiveness of maternal influenza immunization in mothers and infants," *The New England Journal of Medicine*, vol. 359, no. 15, pp. 1555–1564, 2008.

[25] M. C. Steinhoff, S. B. Omer, E. Roy et al., "Neonatal outcomes after influenza immunization during pregnancy: a randomized controlled trial," *Canadian Medical Association Journal*, vol. 184, no. 6, pp. 645–653, 2012.

[26] R. A. Bednarczyk, D. Adjaye-Gbewonyo, and S. B. Omer, "Safety of influenza immunization during pregnancy for the fetus and the neonate," *American Journal of Obstetrics and Gynecology*, vol. 207, no. 3, pp. S38–S46, 2012.

[27] F. M. Munoz, "Safety of influenza vaccines in pregnant women," *The American Journal of Obstetrics and Gynecology*, vol. 207, no. 3, pp. S33–S37, 2012.

[28] P. D. Tamma, K. A. Ault, C. del Rio, M. C. Steinhoff, N. A. Halsey, and S. B. Omer, "Safety of influenza vaccination during pregnancy," *American Journal of Obstetrics and Gynecology*, vol. 201, no. 6, pp. 547–552, 2009.

[29] J. R. Ortiz, K. M. Neuzil, V. I. Ahonkhai et al., "Translating vaccine policy into action: a report from the Bill & Melinda Gates Foundation Consultation on the prevention of maternal and early infant influenza in resource-limited settings," *Vaccine*, vol. 30, no. 50, pp. 7134–7140, 2012.

[30] E. Bhaskar, S. Thobias, S. Anthony, V. Kumar, and N. Navaneethan, "Vaccination rates for pandemic influenza among pregnant women: an early observation from Chennai, South India," *Lung India*, vol. 29, no. 3, pp. 232–235, 2012.

[31] P. A. Koul, N. K. Bali, S. Ali et al., "Poor uptake of influenza vaccination in pregnancy in northern India," *International Journal of Gynecology & Obstetrics*, vol. 127, no. 3, pp. 234–237, 2014.

[32] R. K. Chudasama, U. V. Patel, and P. B. Verma, "Hospitalizations associated with 2009 influenza A (H1N1) and seasonal influenza in Saurashtra region, India," *Journal of Infection in Developing Countries*, vol. 4, no. 12, pp. 834–841, 2010.

[33] P. Gunasekaran, "Influenza A/H1N1 2009 in pregnancy—experience in Tamilnadu, India," *Indian Journal of Scientific Research*, vol. 3, pp. 31–35, 2012.

[34] A. Pramanick, S. Rathore, J. V. Peter, M. Moorthy, and J. Lionel, "Pandemic (H1N1) 2009 virus infection during pregnancy in South India," *International Journal of Gynecology and Obstetrics*, vol. 113, no. 1, pp. 32–35, 2011.

[35] A. Puvanalingam, C. Rajendiran, K. Sivasubramanian, S. Ragunanthanan, S. Suresh, and S. Gopalakrishnan, "Case series study of the clinical profile of H1N1 swine flu influenza," *Journal of Association of Physicians of India*, vol. 59, no. 1, pp. 14–18, 2011.

[36] K. Ramakrishna, S. Sampath, J. Chacko et al., "Clinical profile and predictors of mortality of severe pandemic (H1N1) 2009 virus infection needing intensive care: a multi-centre prospective study from South India," *Journal of Global Infectious Diseases*, vol. 4, no. 3, pp. 145–152, 2012.

[37] S. Mathur, T. Dubey, M. Kulshrestha et al., "Clinical profile and mortality among novel influenza A (H1N1) infected patients: 2009-2010 Jodhpur, Rajasthan pandemic," *Journal of Association of Physicians of India*, vol. 61, no. 9, pp. 627–632, 2013.

[38] A. A. Mehta, V. A. Kumar, S. G. Nair, F. K. Joseph, G. Kumar, and S. K. Singh, "Clinical profile of patients admitted with swine-origin influenza A (H1N1) virus infection: an experience from a tertiary care hospital," *Journal of Clinical and Diagnostic Research*, vol. 7, no. 10, pp. 2227–2230, 2013.

[39] V. Sharma, P. K. Verma, S. Gupta, and A. Sharma, "Mortality from influenza A/H1N1 in a tertiary care teaching institution in North India," *Journal of Infection in Developing Countries*, vol. 4, no. 8, pp. 468–471, 2010.

[40] G. Dubar, E. Azria, A. Tesnière et al., "French experience of 2009 A/H1N1v influenza in pregnant women," *PLoS ONE*, vol. 5, no. 10, Article ID e13112, 2010.

[41] E. Maraví-Poma, I. Martin-Loeches, E. Regidor et al., "Severe 2009 A/H1N1v influenza in pregnant women in Spain," *Critical Care Medicine*, vol. 39, no. 5, pp. 945–951, 2011.

[42] S. Hewagama, S. P. Walker, R. L. Stuart et al., "2009 H1N1 influenza A and pregnancy outcomes in Victoria, Australia," *Clinical Infectious Diseases*, vol. 50, no. 5, pp. 686–690, 2010.

[43] R. Zarychanski, T. L. Stuart, A. Kumar et al., "Correlates of severe disease in patients with 2009 pandemic influenza (H1N1) virus infection," *Canadian Medical Association Journal*, vol. 182, no. 3, pp. 257–264, 2010.

[44] B. B. Sharma and V. Singh, "Flu and pulmonary fibrosis," *Lung India*, vol. 30, no. 2, pp. 95–96, 2013.

[45] M. L. Lim, "2009/H1N1 infection in pregnancy association with adverse perinatal outcomes," *Evidence-Based Nursing*, vol. 15, no. 1, pp. 11–12, 2012.

[46] S.-L. Liu, J. Wang, X.-H. Yang et al., "Pandemic influenza A(H1N1) 2009 virus in pregnancy," *Reviews in Medical Virology*, vol. 23, no. 1, pp. 3–14, 2013.

[47] P. Koul, U. Khan, K. Bhat et al., "Recrudescent wave of A/H1N1pdm09 influenza viruses in Winter 2012-2013 in Kashmir, India," *PLoS Current Outbreaks*, vol. 5, 2013.

[48] Ministry of Health and Family Welfare, Influenza A(H1N1) Swine flu updates, http://mohfw.nic.in/index3.php?lang=1&level=0&deptid=115.

17

Efforts to Improve Immunization Coverage during Pregnancy among Ob-Gyns

Katherine M. Jones,[1,2] Sarah Carroll,[3] Debra Hawks,[3] Cora-Ann McElwain,[1] and Jay Schulkin[1]

[1]Department of Research, American College of Obstetricians and Gynecologists, 409 12th Street SW, Washington, DC 20024, USA
[2]Department of Psychology, American University, 4400 Massachusetts Avenue NW, Washington, DC 20016, USA
[3]Practice Division, American College of Obstetricians and Gynecologists, 409 12th Street SW, Washington, DC 20024, USA

Correspondence should be addressed to Jay Schulkin; jschulkin@acog.org

Academic Editor: Faustino R. Perez-Lopez

Background. Influenza and Tdap vaccines are vital factors for improving maternal and neonatal health outcomes. *Methods.* A prospective, longitudinal study was conducted to determine whether the American College of Obstetricians and Gynecologists' (ACOG's) efforts to increase ob-gyn use of their immunization toolkits and vaccination administration were successful. Pre- and postintervention questionnaires were mailed to a random sample of 1,500 ACOG members between August 2012 and July 2015. *Results.* Significantly more postintervention survey ob-gyns reported that they received the immunization toolkits than preintervention survey ob-gyns (84.5% versus 67.0%, $p < .001$). The large majority of ob-gyns from both surveys (76.9% versus 78.9%) reported that they offered or planned to offer influenza vaccinations to their patients for the 2012-2013 and 2014-2015 flu seasons. Postintervention survey respondents were significantly more likely than preintervention survey participants to report that they routinely offer Tdap vaccinations to all patients during pregnancy (76.8% versus 59.3%, $p < .001$). *Conclusion.* ACOG's efforts to improve ob-gyn use of immunization toolkits and vaccine administration appear to have been successful in several ways. ACOG's toolkits are an example of an effective intervention to overcome barriers to offering vaccines and help improve influenza and Tdap immunization coverage for pregnant women.

1. Introduction

Vaccinations are essential components of preconception, prenatal, and postpartum care and of improving maternal and neonatal health for a number of infectious diseases. The Centers for Disease Control and Prevention (CDC) Advisory Committee on Immunization Practices (ACIP) and the American College of Obstetricians and Gynecologists (ACOG) currently recommend two immunizations for all pregnant women without contraindication, inactivated influenza and adult-type tetanus toxoid, reduced diphtheria toxoid, and acellular pertussis (Tdap) [1, 2]. Additionally, ACIP and ACOG advise other family members and individuals in close contact with the newborn to receive influenza and Tdap vaccination ("cocooning") to further protect the infant [2, 3].

Pregnant women and infants are at increased risk of influenza-related morbidity and mortality and adverse pregnancy outcomes [4]. Influenza vaccination during pregnancy, regardless of pregnancy trimester, can significantly help prevent influenza virus infection among pregnant women and their infants younger than six months of age [5, 6]. Despite public health recommendations, national estimates for influenza immunization coverage during pregnancy have been historically low [5, 7]. According to the CDC, only 52.2% of women reported receiving influenza vaccination before or during pregnancy throughout the 2013-2014 influenza season [6].

Pertussis (whopping cough) is an acute, prolonged respiratory illness caused by the organism *Bordetella pertussis*. Rates of pertussis in the United States have been gradually increasing since 1976, with major epidemics of pertussis occurring over the last several years [2]. Waning vaccine-induced immunity is the key contributing factor to the persistence of the disease, particularly in adults and adolescents [8]. However, those at the greatest risk are young infants who have the highest rates of morbidity, complication, hospitalization, and mortality associated with the disease [9, 10]. Studies have shown that parents, older siblings, other family members and relatives living in the household, and individuals who were close contacts were the source of pertussis transmission to young infants in 75%–85% of the cases. Parents, particularly mothers, were the transmission source more than 50% of the time [11]. Immunity against pertussis does not develop until infants have received three doses of diphtheria and tetanus toxoids and acellular pertussis (DTaP) vaccine, usually by six months of age. Thus, infants under the age of six months rely on passively acquired maternal antibodies for protection [12]. In order for the infant to receive adequate levels of pertussis antibodies, ACIP and ACOG recommend Tdap vaccination to all pregnant women during each pregnancy, regardless of prior Tdap vaccination, between 27 and 36 weeks of gestation, and to other family members and individuals in close contact with the newborn [1, 2, 13]. If Tdap vaccination is not given during pregnancy, and the woman has never received Tdap, it should be given postpartum. National estimates indicate that only 9.8% of pregnant women report receiving Tdap vaccination [14].

Physician recommendations for and administration of vaccines have been shown to be the strongest predictors of vaccine receipt among patients [15]. As the primary health care provider for most women during pregnancy, obstetrician-gynecologists (ob-gyns) can and should play a critical role in administering influenza and Tdap vaccinations to women during pregnancy [1, 3, 5]. Previous studies demonstrate that the majority of ob-gyns believe screening for vaccine-preventable diseases and offering immunizations to pregnant women are within their professional responsibilities [16]. Moreover, the majority of ob-gyns know that influenza and Tdap immunizations (89.9% and 58.6%, resp.) are safe to administer during pregnancy, and most ob-gyns (84.5%) agree that pregnant women should receive annual influenza vaccination [16]. Despite ob-gyns' overall positive attitudes toward immunizations, reported rates of influenza and Tdap vaccination coverage vary widely among ob-gyns (66.8%–79.6% and 29.9%, resp.) [17]. Of even greater concern, national estimates indicate that a much smaller percentage of pregnant women report having received influenza and Tdap vaccinations compared to the percentage of ob-gyns who report having offered the vaccines [14], thus warranting further investigation. One study examining ob-gyns' immunization practices found that the majority of ob-gyn respondents (79.6%) believed educational tools for clinicians and patient educational materials should be a priority for ACOG [18].

In an effort to increase the efficacy of these immunization toolkits and ob-gyn use of toolkit materials and immunization administration, ACOG recently revised and revamped its toolkits based on feedback received from four focus groups that met at the 2013 and 2014 ACOG Annual Meeting. The purpose of this pre- and postintervention questionnaire study was to examine whether ACOG's efforts to improve the usefulness of its immunization toolkits were successful.

2. Method

2.1. Sample and Study Design. A prospective, longitudinal study was conducted to assess the impact of ACOG's efforts to increase ob-gyn use of ACOG's immunization toolkits and vaccination administration. Between August 2012 and March 2013, the ACOG Immunization Department distributed three immunization toolkits to ACOG's general membership. Following the distribution of the third toolkit, a preintervention questionnaire was sent out to a random sample of 1,500 ACOG members. After data collection concluded for the preintervention questionnaire, three revised toolkits (the "intervention") were sent to ACOG's general membership between September 2013 and September 2014. In October 2014, following the distribution of the third revised toolkit, a postintervention questionnaire was sent to 1,370 participants of the original 1,500 sample.

Revisions to the toolkits included updating the clinical information and revising the wording of some materials based on feedback from focus groups with ACOG members. ACOG also increased the promotion to members through electronic notifications such as e-mail, ACOG newsletters, and ACOG's Immunization for Women website in addition to promotion through partner organizations. These toolkit revisions were expected to provide supplemental information to ob-gyns, who administer influenza and Tdap vaccinations, in order to improve the usefulness of the immunization toolkits.

A questionnaire on ob-gyn practices and opinions related to immunizations was developed by a team of researchers in the Immunization Department at ACOG familiar with this subject. The preintervention questionnaire contained 24 questions regarding physicians' receipt and use of ACOG's immunization toolkits, immunization resources needed, general immunization practice patterns, barriers to offering vaccinations, and physician use of ACOG's Immunization for Women website. Demographic questions included gender, year of birth, and state/territory of primary practice. Some items were added to the postintervention questionnaire to gather more detailed information regarding participants' demographic background, their patient population, and their use of ACOG's most recently distributed immunization toolkits. New demographic questions included the participants' number of years in practice, type of practice, primary medical specialty, practice location, primary race/ethnicity of patient population, and primary type of patient insurance. The revised postintervention questionnaire contained a total of 34 questions. Questions included yes/no, check boxes, forced choice, and Likert-scales. The questionnaire was constructed to be completed in approximately 5–10 minutes.

The ACOG Immunization Department has been distributing toolkits on vaccinations to its members since 2011 and has sent a total of seven toolkits to date. These toolkits contain resources to help educate ob-gyns and their patients on immunizations for influenza, Tdap, and human papillomavirus (HPV) and to provide physicians with tools for integrating immunizations into routine care. Each toolkit is designed based upon existing ACOG guidance primarily derived from ACOG Committee Opinions. Toolkits feature corresponding materials, including a letter from ACOG's Vice President of Practice Activities, encouraging providers to use the resources in the toolkit; frequently asked questions (FAQs) handouts for patients; a Physician Script; coding information relevant to specific vaccines; and partner materials such as Vaccine Information Statements and sample standing orders from the CDC and Immunization Action Coalition (IAC).

2.2. Preintervention Study. ACOG membership includes 95% of board-certified obstetrician-gynecologists in the United States. In January 2013, a random sample of 1,500 active ACOG members was selected to participate in this study. Participation was voluntary, with no compensation offered to participants. Participants were sent an electronic flyer alerting them that they would shortly receive an invitation to participate in an electronic questionnaire on ob-gyns' immunization practices. The online survey was conducted using Real Magnet®, and the purpose, risks, and benefits of the study were outlined in an e-mail containing the live survey link. Up to six reminder e-mails including a link to the electronic questionnaire were sent between February and March 2013 to nonresponders. Participants were not provided with supplementary information regarding the topic of the survey and were instructed not to look up any additional information.

In April 2013, a paper questionnaire was mailed to all nonresponders of the electronic survey (n = 1,403). The purpose, risks, and benefits of the study were outlined in an accompanying cover letter. Two subsequent mailings were sent to nonresponders between May and June 2013. Finally, a shortened letter version of the questionnaire, which contained 10 of the original survey items, was sent to a randomly selected sample of nonresponders (n = 300) in September 2013. The letter responses were used to assess a potential nonresponse bias and were not included in data analysis. The electronic questionnaire remained open until data collection for the paper mailing ended in October 2013; thus, participants who received the paper questionnaire could elect to complete either the online or paper survey. Participants were instructed to only complete the survey one time, and responses were tracked using deidentified participant ID numbers.

2.3. Postintervention Study. In October 2014, 1,370 participants from the original sample were sent an electronic flyer alerting them that they would receive an invitation to participate in the follow-up study (otherwise known as "postintervention study") on immunization practices among ob-gyns. One hundred thirty participants from the original sample were not included in the follow-up study because they were no longer active members of ACOG. Members who did not participate in the preintervention questionnaire were permitted to participate in the postintervention questionnaire. The online survey was conducted using Real Mail®,

and the purpose, risks, and benefits of the study were outlined in an e-mail containing a live link to the survey. Up to six reminder e-mails including a link to the online survey were sent between October and December 2014 to nonresponders. Participants were not provided with supplementary information regarding the topic of the survey and were instructed not to look up any additional information.

In February 2015, a paper questionnaire was mailed to all nonresponders of the electronic survey (n = 1,245). The purpose, risks, and benefits of the study were outlined in an accompanying cover letter. Two subsequent mailings were sent to nonresponders between April and May 2015. Finally, a shortened letter version of the questionnaire, identical to the one used in the preintervention study, was sent to a randomly selected sample of nonresponders (n = 300) in June 2015. The letter responses were used to assess for potential nonresponse bias and were not included in data analysis. The electronic questionnaire remained open until data collection for the paper mailings ended in July 2015; thus, participants who received the paper survey could elect to complete either the online or paper questionnaire. Participants were instructed to only complete the survey one time, and responses were tracked using deidentified participant ID numbers. In the follow-up study, all participants were given the option to opt out of completing the survey, and these participants were removed from the total sample size.

2.4. Data Analysis. Data were analyzed using a statistical software package (IBM SPSS Statistics® 20.0, IBM Corp©, Armonk, NY). The study was approved by the ACOG Institutional Review Board. Completion of the online survey or return of the completed paper questionnaire indicated informed consent to participate in the study. Descriptive statistics were computed for measures used in the analyses and reported as mean values ± standard deviation. Chi-square tests were performed for categorical and comparative analyses. One-way analysis of variance (ANOVA) was used to compare group means of continuous variables. Nonparametric statistics were computed for comparative analyses of Likert-scale variables. Comparative results were reported as preintervention study % versus postintervention study %. Findings were reported as significant at $p < .05$.

3. Results

3.1. Preintervention Study. One hundred thirty-one participants completed the electronic survey, 272 participants returned the paper questionnaire, and 31 participants completed the shortened letter version questionnaire, resulting in a total response rate of 29.3%. Nineteen questionnaires were judged invalid (i.e., provider retired or provider was unreachable by mail); these participants were thus excluded from analysis. Responses to the letter questionnaire did not differ significantly from those of the electronic or paper surveys. Letter responses were excluded from data analysis because of the abbreviated questions found in the letter.

ACOG's total membership in 2013 consisted of 30,015 female members (52.5%) and 27,160 male members (47.5%).

Among respondents, 203 were female (59.0%) and 141 were male (41.0%). Males were significantly older than females (males, mean age = 55.19 years ± 10.29 years; females, mean age = 45.19 years ± 9.75 years; $F(1, 337) = 81.90$, $p < .001$). Respondents were from the District of Columbia, Puerto Rico, and every state in the United States except Delaware, North Dakota, and Wyoming.

3.2. Postintervention Study. One hundred and one participants completed the electronic survey, 186 participants returned the paper questionnaire, and 12 participants completed the shortened letter version questionnaire, resulting in a total response rate of 24.0%. Forty-seven questionnaires were judged invalid (i.e., provider retired, provider opted out, or provider was unreachable by mail); these participants were thus excluded from analysis. Responses to the letter questionnaire did not differ significantly from those of the electronic or paper surveys. Letter responses were excluded from data analysis because of the abbreviated questions found in the letter.

Among respondents, 182 were female (64.1%) and 102 were male (35.9%). Males were significantly older than females (males, mean age = 55.51 years ± 9.63 years; females, mean age = 46.18 years ± 9.05 years; $F(1, 279) = 65.77$, $p < .001$). Respondents were from the District of Columbia and every state in the United States except Alaska, Delaware, New Hampshire, New Mexico, North Dakota, and Wyoming. Additional demographic information for postintervention study participants can be found in Table 1. The demographic information provided by the postintervention study is similar to the demographic characteristics of ACOG's full membership [19].

3.3. Pre- versus Postintervention Study Comparative Analysis

3.3.1. ACOG Immunization Toolkits. Significantly more obgyns from the postintervention study (84.5%) reported that they received the immunization toolkits than ob-gyns from the preintervention study (67.0%) (χ^2 (2, $N = 681$) = 26.77, $p < .001$). Of those who indicated that they had received the toolkits, an average of 87.3% of respondents from both studies reported that they reviewed the toolkit materials. Among postintervention study participants, obgyns in group practice (90.3%) were significantly more likely to report that they received the toolkits mailings compared to those in private practice (59.5%) or other types of practice (85.3%) (e.g., community hospital or university faculty and practice) (χ^2 (4, $N = 282$) = 25.57, $p < .001$).

Providers were asked to indicate the extent to which they planned to use the immunization toolkit resources. Participant responses from both studies are detailed in Table 2. More postintervention study than preintervention study obgyns reported already using all of the toolkit resources, except the ACOG Immunization for Women website; however, these results did not reach statistical significance.

Physicians' frequency of toolkit use was assessed. The most frequently used (i.e., "weekly use") toolkit items reported in pre- and postintervention studies were the Flu

TABLE 1: Demographic characteristics of postintervention study respondents.

Characteristics	Percentage (%)
Years since completion of residency	
21–30 years	33.6
11–20 years	28.7
5–10 years	16.1
<5	11.9
Type of practice	
Large group (4+ partners)	43.2
Solo private practice	14.7
University full-time faculty & practice	13.3
Small group (2-3 partners)	10.9
Community hospital full-time	7.7
One partner	3.9
Others	3.9
Community hospital part-time	1.4
Military/government	1.1
Primary medical specialty	
General ob-gyn	74.8
Gynecology only	8.0
Maternal/fetal medicine	7.3
Reproductive endocrinology/infertility	5.6
Gynecologic oncology	2.4
Obstetrics only	1.4
Urogynecology	0.3
Practice location	
Suburban	47.9
Urban, noninner city	25.9
Urban, inner city	15.0
Rural	10.8
Military	0.3
Professional self-identification	
Both primary care physician and specialist	47.9
Specialist	46.9
Primary care physician	5.2
Patient race	
White, non-Hispanic	63.7
Multiracial	16.5
White, Hispanic	10.2
African American, non-Hispanic	3.2
African American, Hispanic	2.1
Asian/Pacific Islander	1.1
American Indian/Alaska native	0.7
Patient insurance	
Private (including HMO, IPO, military)	70.9
Medicaid/Medicare	26.3
Uninsured	2.8

FAQ Tear Pad (28.9% versus 31.2%) and the Tdap FAQ Tear Pad (26.7% versus 31.0%). The least frequently used (i.e., "never use") toolkit resources reported were the Physician Script (58.7% versus 59.2%), Coding Guide (51.3% versus

TABLE 2: The extent to which ob-gyns plan to use immunization toolkit resources.

	Already use (%)		Plan to use (%)		Will not likely use (%)		Definitely will not use (%)	
	Pre	Post	Pre	Post	Pre	Post	Pre	Post
Flu FAQ Tear Pad	37.7	44.5	30.0	21.6	21.8	23.3	10.5	10.6
Tdap FAQ Tear Pad	36.1	44.7	31.0	20.8	22.4	23.9	10.6	10.6
Vaccine Safety Tear Pad	30.7	36.5	32.7	21.6	26.0	29.7	10.6	12.2
Immunization for Women website	17.3	15.6	40.3	30.7	31.9	39.9	10.5	13.8
Coding Guide	14.2	16.0	27.6	21.1	40.2	40.8	18.0	22.1
Physician Script	12.4	18.4	21.8	13.2	46.2	46.2	19.7	22.2

FAQ, frequently asked question; Tdap, tetanus-diphtheria-acellular pertussis.

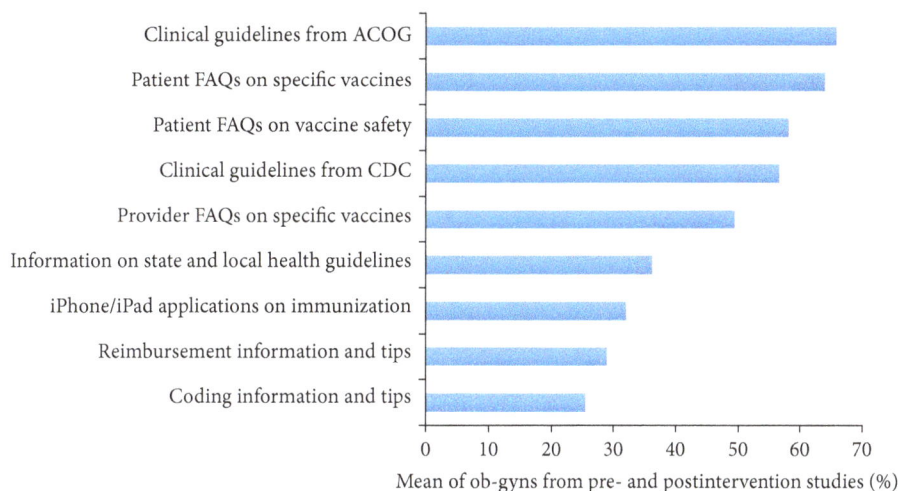

FIGURE 1: Resources ob-gyns indicated would be most valuable in ACOG's next immunization toolkit.

56.3%), and Immunization for Women website (45.9% versus 52.6%).

3.3.2. Immunization Resources.

Providers were asked about their opinions regarding which immunization resources they would find most useful in future immunization toolkits. The immunization resources most frequently selected as valuable in both pre- and postintervention studies were clinical guidelines from ACOG (71.2% versus 58.0%), patient FAQs on specific vaccines (61.3% versus 67.7%), patient FAQs on vaccine safety (54.9% versus 62.6%), and clinical guidelines from the CDC (58.8% versus 53.3%) (Figure 1). Three statistically significant differences were found between these pre- and postintervention study responses (Table 3). The immunization resources reported the least frequently as valuable in the pre- and postintervention studies were not identical; thus, the combined mean responses are reported: videos on immunization (4.4%), webinars on immunization (5.1%), CD-ROMS on vaccinations (5.2%), postgraduate courses (6.6%), and information provided at ACOG Annual District Meetings (6.6%).

3.3.3. Immunization Practices Patterns.

Ob-gyns' immunization practice patterns were examined. The use of standing orders for immunizations and the routine administration of Tdap vaccinations during pregnancy appear to be improving.

Significantly more providers from the postintervention study (46.6%) than the preintervention study (36.5%) reported that they use standing orders for immunizations in their practices (χ^2 (1, $N = 627$) = 6.55, $p = .011$). Additionally, postintervention study respondents (76.8%) were significantly more likely than preintervention study participants (59.3%) to report that they routinely offer Tdap vaccinations to all patients during pregnancy (χ^2 (4, $N = 612$) = 30.55, $p < .001$). Among providers who did not report offering Tdap to all pregnant patients, the majority indicated that they either offer Tdap to their patients postpartum (10.5%) or recommend and refer patients to other local providers (18.3%).

Approximately one-quarter of pre- and postintervention study respondents reported that they have assigned a staff member to be the vaccine coordinator of their practice (23.0% versus 26.1%) or always use a needs assessment with patients to determine what vaccinations they need at the time of their appointment (20.4% versus 27.0%). The large majority of ob-gyns from both studies reported that they offered or planned to offer influenza vaccinations to their patients for the 2012-2013 and 2014-2015 flu seasons (76.9% versus 78.9%). Among physicians who did not offer or plan to offer influenza vaccinations, 97.2% of preintervention study providers and 92.9% of postintervention study providers reported that they would recommend them to their patients or refer patients to local vaccine clinics or providers. Participants were also

TABLE 3: Statistically significant differences between pre- and postintervention study providers.

Variable	Preintervention study (%)	Postintervention study (%)	p value
Received ACOG's immunization toolkit mailings[†]	67.0	84.5	<.001
Valuable immunization resources to include in future toolkit mailings			
Clinical guidelines from ACOG[†]	71.2	58.0	.001
Coding information and tips[†]	30.7	18.0	<.001
Reimbursement information and tips[†]	15.2	9.4	<.001
Barriers to offering immunizations			
Cost[†]	45.5	34.8	.006
Time[*]	25.4	33.0	.036
Lack of access to patient records[*]	7.5	3.7	.048
Lack of patient interest[*]	29.9	37.5	.043
Use standing orders for immunizations[*]	36.5	46.6	.011
Routinely offer Tdap to all pregnant patients[†]	59.3	76.8	<.001
Common reasons patients decline vaccinations			
They do not think they need vaccines[†]	70.4	80.6	.003
Percentage of patients that decline vaccinations			
Less than one-third[†]	64.4	76.5	.001
Receive annual influenza vaccination themselves[*]	90.7	96.1	.024
Require staff to receive annual influenza vaccination[*]	78.1	86.2	.011

ACOG, American College of Obstetricians and Gynecologists; Tdap, tetanus-diphtheria-acellular pertussis.
[*]$p < .05$, [†]$p < .01$.

asked whether they receive annual influenza vaccination. Significantly more respondents from the postintervention study (96.1%) than the preintervention study (90.7%) indicated that they receive an annual flu vaccine (χ^2 (2, $N = 678$) = 7.44, $p = .024$).

Preintervention study physicians who reported that they annually receive a flu vaccine were significantly more likely to offer Tdap immunizations to all of their pregnant patients (62.5%) (χ^2 (8, $N = 342$) = 42.09, $p < .001$) compared to physicians who reported that they do not receive annual influenza vaccination. These differences were not present in the postintervention study. However, significant differences based on practice type and primary medical specialty were noted in the postintervention study. Providers in solo practice were less likely to offer Tdap vaccination to all patients during pregnancy (55.9%), administer flu vaccines (53.7%), and use standing orders for immunizations (12.8%) compared with providers in group ob-gyn practice (78.3%, 81.0%, and 46.5%, resp.) or providers practicing in other settings (e.g., university faculty and practice, community hospitals) (84.1%, 87.7%, and 59.5%, resp.) ($p = .002$, $p < .001$, and $p < .001$, resp.). Additionally, physicians who identified their primary medical specialty as general obstetrics and gynecology and obstetrics only were more likely to administer influenza vaccines to their patients (85.6% and 75.0%, resp.) and use standing orders for immunizations (51.5% and 66.7%, resp.) than providers who identified their primary medical specialty as gynecology only (50.0% and 22.7%, resp.) or "other" (i.e., reproductive endocrinology/infertility, maternal/fetal medicine, urogynecology, and gynecologic oncology) (64.4% and 29.5%, resp., $p < .001$).

Lastly, ob-gyns were surveyed about whether they require their staff to receive immunizations for influenza, Hepatitis B, and Tdap. Postintervention study physicians (86.2%) were significantly more likely than preintervention study physicians (78.1%) to report that they required their staff to receive an annual influenza vaccine (χ^2 (2, $N = 641$) = 6.52, $p = .011$). Responses to the other vaccination questions did not differ significantly between pre- and postintervention study providers. The majority of participants from both studies reported that they require their staff to receive Hepatitis B immunization (62.4% versus 62.1), while slightly less than half of the providers require their staff to receive Tdap vaccination (42.5% versus 49.1%).

3.3.4. Barriers to Offering Immunizations. Ob-gyns were asked to rank their top three barriers to offering immunizations in their offices and the top two most common reasons their patients provide for declining vaccinations. While the top three most frequently reported barriers remained the same for pre- and postintervention studies (inadequate reimbursement, cost, and lack of patient interest), several significant differences were found between the two studies regarding the percentage of respondents who endorsed some of the listed barriers (Table 4). Preintervention study providers were significantly more likely than those of the postintervention study to indicate that cost and lack of access to patient records were barriers to providing immunizations, while postintervention study respondents were more likely to report that time and lack of patient interest were barriers.

Several other demographic differences were observed in the postintervention study. A larger number of ob-gyns who

TABLE 4: Barriers to offering immunizations among ob-gyns.

Barrier	Overall % of ob-gyns who agreed		
	Preintervention study	Postintervention study	p value
Inadequate reimbursement	51.4	44.6	.085
Cost†	45.5	34.8	.006
Lack of interest from patients*	29.9	37.5	.043
Lack of time*	25.4	33.0	.036
Lack of storage for vaccine/supplies	24.2	18.0	.059
Concerns about vaccine safety	18.5	18.4	.959
Lack of staff	16.7	19.5	.363
Participating in immunization registries	10.5	9.0	.514
Lack of access to patient records*	7.5	3.7	.048

$^*p < .05, ^†p < .01.$

reported practicing in suburban and rural locations indicated that cost (44.7% and 48.4%, $p < .001$) and inadequate reimbursement (52.8% and 51.6%, $p = .012$) were obstacles than clinicians who reported practicing in urban locations (20.7% and 34.2%). Significant demographic differences based upon practice type and primary medical specialty were also found for reported barriers to offering immunization and common reasons patients decline vaccinations. Providers in solo practice were more likely to report cost (48.8%, $p = .005$) and inadequate reimbursement (70.7%, $p < .001$) and least likely to report inadequate time (17.1%, $p = .038$) and concerns about vaccine safety (2.4%, $p = .013$) as barriers than providers in group practice (38.1%, 47.1%, 33.5%, and 22.6%, resp.) or other types of practices (e.g., university faculty and practice, community hospitals) (20.3%, 24.6%, 40.6%, and 18.8%, resp.). Providers who identified their primary medical specialty as obstetrics only (66.7%, $p = .037$) were more likely to report lack of staff as a barrier than providers who identified their primary medical specialty as general obstetrics and gynecology (16.9%), gynecology only (13.6%), or "other" (30.0%) (i.e., reproductive endocrinology/infertility, maternal/fetal medicine, urogynecology, and gynecologic oncology).

According to pre- and postintervention study participants, the top two most common reasons patients provide for declining vaccinations are safety concerns (84.2% versus 78.5%; (χ^2 (1, $N = 659$) = 3.48, $p = .062$)) and the belief that they do not need vaccines (70.4% versus 80.6%; (χ^2 (1, $N = 658$) = 8.77, $p = .003$)). While ob-gyns indicated that their patients express concerns over vaccine safety, the majority of respondents from both studies (64.4% versus 76.5%; (χ^2 (1, $N = 617$) = 10.42, $p = .001$)) estimated that less than one-third of their patients decline vaccinations after their recommendations. Responses from

both of these questions suggest that the described concerns are mostly patient concerns; 96.1% of preintervention study providers and 93.9% of postintervention study providers who reported concerns for vaccine safety as a barrier to offering immunizations also selected it as a common reason that patients decline vaccinations.

3.3.5. Immunization for Women Website and Text4baby Program. Ob-gyn awareness and use of the ACOG Immunization for Women website and the Text4baby program were assessed. Text4baby is a free mobile educational service designed for pregnant women to promote maternal and child health through text messaging. No significant differences were found between pre- and postintervention study respondents for any of these variables. Less than one-quarter of pre- (19.0%) and post- (22.1%) intervention study providers reported that they had ever visited ACOG's Immunization for Women website. The majority of pre- and postintervention study ob-gyns reported that they never refer staff (77.3% versus 74.1%), fellow ob-gyns (82.1% versus 80.8%), or patients (76.3% versus 68.4%) to ACOG's Immunization for Women website. Responses to this question did not differ by physician age or gender. Similarly, most ob-gyns were unfamiliar with the Text4baby program (72.7% versus 69.5%). Younger physicians (pre (χ^2 (4, $N = 326$) = 24.83, $p < .001$); post (χ^2 (4, $N = 275$) = 22.61, $p < .001$)) and female physicians (pre (χ^2 (1, $N = 333$) = 6.00, $p = .014$); post (χ^2 (1, $N = 276$) = 4.15, $p = .042$)) were more likely to be familiar with Text4baby. Among ob-gyns who were familiar with Text4baby, slightly less than half of the pre- and postintervention study respondents (47.1% versus 41.7%) recommended the program to patients who are pregnant or have children.

4. Discussion

Findings from this study indicate that ACOG's efforts to improve their immunization resources were successful in many ways. More ob-gyns from the postintervention study reported receiving the immunization toolkits than respondents from the preintervention study. This may be attributed to the more robust promotional campaign that accompanied the second round of immunization toolkits. It is also possible that the increase of postintervention respondents resulted from some type of Hawthorne effect whereby ob-gyns were made aware of the toolkit purely by participating in the preintervention study. Additionally, a greater number of postintervention study providers reported already using all of the immunization toolkit resources (except the Immunization for Women website); however, these results were not statistically significant. The most frequently used toolkit materials reported in both studies were the Flu FAQ Tear Pad and the Tdap FAQ Tear Pad.

The percentage of physicians who reported offering Tdap vaccination to all women during pregnancy increased significantly from 59% to 77% between pre- and postintervention studies. However, these numbers are much higher than those found in the existing literature (30%), indicating that further research is warranted to clarify accurate estimates of Tdap coverage among ob-gyns [18]. The large majority of providers in both studies reported offering influenza vaccines to their patients during the 2013-2014 and 2014-2015 influenza seasons. While our findings align with previously reported rates of influenza administration among ob-gyns [17, 20], an important discrepancy should be noted. According to previously reported national estimates, far fewer pregnant women report receiving influenza and Tdap immunizations than the number of ob-gyns in our study who reported offering them [14, 15]. However, published numbers specifically on Tdap immunization rates are several years old and reflect the rates before ACOG published its recommendations in 2013 to offer the vaccine during every pregnancy [1]. More recent data in states like Wisconsin demonstrate much higher rates of Tdap vaccination during pregnancy than the dreadful "2.6%" that is so commonly referenced [14, 21]. It is possible that ob-gyn respondents are overestimating the proportion of pregnant patients being vaccinated or that ob-gyns respondents of our questionnaires were more likely to routinely administer influenza vaccination or recommend and refer their patients to receive it compared to ob-gyns who did not respond to this study. This discrepancy may also be partially explained by a small percentage of pregnant women who refuse vaccine administration, although research shows that when women are offered vaccination, the majority tends to accept it [15, 22].

Several barriers to offering immunizations were identified by participants. In support of previous findings [16–18], frequently reported obstacles to vaccine administration were financial concerns (cost and inadequate reimbursement), lack of patient interest, lack of time, and inadequate storage for vaccines and supplies. Efficacious interventions are necessary to combat these barriers and improve influenza and Tdap immunization coverage for pregnant women. ACOG recommends several strategies to help ob-gyns prevent missed opportunities for vaccination among pregnant women. These include designating a vaccine coordinator and backup coordinator in their practices to order and receive vaccines, ensure proper storage of vaccines, and be familiar with appropriate billing codes for reimbursement; incorporate needs assessments to determine each pregnant woman's immunization status and administration of indicated vaccinations; and use standing orders to ensure that indicated vaccinations can be administered to all pregnant women without an individual physician order [1]. Discouragingly, less than half of the ob-gyns from the pre- and postintervention studies reported using standing orders for immunizations, and less than one-quarter of participants indicated that they use needs assessments or have assigned a vaccine coordinator within their practices. Other strategies that have been shown to improve immunization rates include educating pregnant women about the maternal and neonatal benefits of immunizations, recommending and offering on-site vaccine administration during pregnancy, and utilizing prompts to help providers and their staff easily identify vaccine-eligible obstetric patients [1, 15, 17, 23]. Improvements in health care policies are essential to help deliver reliable reimbursement to vaccine providers and to curb the high costs of ordering and storing immunizations [24].

One of the limitations to this study is the relatively low response rate. The low response rate may indicate a lack of physician interest in this topic. In order to increase the response rate, multiple mailings and a simplified questionnaire were utilized. It is also possible that characteristics of respondents are different from those of nonrespondents, although nonresponse bias analysis did not reveal statistically significant differences for comparison variables. The simplified questionnaire offered a sufficient amount of content-relevant questions that would assert that those who responded and those who did not respond held similar attitudes towards vaccination during pregnancy. Lastly, these data are based on physician recall and could not be checked through chart review or other methods.

Improving immunization coverage among pregnant women has numerous health benefits for mothers, their infants, and society. While it appears that influenza and Tdap administration rates are increasing among ob-gyns, several barriers to offering immunizations persist. It is crucial to help providers overcome these obstacles in order to ensure that these vaccinations become a routine part of obstetric health care.

Disclaimer

The study's contents are solely the responsibility of the authors and do not necessarily represent the official views of the Centers for Disease Control and Prevention.

Conflict of Interests

The authors declare that there is no conflict of interests regarding the publication of this paper.

Acknowledgment

This study was supported by Cooperative Agreement 5U66IP000667 from the Centers for Disease Control and Prevention.

References

[1] American College of Obstetricians and Gynecologists, "ACOG committee opinion no. 558: integrating immunizations into practice," *Obstetrics and Gynecology*, vol. 121, pp. 897–903, 2013.

[2] Centers for Disease Control and Prevention, "Prevention of pertussis, tetanus, and diphtheria among pregnant and postpartum women and their infants recommendations of the Advisory Committee on Immunization Practices (ACIP)," *MMWR Recommendations and Reports*, vol. 57, no. 4, pp. 1–51, 2008.

[3] American College of Obstetricians and Gynecologists, "Update on immunization and pregnancy: tetanus, diphtheria, and pertussis vaccination [Committee Opinion No. 566]," *Obstetrics & Gynecolog*, vol. 121, pp. 1411–1414, 2013.

[4] A. L. Naleway, W. J. Smith, and J. P. Mullooly, "Delivering influenza vaccine to pregnant women," *Epidemiologic Reviews*, vol. 28, no. 1, pp. 47–53, 2006.

[5] American College of Obstetricians and Gynecologists, "Influenza vaccination during pregnancy. Committee opinion no. 608," *Obstetrics and Gynecology*, vol. 124, pp. 648–651, 2014.

[6] Centers for Disease Control and Prevention, "Prevention and control of influenza with vaccines: recommendations of the Advisory Committee on Immunization Practices (ACIP), United States, 2013-14," *Morbidity and Mortality Weekly Report*, vol. 62, no. 7, pp. 1–43, 2013.

[7] P. Lu, C. B. Bridges, G. L. Euler, and J. A. Singleton, "Influenza vaccination of recommended adult populations, U.S., 1989–2005," *Vaccine*, vol. 26, no. 14, pp. 1786–1793, 2008.

[8] D. Güriş, P. M. Strebel, B. Bardenheier et al., "Changing epidemiology of pertussis in the United States: increasing reported incidence among adolescents and adults, 1990–1996," *Clinical Infectious Diseases*, vol. 28, no. 6, pp. 1230–1237, 1999.

[9] Centers for Disease Control and Prevention, "Pertussis—United States, 1997–2000," *Morbidity and Mortality Weekly Report*, vol. 51, no. 4, pp. 73–76, 2002.

[10] M. Tanaka, C. R. Vitek, F. B. Pascual, K. M. Bisgard, J. E. Tate, and T. V. Murphy, "Trends in pertussis among infants in the in the United States, 1980–1999," *The Journal of the American Medical Association*, vol. 290, no. 22, pp. 2968–2975, 2003.

[11] A. M. Wendelboe, E. Njamkepo, A. Bourillon et al., "Transmission of *Bordetella pertussis* to young infants," *Pediatric Infectious Disease Journal*, vol. 26, no. 4, pp. 293–299, 2007.

[12] T. Q. Tan and M. V. Gerbie, "Pertussis, a disease whose time has come: what can be done to control the problem?" *Obstetrics & Gynecology*, vol. 122, no. 2, part 1, pp. 370–373, 2013.

[13] Centers for Disease Control and Prevention, "Updated recommendations for use of tetanus toxoid, reduced diphtheria toxoid and acellular pertussis vaccine (Tdap) in pregnant women and persons who have or anticipate having close contact with an infant aged <12 months—Advisory Committee on Immuniza," *Morbidity and Mortality Weekly Report*, vol. 60, no. 41, pp. 1424–1426, 2011.

[14] Centers for Disease Control and Prevention, "Updated recommendations for use of tetanus toxoid, reduced diphtheria toxoid and acellular pertussis vaccine (Tdap) in pregnant women—Advisory Committee on Immunization Practices (ACIP), 2012," *Morbidity and Mortality Weekly Report*, vol. 62, no. 7, pp. 131–135, 2013.

[15] Centers for Disease Control and Prevention, "Influenza vaccination coverage among pregnant women, United States. 2013-14 Influenza season," *Morbidity and Mortality Weekly Report*, vol. 63, no. 37, pp. 816–821, 2014.

[16] M. A. Leddy, B. L. Anderson, M. L. Power, S. Gall, B. Gonik, and J. Schulkin, "Changes in and current status of obstetrician-gynecologists' knowledge, attitudes, and practice regarding immunization," *Obstetrical and Gynecological Survey*, vol. 64, no. 12, pp. 823–829, 2009.

[17] D. M. Kissin, M. L. Power, E. B. Kahn et al., "Attitudes and practices of obstetrician-gynecologists regarding influenza vaccination in pregnancy," *Obstetrics and Gynecology*, vol. 118, no. 5, pp. 1074–1080, 2011.

[18] M. L. Power, M. A. Leddy, B. L. Anderson, S. A. Gall, B. Gonik, and J. Schulkin, "Obstetrician-gynecologists' practices and perceived knowledge regarding immunization," *American Journal of Preventive Medicine*, vol. 37, no. 3, pp. 231–234, 2009.

[19] American College of Obstetricians and Gynecologists, *2013 Socioeconomic Survey of ACOG Fellows*, American College of Obstetricians and Gynecologists, 2013, https://www.acog.org/-/media/Departments/Practice-Management-and-Managed-Care/2013SocioeconomicSurvey.pdf.

[20] K. L. Murtough, M. L. Power, and J. Schulkin, "Knowledge, attitudes, and practices of obstetrician-gynecologists regarding influenza prevention and treatment following the 2009 H1N1 pandemic," *Journal of Women's Health*, vol. 24, no. 10, pp. 849–854, 2015.

[21] Centers for Disease Control and Prevention, "Pertussis and influenza vaccination among insured pregnant women—Wisconsin, 2013-2014," *Morbidity and Mortality Weekly Report*, vol. 64, no. 27, pp. 746–750, 2015.

[22] B. Gonik, T. Jones, D. Contreras, N. Fasano, and C. Roberts, "The obstetrician-gynecologist's role in vaccine-preventable diseases and immunization," *Obstetrics and Gynecology*, vol. 96, no. 1, pp. 81–84, 2000.

[23] M. H. Moniz and R. H. Beigi, "Maternal immunization," *Human Vaccines & Immunotherapeutics*, vol. 10, no. 9, pp. 2562–2570, 2014.

[24] B.-K. Yoo, "How to improve influenza vaccination rates in the U.S.," *Journal of Preventive Medicine and Public Health*, vol. 44, no. 4, pp. 141–148, 2011.

18

Maternal Lopinavir/Ritonavir Is Associated with Fewer Adverse Events in Infants than Nelfinavir or Atazanavir

Christiana Smith,[1] Adriana Weinberg,[1,2,3] Jeri E. Forster,[4] Myron J. Levin,[1,2] Jill Davies,[5,6] Jennifer Pappas,[7] Kay Kinzie,[7] Emily Barr,[1] Suzanne Paul,[1] and Elizabeth J. McFarland[1]

[1]Division of Infectious Diseases, Department of Pediatrics, University of Colorado School of Medicine and Children's Hospital Colorado, Aurora, CO 80045, USA
[2]Department of Medicine, University of Colorado School of Medicine, Aurora, CO 80045, USA
[3]Department of Pathology, University of Colorado School of Medicine, Aurora, CO 80045, USA
[4]Department of Biostatistics and Informatics, Colorado School of Public Health, Aurora, CO 80045, USA
[5]Department of Obstetrics and Gynecology, University of Colorado School of Medicine, Aurora, CO 80045, USA
[6]Denver Health Medical Center, Denver, CO 80204, USA
[7]Children's Hospital Colorado, Aurora, CO 80045, USA

Correspondence should be addressed to Christiana Smith; christiana.smith@childrenscolorado.org

Academic Editor: Bryan Larsen

Combination antiretroviral therapy (cART) is successfully used for prevention of perinatal HIV transmission. To investigate safety, we compared adverse events (AE) among infants exposed to different maternal cART regimens. We reviewed 158 HIV-uninfected infants born between 1997 and 2009, using logistic regression to model grade ≥ 1 AE and grade ≥ 3 AE as a function of maternal cART and confounding variables (preterm, C-section, illicit drug use, race, ethnicity, infant antiretrovirals, and maternal viremia). Frequently used cART regimens included zidovudine (63%), lamivudine (80%), ritonavir-boosted lopinavir (37%), nelfinavir (26%), and atazanavir (10%). At birth, anemia occurred in 13/140 infants (9%), neutropenia in 27/107 (25%), thrombocytopenia in 5/133 (4%), and liver enzyme elevation in 21/130 (16%). Corresponding rates of AE at 4 weeks were 59/141 (42%), 54/130 (42%), 3/137 (2%), and 3/104 (3%), respectively. Serious AE (grade ≥ 3) exceeded 2% only for neutropenia (13% at birth; 9% at 4 weeks). Compared with infants exposed to maternal lopinavir/ritonavir, infants exposed to nelfinavir and atazanavir had a 5-fold and 4-fold higher incidence of AE at birth, respectively. In conclusion, hematologic and hepatic AE were frequent, but rarely serious. In this predominantly protease inhibitor-treated population, lopinavir/ritonavir was associated with the lowest rate of infant AE.

1. Introduction

The prevention of perinatal transmission of HIV is one of the most successful public health interventions of the last few decades. The use of maternal combination antiretroviral therapy (cART), when combined with infant postnatal prophylaxis, has reduced transmission rates to less than 1% in developed countries [1, 2]. This is a remarkable achievement, but concerns remain regarding toxicity in these infants after exposure to multiple antiretrovirals (ARV) in utero, during delivery, and in early infancy [3].

Spontaneous preterm delivery and low birth weight have been associated with HIV infection during pregnancy.

Although not a uniform finding across studies, the use of protease inhibitors (PI) during pregnancy may increase the incidence of preterm delivery [4–6]. Mitochondrial and nuclear genotoxicity are associated with in utero exposure to nucleoside reverse transcriptase inhibitors (NRTI) [7, 8]. In addition, laboratory adverse events (AE) have been described in ARV-exposed infants, including hematologic cytopenias and disruption of liver function. The NRTI are known to alter in vitro hematopoiesis [9, 10]. Transient macrocytic anemia was the most common side effect in infants exposed to zidovudine (ZDV) pre- and postnatally in the landmark PACTG 076 study [11, 12], and several reports describe profound neonatal anemia after ARV exposure in utero [13, 14]. Other studies have confirmed the link between ARV exposure and neonatal neutropenia, lymphopenia, and thrombocytopenia [15–20]. Liver dysfunction is described less frequently, although several studies have demonstrated elevated neonatal aspartate aminotransferase (AST), alanine aminotransferase (ALT), and bilirubin after exposure to perinatal ARV [21–25]. Increasing complexity of maternal cART correlates with an increased risk for hematologic and hepatic AE [15, 17, 21, 22, 26–28].

As new ARV and more complex cART regimens are administered for the prevention of perinatal HIV transmission, it is important to identify the toxicities associated with both established and novel regimens in order to inform best choices [29–31]. Prior studies have compared infant AE after exposure to different classes of ARV, for example, nonnucleoside reverse transcriptase inhibitor- (NNRTI-) based cART and PI-based cART [22, 27]. In this study, we examine infant AE after exposure to different maternal drugs within ARV classes.

2. Materials and Methods

2.1. Study Design. This study was approved by the Colorado Multiple Institutional Review Board and exempted from informed consent. This was a retrospective chart review of 190 pregnancies complicated by HIV infection that were managed by the Children's Hospital Immunodeficiency Program (CHIP) in Denver. CHIP is the reference center for the care of HIV-infected pregnant women in Colorado and neighboring states. Data were abstracted for all pregnancies from 1997 to 2009 that resulted in a live infant birth. Maternal data collected included demographics, ARV use, illicit drug use, mode of delivery, hematologic and hepatic laboratory values, CD4 count, and viral load. Undetectable viral load was defined as <400 copies/mL, as this was the lower limit of detection for the earliest data. Duration of maternal viremia during pregnancy was defined as the number of days from the estimated conception date until either the date of the first undetectable viral load measurement after which all subsequent viral load measurements were undetectable or, if there was no sustained viral suppression, the number of days between the estimated conception date and the date of infant birth. The estimated conception date was calculated from infant gestational age determined at birth. Infant data collected included gestational age (preterm defined as <37 weeks), birth weight (small for gestational age (SGA) defined as <3rd percentile of expected weight for gestational age), postnatal ARV prophylaxis, laboratory values (hemoglobin, neutrophil count, platelets, AST, ALT, and total bilirubin), and hospitalizations or illnesses. Infant complete blood count and liver function panel was assessed at birth (age 0–7 days) and at 4 weeks (±2 weeks). Laboratory toxicities were graded using the Division of AIDS Table for Grading the Severity of Adult and Pediatric Adverse Events [32]. If the medical record did not specify an upper limit of normal for AST and ALT, the limits imposed were 60 IU/L and 65 IU/L for AST and ALT, respectively, as these are the limits used by the Children's Hospital Colorado Laboratory. Infant infection status was monitored using HIV RNA and/or DNA PCR at

birth, 2 weeks, 4 weeks, 6 weeks, and 4 months of age and HIV antibody testing starting at 12 months of age and repeated every 3–6 months until seroreversion was demonstrated.

2.2. Prophylaxis Regimens. Pregnant women received a clinician-prescribed antenatal ARV regimen that consisted of cART (≥3 ARV from ≥2 ARV classes) in most cases; modifications during the pregnancy were based on viral genotype, virologic response, safety, and tolerability, as previously described [33–35]. PI serum levels were routinely monitored and doses adjusted to achieve a trough above the 25th percentile for nonpregnant adults. Infant ARV exposure was assigned based on the maternal ARV received for ≥28 days during the 35 days immediately prior to delivery, thereby setting a minimum period of in utero drug exposure occurring near the time of infant laboratory assessment. Other maternal ARV received before the 35 days immediately prior to delivery was not accounted for in the analysis.

Most infants were prescribed postnatal prophylaxis consisting of six weeks of ZDV. In some infants, ZDV was replaced by stavudine (d4T) due to anemia, neutropenia, or both. In situations where the risk of perinatal transmission was increased, infants received two- or three-drug ARV. A detailed description of the infant postnatal prophylaxis prescribed and associated adverse events has been previously reported [36].

2.3. Statistical Analysis. The analysis included infants with at least one laboratory value at either birth or 4 weeks. The statistical analyses require that all observations (infants) are independent of one another or the results may be biased. Given that twins have identical exposure in utero and in order not to underestimate associations between AE and ARV, the twin with the lower grade toxicity was excluded from each pair. Maternal and infant characteristics were compared using t-tests, chi-square tests, and Fisher's exact tests, as appropriate. Because most infants were exposed to an antenatal ARV regimen containing two NRTI and a PI, AE were compared between infants exposed to different NRTI and between infants exposed to different PI. The number of infants exposed to nevirapine ($n = 10$) was too small for comparison. Rates of preterm birth and SGA were compared as a univariate analysis. Logistic regression was used to model grade ≥1 laboratory AE and grade ≥3 laboratory AE (yes/no) as a function of maternal ARV received for ≥28 days during the 35 days immediately prior to delivery and any confounding variable that changed the odds ratio (OR, 95% confidence interval) by >20%. Confounding variables used in the multivariate analyses include preterm birth, infant exposure to ZDV monoprophylaxis versus combination prophylaxis, mechanism of delivery, maternal race and ethnicity, maternal illicit drug use, and duration of maternal viremia during the pregnancy. Statistical significance was defined by $p \leq 0.05$.

3. Results

3.1. Maternal Characteristics and Antiretroviral Regimens. One hundred and sixty-five mothers were managed at CHIP

TABLE 1: Infant demographics and select obstetrical characteristics.

Characteristic	Number of infants/number evaluated[a] (%)[b]
Race[c]	
Caucasian	92/158 (58%)
African American	53/158 (34%)
American Indian/Alaskan Native	2/158 (1%)
Other/unknown	11/158 (7%)
Ethnicity[c]	
Hispanic	55/158 (34%)
Not Hispanic	94/158 (60%)
Other/unknown	10/158 (6%)
Sex, male	81/152 (53%)
Entry maternal CD4 count[d]	
<200 cells/mm^3	7/101 (7%)
200–500 cells/mm^3	40/101 (40%)
>500 cells/mm^3	54/101 (53%)
Entry median maternal HIV RNA copies/mL in plasma[d] (range) $N = 109$	2120 (<20–213,191)
Antiretrovirals initiated before conception	44/152 (29%)
Maternal illicit drug use	19/158 (12%)
Mean gestational age in weeks (range) $N = 150$	37.7 (25–41.7)
Preterm deliveries	26/150 (17%)
Deliveries via Cesarean section	64/158 (41%)

[a]Denominator represents the number of infants with available data.
[b]Unless units of measurement are otherwise indicated.
[c]Infant race and ethnicity determined by maternal self-report.
[d]From earliest known maternal laboratory values during pregnancy.

for 190 pregnancies, resulting in 196 live births. Of these, 163 infants (5 twins) had at least one laboratory value available for analysis. The analysis cohort consisted of 158 mother/infant pairs after excluding one infant from each twin pair. There were no perinatal transmissions of HIV. The infant demographics and maternal HIV and obstetrical characteristics are reported in Table 1. Severe maternal immune suppression was rare; only 7% of women had a CD4 count <200 cells/mm^3 in early pregnancy. One hundred twenty-seven women (80%) received cART for at least 28 days prior to delivery. Fifteen women received cART for less than 28 days prior to delivery. Sixteen women received a less intensive ARV regimen. Maternal ARV received in the last month of pregnancy are detailed in Table 2. PI-based cART was received by 77% of women, including lopinavir with ritonavir (LPV/r, 37%), nelfinavir (NFV, 26%), atazanavir (ATV, 10%, including 2% without ritonavir), and saquinavir (4%). The majority of women received ZDV (63%), but 13%, 9.5%, and 4% received d4T, tenofovir (TDF), and abacavir (ABC), respectively. There were few differences in maternal and infant characteristics between the two largest treatment groups, LPV/r versus NFV (Supplementary Table 1 in the Supplementary Material available online at http://dx.doi.org/10.1155/2016/9848041).

3.2. Overall Frequency of Adverse Events. Laboratory AE in the first four weeks of life were common, with three quarters of infants having an AE (any grade) at either birth or 4 weeks. The frequency of an AE grade ≥3 in any laboratory category

was 12% at birth and 16% at 4 weeks. Neutropenia was most common, with 25% and 42% of infants having any grade AE, and 13% and 9% having grade ≥3 AE, at birth and 4 weeks, respectively (Figure 1). Anemia was the next most common, with 9% and 42% of infants having any grade AE, but only 1% and 0% having grade ≥3 AE, at birth and 4 weeks, respectively. Rates of AST AE fell from 16% at birth to 3% at 4 weeks. Rates of ALT AE and thrombocytopenia were low at birth and at 4 weeks. No infants had hyperbilirubinemia at birth.

The 26 (17%) infants born preterm were more likely than term infants to develop an AE of any grade (93% versus 71%, $p = 0.03$) or grade ≥3 (46% versus 17%, $p = 0.003$) at either birth or 4 weeks. Four preterm infants required blood transfusions due to severe anemia. No infants suffered a serious bacterial infection or a bleeding disorder as a complication of neutropenia or thrombocytopenia, and no infants developed liver failure as a result of hepatic inflammation. No infants developed renal or cardiac dysfunction.

3.3. Association of Maternal ARV with Infant Adverse Events. Rates of infant laboratory AE relative to antenatal exposure to maternal ARV were compared in a multivariate analysis. At birth, infants exposed to maternal NFV compared to LPV/r had a higher rate of anemia (OR 7.4 (95% CI 1.4–39.0), $p = 0.02$), neutropenia (OR 10.6 (95% CI 1.7–66.4), $p = 0.01$), and any AE (OR 5.3 (95% CI 1.9–14.9), $p = 0.002$) (Figure 2). This association was maintained when limited to infants exposed to the same maternal NRTI backbone (ZDV

TABLE 2: Antenatal antiretroviral exposure of infants.

Drug[a]	Number exposed (%) N = 158
Nucleoside reverse transcriptase inhibitors	
Abacavir	7 (4%)
Emtricitabine	15 (9.5%)
Lamivudine	126 (80%)
Stavudine	21 (13%)
Tenofovir	15 (9.5%)
Zidovudine	99 (63%)
Nonnucleoside reverse transcriptase inhibitors	
Nevirapine	10 (6%)
Protease inhibitors	
Atazanavir ± ritonavir[b]	16 (10%)
Lopinavir + ritonavir	59 (37%)
Nelfinavir	41 (26%)
Saquinavir ± ritonavir	7 (4%)

[a] Maternal treatment administered for ≥28 days of the 35 days immediately preceding delivery.
[b] Thirteen of sixteen women received ritonavir-boosted atazanavir.

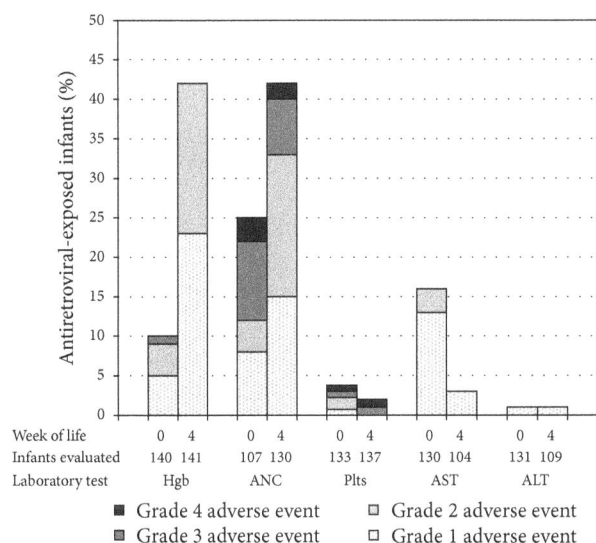

FIGURE 1: Frequency of infant adverse events. Bars represent percentages of infants with laboratory adverse events at birth (age 0–7 days) and at 4 weeks (±2 weeks). Hgb, hemoglobin; ANC, absolute neutrophil count; plts, platelet count; AST, aspartate aminotransferase; ALT, alanine aminotransferase.

and lamivudine) (Table 3). The difference was primarily the result of grade 1 AE; rates of grade ≥3 AE remained relatively low in both groups (9% versus 14% of LPV/r-exposed versus NFV-exposed infants, resp.; Figure 2). Exposure to maternal ATV was also associated with a higher rate of any laboratory AE compared to LPV/r (OR 4.2 (95% CI 1.0–17.5), $p = 0.046$) with the difference primarily due to higher rates of neutropenia (OR 18.3 (95% CI 1.2–267.8), $p = 0.03$) (Figure 2). At 4 weeks, there were no longer significant

differences in AE between infants exposed to different PI (Table 4).

Additional maternal and infant characteristics were examined to determine whether variables not included in the multivariate analysis might contribute to differences in infant AE at birth for the NFV and LPV/r groups, which had a sample size large enough for analysis (Supplementary Table 1). The mean estimated duration of maternal viremia was longer in the NFV-exposed group than in the LPV/r-exposed group (172 versus 125 days, $p = 0.05$). However, the association of infant AE with NFV versus LPV/r exposure remained significant when duration of maternal viremia was included as a covariate in the multivariate analysis (OR 7.9 (95% CI 2.4–26.2), $p = 0.0007$). In addition, a univariate analysis demonstrated that the duration of maternal viremia did not correlate with the frequency of infant AE (OR 1.0 (95% CI 0.99–1.0), $p = 0.57$). An anticipated difference between the treatment groups was the year of delivery. NFV was prescribed in an earlier time period (1997–2007); LPV/r was first prescribed in 2003 and surpassed NFV as the most commonly used PI at our center by 2004. Other variables did not differ including the duration of antenatal exposure to NFV or LPV/r or the proportion of women who received the PI prior to conception (Supplementary Table 1).

Most women were treated with ZDV, but a substantial number received ABC, d4T, or TDF; therefore, rates of infant AE were compared between these groups. There were no significant differences at birth in rates of anemia, neutropenia, thrombocytopenia, or liver enzyme elevation between infants exposed to maternal ZDV compared with ABC, d4T, or TDF (Supplementary Table 2).

Rates of preterm birth and SGA for infants exposed to different maternal PI were compared in a univariate analysis. No significant differences were found in rates of preterm birth (5/16 (31%), 9/58 (16%), and 5/37 (14%), $p = 0.26$)

TABLE 3: Infant adverse events at birth associated with maternal lopinavir/ritonavir versus nelfinavir, in combination with zidovudine and lamivudine[a].

Laboratory test[b]	Lopinavir/ritonavir[c]	Nelfinavir[c]	Odds ratio (95% CI) p value
Hgb	2/34 (6%)	6/29 (21%)	6.3 (1.01–39.8) p = 0.049
ANC	2/22 (9%)	7/25 (28%)	N/A[d] p = 0.14
AST	4/34 (12%)	7/25 (28%)	3.5 (0.73–16.7) p = 0.12
Highest grade AE, all tests	10/35 (29%)	17/29 (59%)	4.9 (1.6–15.4) p = 0.006

Hgb, hemoglobin; ANC, absolute neutrophil count; AST, aspartate aminotransferase.
[a]Multivariate analysis using logistic regression was used to model grade ≥1 AE (yes/no) as a function of maternal antiretroviral treatment. Groups restricted to infants born to mothers treated with zidovudine/lamivudine in combination with either lopinavir/ritonavir or nelfinavir.
[b]There were no adverse events for bilirubin, 1 adverse event for alanine aminotransferase in the lopinavir/ritonavir group, and 3 adverse events for platelet count in the nelfinavir group, not shown separately but included in the maximum adverse events.
[c]Number of infants with adverse event/number of infants exposed (%).
[d]Fisher's exact test reported.

TABLE 4: Infant adverse events at 4 weeks associated with exposure to maternal lopinavir/ritonavir versus nelfinavir or atazanavir[a].

Laboratory test[b]	Lopinavir/ritonavir[c]	Nelfinavir[c]	Odds ratio (95% CI) p value[d]	Atazanavir[c]	Odds ratio (95% CI) p value[e]
Hgb	19/53 (36%)	14/34 (41%)	1.3 (0.52–3.0) p = 0.62	6/14 (43%)	1.3 (0.41–4.4) p = 0.63
ANC	24/48 (50%)	11/30 (37%)	0.58 (0.23–1.5) p = 0.25	5/14 (36%)	0.56 (0.16–1.9) p = 0.35
Bili	11/52 (21%)	9/26 (35%)	2.5 (0.75–8.1) p = 0.14	3/7 (43%)	2.0 (0.35–11.4) p = 0.44
Highest grade AE, all tests	38/55 (69%)	22/35 (63%)	0.76 (0.31–1.8) p = 0.54	9/14 (64%)	0.62 (0.16–2.4) p = 0.49

Hgb, hemoglobin; ANC, absolute neutrophil count; Bili, total bilirubin; AE, adverse event.
[a]Multivariate analysis using logistic regression was used to model grade ≥1 AE (yes/no) as a function of maternal antiretroviral treatment. No significant differences were found.
[b]There were no adverse events for alanine aminotransferase, 1 adverse event each for aspartate aminotransferase in the lopinavir/ritonavir and atazanavir groups, and 1 adverse event for platelet count in each group, not shown separately but included in the maximum adverse events.
[c]Number of adverse events/number exposed (%).
[d]Lopinavir/ritonavir versus nelfinavir.
[e]Lopinavir/ritonavir versus atazanavir.

or SGA (2/16 (13%), 7/56 (13%), and 4/35 (11%), p > 0.99) between infants exposed to ATV, LPV/r, and NFV, respectively, although the small sample size limited the power to detect a difference.

4. Discussion

Low-grade laboratory AE were common at birth and 4 weeks in the cART-exposed infants, but grade ≥3 AE were rare. Anemia and neutropenia made up the majority of AE, and neutropenia comprised nearly all grade ≥3 AE. Our results are in agreement with those of previous studies, which showed frequent, but low-grade, hematologic abnormalities among ARV-exposed infants. Pacheco et al. reported significantly decreased infant hemoglobin and neutrophil values, and Mussi-Pinhata et al. described anemia at hospital discharge in 24% of ARV-exposed infants, although in both studies nearly all AE were of grade 1 or 2 [17, 23]. Read et al. described grade

≥3 anemia or neutropenia in less than 10% of ARV-exposed infants in the first six weeks of life [19]. Four infants in our study required a blood transfusion due to anemia, all of whom were born at ≤32 weeks of gestation. Preterm infants are likely to require blood transfusion even when unexposed to ARV, with about 80% of US infants with birth weight <1500 grams requiring at least one transfusion [37]. None of the infants born ≥37 weeks of gestation in this study developed clinically significant AE. Although the majority of AE in these HIV- and ARV-exposed infants were of low grade, the mechanism underlying the AE is not fully understood and the long term effects of these early toxicities are unknown.

We found increased infant laboratory AE at birth associated with exposure to maternal NFV and ATV compared with LPV/r. The difference was observed even when the analysis was restricted to mother/infant pairs with the same NRTI background. At 4 weeks, no difference was detectable between these groups, suggesting that the effect is either

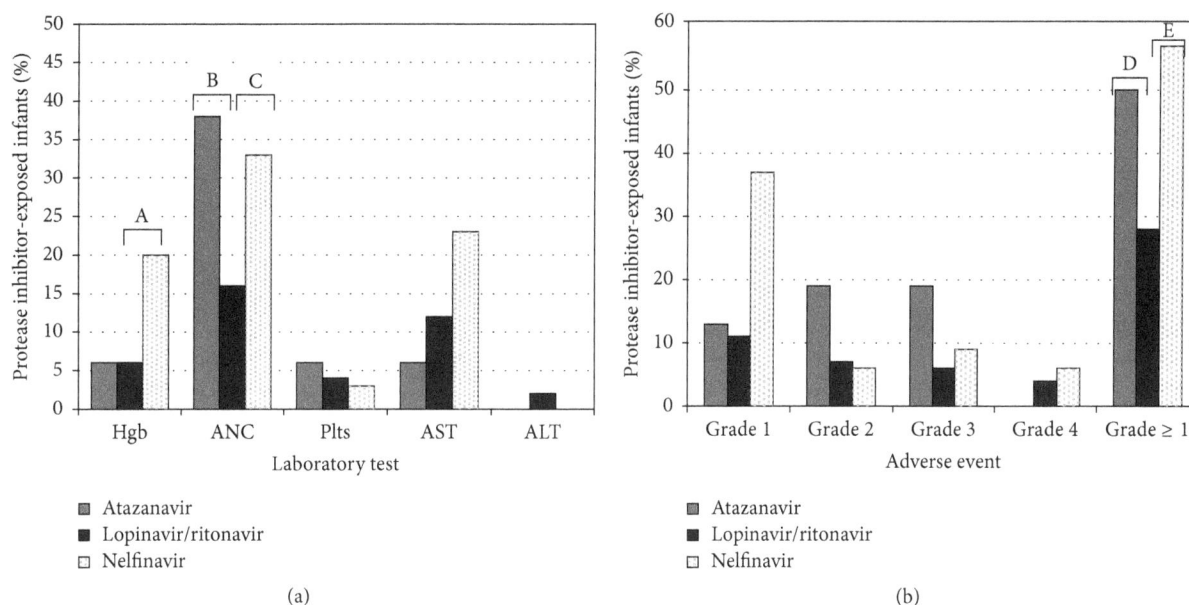

FIGURE 2: Frequency of infant adverse events at birth by maternal protease inhibitor. Bars represent the percentage of infants with a laboratory adverse event of any grade (a) or the percentage of infants whose most severe adverse event was represented by that particular grade (b). Number of infants per group: atazanavir ± ritonavir (16), lopinavir/ritonavir (54), and nelfinavir (35). Hgb, hemoglobin; ANC, absolute neutrophil count; plts, platelet count; AST, aspartate aminotransferase; ALT, alanine aminotransferase. [A]OR = 7.4 (95% CI 1.4–39.0), $p = 0.02$; [B]OR = 18.3 (95% CI 1.2–267.8), $p = 0.03$; [C]OR = 10.6 (95% CI 1.7–66.4), $p = 0.01$; [D]OR = 4.2 (95% CI 1.0–17.5), $p = 0.046$; [E]OR = 5.3 (95% CI 1.9–14.9), $p = 0.002$.

transient or masked by the effect of postnatal ARV. Our multivariate analysis controlled for exposure to postnatal ZDV monoprophylaxis versus combination prophylaxis. The association of laboratory AE with particular antenatal ARV within the PI class is reported here for the first time. Of note, Bellon Cano et al. described increased anemia, thrombocytopenia, and liver enzyme elevation after exposure to PI-based cART (of which most regimens contained NFV) compared with two or three NRTI or NNRTI-based cART [22].

The mechanism of the PI effect on hematologic AE is unclear. Fetal hematopoiesis may be more susceptible to the effects of PI, as it occurs mainly in the liver and peripheral lymphoid tissues. PI cross the placenta to some degree; albeit due to their large molecular weight and high protein binding capacity, they do not reach therapeutic levels in cord blood. Cord blood to maternal plasma ratios for ATV, NFV, and LPV range between 0.13–0.24, 0.16–0.22, and 0–0.49, respectively [38]. Amniotic fluid to maternal plasma ratios have been described for NFV (0.14–0.44) and LPV (0.08) [39, 40]. Although serum levels for some PI may be low during pregnancy [41], in this cohort plasma PI levels were routinely monitored during pregnancy and doses adjusted to achieve a trough above the 25th percentile for nonpregnant adults. Therefore, the difference in infant AE is not likely attributable to differences in maternal PI drug levels.

Because this was a retrospective study, it is possible that the maternal receipt of various PI could be a marker for another confounding variable that contributed to infant AE. Examination for potential confounding variables between the NFV and LPV/r groups identified that on average women

receiving NFV had a longer duration of viremia than women receiving LPV/r. However, viremia did not correlate with increased risk of infant AE, and inclusion of maternal viremia as a covariate did not alter the relationship of infant AE with exposure to NFV versus LPV/r.

Owing to its limited antiviral activity, NFV is no longer recommended for use in pregnant women [42]. However, there may be rare clinical scenarios in which NFV use might be considered, such as for patients who cannot tolerate or have resistance to other ARV that are included in the preferred and alternative regimens for pregnancy. The results of this study may be further rationale to avoid NFV during pregnancy.

We found that ATV exposure was associated with a higher incidence of neutropenia compared with LPV/r. However, infants in this study who were exposed to ATV did not show increased rates of liver enzyme elevation or hyperbilirubinemia compared with infants exposed to other PI. These findings are in contrast to those of Mandelbrot et al. who described a series of twenty-three infants exposed in utero to ATV, nine of whom developed elevated serum bilirubin concentrations at birth and five required phototherapy in the first three days of life [25]. Notably, a subsequent study found no association between ATV exposure and neonatal hyperbilirubinemia [43]. Our data need to be further confirmed in larger studies, because they were derived from only sixteen infants exposed to ATV, resulting in an OR with relatively large confidence intervals.

Although ZDV is commonly associated with hematologic side effects in exposed infants, we did not find more hematologic AE at birth among infants exposed to antenatal

ZDV compared with those exposed to ABC, d4T, or TDF, but the number of infants exposed to the alternative NRTI was small. Few studies compare infant toxicities after in utero exposure to different NRTI, although Vivanti et al. demonstrated decreased genotoxicity in cord blood of infants exposed in utero to TDF versus ZDV [44].

Preterm birth has been described previously in association with in utero exposure to PI [4–6]. We did not find an association of preterm birth or SGA with LPV/r, NFV, or ATV, but the power to detect differences was limited by our small sample size. In addition, data describing other risk factors for preterm birth or SGA were not available in our data set. Perry et al. recently showed no differences in preterm birth or birth weight in infants exposed to maternal LPV/r versus ATV; this study did not report infant laboratory outcomes [45].

We acknowledge several limitations in this study. The sample size was relatively small. Mothers and infants were not randomized to various ARV in our study; they received a regimen that was clinically appropriate based on severity of disease, tolerability, viral response to therapy, and risk of perinatal HIV transmission. Although two groups of infants for whom we found a significant difference in AE (those exposed to LPV/r and NFV) were cared for in different time periods, we also found differences between the effect of LPV/r and ATV exposure, whose use was roughly contemporaneous. Despite these limitations, this study permits comparison of infant AE within classes of ARV, whereas most similar studies have compared between classes of ARV. It also provides data on newer ARV used for prevention of perinatal transmission.

5. Conclusions

In summary, when used in maternal cART for prevention of perinatal transmission of HIV, NFV and ATV were associated with increased infant AE compared to LPV/r. As ATV use in pregnant women is increasing, larger, preferably randomized studies of infants exposed to LPV/r versus ATV/r are needed to evaluate laboratory AE and to clarify any association with prematurity. Investigations into the safest maternal ARV regimens and timing of ARV initiation are important for optimizing outcomes for HIV-exposed infants, especially those with higher risk of hematologic and hepatic toxicity, such as preterm infants and infants in resource-limited settings.

Disclosure

These data were presented in part at the 49th annual meeting of the Infectious Diseases Society of America (poster presentation), Boston, MA, October 2011.

Competing Interests

This work was partially supported by funding from Colorado HIV-1 Research Training Program Fellowship Position (Grant T32AI007447-23) and by contributions from Pfizer (Project no. 2580628) and Abbott (Project no. 2580614). Dr. Weinberg receives research funds from MedImmune, Becton Dickinson, Roche, Cepheid, Diagnostic Hybrids, and Sanofi Pasteur. Dr. Levin receives research funds, fees for consultation, and royalties from Patent no. 5,997,880, entitled "Method for Alleviating Varicella Related Post-Herpetic Neuralgia" from Merck & Co. Dr. Levin also receives research funds from and sits on the adjudication committee for GlaxoSmithKline. Dr. McFarland receives research funds from Gilead. In addition, Drs. Levin and Weinberg share competing interests due to their marital association. For the remaining authors, none were declared.

Acknowledgments

The authors would like to thank Carol Salbenblatt and Annie Vasquez for their assistance with data entry and Jessica Peterson for her assistance with record retrieval.

References

[1] J. C. Forbes, A. M. Alimenti, J. Singer et al., "A national review of vertical HIV transmission," *AIDS*, vol. 26, no. 6, pp. 757–763, 2012.

[2] L. Navér, S. Lindgren, E. Belfrage et al., "Children born to HIV-1-infected women in Sweden in 1982–2003: trends in epidemiology and vertical transmission," *Journal of Acquired Immune Deficiency Syndromes*, vol. 42, no. 4, pp. 484–489, 2006.

[3] L. M. Mofenson, "Editorial commentary: new challenges in the elimination of pediatric HIV infection: the expanding population of HIV-exposed but uninfected children," *Clinical Infectious Diseases*, vol. 60, no. 9, pp. 1357–1360, 2015.

[4] D. H. Watts, P. L. Williams, D. Kacanek et al., "Combination antiretroviral use and preterm birth," *The Journal of Infectious Diseases*, vol. 207, no. 4, pp. 612–621, 2013.

[5] European Collaborative Study, "Exposure to antiretroviral therapy in utero or early life: the health of uninfected children born to HIV-infected women," *Journal of Acquired Immune Deficiency Syndromes*, vol. 32, no. 4, pp. 380–387, 2003.

[6] J. Sibiude, J. Warszawski, R. Tubiana et al., "Premature delivery in HIV-infected women starting protease inhibitor therapy during pregnancy: role of the ritonavir boost?" *Clinical Infectious Diseases*, vol. 54, no. 9, pp. 1348–1360, 2012.

[7] I. André-Schmutz, L. Dal-Cortivo, E. Six et al., "Genotoxic signature in cord blood cells of newborns exposed in utero to a zidovudine-based antiretroviral combination," *Journal of Infectious Diseases*, vol. 208, no. 2, pp. 235–243, 2013.

[8] S. Blanche, M. Tardieu, V. Benhammou, J. Warszawski, and P. Rustin, "Mitochondrial dysfunction following perinatal exposure to nucleoside analogues," *AIDS*, vol. 20, no. 13, pp. 1685–1690, 2006.

[9] N. Dainiak, M. Worthington, M. A. Riordan, S. Kreczko, and L. Goldman, "3′-Azido-3′-deoxythymidine (AZT) inhibits proliferation in vitro of human haematopoietic progenitor cells," *British Journal of Haematology*, vol. 69, no. 3, pp. 299–304, 1988.

[10] M. M. Shah, Y. Li, and R. D. Christensen, "Effects of perinatal zidovudine on hematopoiesis: a comparison of effects on progenitors from human fetuses versus mothers," *AIDS*, vol. 10, no. 11, pp. 1239–1247, 1996.

[11] E. M. Connor, R. S. Sperling, R. Gelber et al., "Reduction of maternal-infant transmission of human immunodeficiency virus type 1 with zidovudine treatment. Pediatric AIDS Clinical

Trials Group Protocol 076 Study Group," *The New England Journal of Medicine*, vol. 331, no. 18, pp. 1173–1180, 1994.

[12] R. S. Sperling, D. E. Shapiro, G. D. McSherry et al., "Safety of the maternal-infant zidovudine regimen utilized in the Pediatric AIDS Clinical Trial Group 076 study," *AIDS*, vol. 12, no. 14, pp. 1805–1813, 1998.

[13] W. J. Watson, T. P. Stevens, and G. A. Weinberg, "Profound anemia in a newborn infant of a mother receiving antiretroviral therapy," *Pediatric Infectious Disease Journal*, vol. 17, no. 5, pp. 435–436, 1998.

[14] S. A. Myers, S. Torrente, D. Hinthorn, and P. L. Clark, "Life-threatening maternal and fetal macrocytic anemia from antiretroviral therapy," *Obstetrics and Gynecology*, vol. 106, no. 5, part 2, pp. 1189–1191, 2005.

[15] M. Bunders, C. Thorne, and M. L. Newell, "Maternal and infant factors and lymphocyte, CD4 and CD8 cell counts in uninfected children of HIV-1-infected mothers," *AIDS*, vol. 19, no. 10, pp. 1071–1079, 2005.

[16] M. E. Paul, C. J. Chantry, J. S. Read et al., "Morbidity and mortality during the first two years of life among uninfected children born to human immunodeficiency virus type 1-infected women: the women and infants transmission study," *Pediatric Infectious Disease Journal*, vol. 24, no. 1, pp. 46–56, 2005.

[17] S. E. Pacheco, K. McIntosh, M. Lu et al., "Effect of perinatal antiretroviral drug exposure on hematologic values in HIV-uninfected children: an analysis of the women and infants transmission study," *Journal of Infectious Diseases*, vol. 194, no. 8, pp. 1089–1097, 2006.

[18] M. Lallemant, G. Jourdain, S. Le Coeur et al., "A trial of shortened zidovudine regimens to prevent mother-to-child transmission of human immunodeficiency virus type 1," *The New England Journal of Medicine*, vol. 343, no. 14, pp. 982–991, 2000.

[19] J. S. Read, Y. Huo, K. Patel, M. Mitchell, and G. B. Scott, "Laboratory abnormalities among HIV-exposed, uninfected infants: IMPAACT protocol P1025," *Journal of the Pediatric Infectious Diseases Society*, vol. 1, no. 2, pp. 92–102, 2012.

[20] European Collaborative Study, "Levels and patterns of neutrophil cell counts over the first 8 years of life in children of HIV-1-infected mothers," *AIDS*, vol. 18, no. 15, pp. 2009–2017, 2004.

[21] L. Mandelbrot, A. Landreau-Mascaro, C. Rekacewicz et al., "Lamivudine-zidovudine combination for prevention of maternal-infant transmission of HIV-1," *Journal of the American Medical Association*, vol. 285, no. 16, pp. 2083–2093, 2001.

[22] J. M. Bellon Cano, S. Sanchez-Ramon, L. Ciria et al., "The effects on infants of potent antiretroviral therapy during pregnancy: a report from Spain," *Medical Science Monitor*, vol. 10, no. 5, pp. CR179–CR184, 2004.

[23] M. M. Mussi-Pinhata, M. A. C. Rego, L. Freimanis et al., "Maternal antiretrovirals and hepatic enzyme, hematologic abnormalities among human immunodeficiency virus type 1-uninfected infants: the NISDI perinatal study," *Pediatric Infectious Disease Journal*, vol. 26, no. 11, pp. 1032–1037, 2007.

[24] T. E. Taha, N. Kumwenda, A. Gibbons et al., "Effect of HIV-1 antiretroviral prophylaxis on hepatic and hematological parameters of African infants," *AIDS*, vol. 16, no. 6, pp. 851–858, 2002.

[25] L. Mandelbrot, F. Mazy, C. Floch-Tudal et al., "Atazanavir in pregnancy: impact on neonatal hyperbilirubinemia," *European Journal of Obstetrics Gynecology and Reproductive Biology*, vol. 157, no. 1, pp. 18–21, 2011.

[26] S. Dryden-Peterson, R. L. Shapiro, M. D. Hughes et al., "Increased risk of severe infant anemia after exposure to maternal HAART, Botswana," *Journal of Acquired Immune Deficiency Syndromes*, vol. 56, no. 5, pp. 428–436, 2011.

[27] C. Feiterna-Sperling, K. Weizsaecker, C. Bührer et al., "Hematologic effects of maternal antiretroviral therapy and transmission prophylaxis in HIV-1-exposed uninfected newborn infants," *Journal of Acquired Immune Deficiency Syndromes*, vol. 45, no. 1, pp. 43–51, 2007.

[28] J. Le Chenadec, M.-J. Mayaux, C. Guihenneuc-Jouyaux, and S. Blanche, "Perinatal antiretroviral treatment and hematopoiesis in HIV-uninfected infants," *AIDS*, vol. 17, no. 14, pp. 2053–2061, 2003.

[29] D. Nurutdinova, N. F. Onen, E. Hayes, K. Mondy, and E. T. Overton, "Adverse effects of tenofovir use in HIV-infected pregnant women and their infants," *Annals of Pharmacotherapy*, vol. 42, no. 11, pp. 1581–1585, 2008.

[30] S. Baroncelli, E. Tamburrini, M. Ravizza et al., "Antiretroviral treatment in pregnancy: a six-year perspective on recent trends in prescription patterns, viral load suppression, and pregnancy outcomes," *AIDS Patient Care and STDs*, vol. 23, no. 7, pp. 513–520, 2009.

[31] R. Griner, P. L. Williams, J. S. Read et al., "In utero and postnatal exposure to antiretrovirals among hiv-exposed but uninfected children in the united states," *AIDS Patient Care and STDs*, vol. 25, no. 7, pp. 385–394, 2011.

[32] Division of AIDS and National Institutes of Health, *Division of AIDS Table for Grading the Severity of Adult and Pediatric Adverse Events*, Division of AIDS, National Institutes of Health, Bethesda, Md, USA, 2004, http://rsc.tech-res.com/safetyandpharmacovigilance/gradingtables.aspx.

[33] A. Weinberg, J. Forster-Harwood, E. J. McFarland et al., "Resistance to antiretrovirals in HIV-infected pregnant women," *Journal of Clinical Virology*, vol. 45, no. 1, pp. 39–42, 2009.

[34] A. Weinberg, J. E. F. Harwood, E. J. McFarland et al., "Kinetics and determining factors of the virologic response to antiretrovirals during pregnancy," *Infectious Diseases in Obstetrics and Gynecology*, vol. 2009, Article ID 621780, 8 pages, 2009.

[35] A. Weinberg, J. Forster-Harwood, J. Davies et al., "Safety and tolerability of antiretrovirals during pregnancy," *Infectious Diseases in Obstetrics and Gynecology*, vol. 2011, Article ID 867674, 6 pages, 2011.

[36] C. Smith, J. E. Forster, M. J. Levin et al., "Serious adverse events are uncommon with combination neonatal antiretroviral prophylaxis: a retrospective case review," *PLoS ONE*, vol. 10, no. 5, Article ID e0127062, 2015.

[37] V. Venkatesh, R. Khan, A. Curley, H. New, and S. Stanworth, "How we decide when a neonate needs a transfusion," *British Journal of Haematology*, vol. 160, no. 4, pp. 421–433, 2013.

[38] S. A. McCormack and B. M. Best, "Protecting the fetus against HIV infection: a systematic review of placental transfer of antiretrovirals," *Clinical Pharmacokinetics*, vol. 53, no. 11, pp. 989–1004, 2014.

[39] A. Gingelmaier, M. Kurowski, R. Kästner et al., "Placental transfer and pharmacokinetics of lopinavir and other protease inhibitors in combination with nevirapine at delivery," *AIDS*, vol. 20, no. 13, pp. 1737–1743, 2006.

[40] C. Bennetto-Hood, Y. J. Bryson, A. Stek, J. King, M. Mirochnick, and E. Acosta, "Zidovudine, lamivudine, and nelfinavir concentrations in amniotic fluid and maternal serum," *HIV Clinical Trials*, vol. 10, no. 1, pp. 41–47, 2009.

[41] A. Colbers, R. Greupink, and D. Burger, "Pharmacological considerations on the use of antiretrovirals in pregnancy," *Current Opinion in Infectious Diseases*, vol. 26, no. 6, pp. 575–588, 2013.

[42] Panel on Treatment of HIV-Infected Pregnant Women and Prevention of Perinatal Transmission, Recommendations for Use of Antiretroviral Drugs in Pregnant HIV-1-Infected Women for Maternal Health and Interventions to Reduce Perinatal HIV Transmission in the United States, 2015.

[43] T. Eley, S.-P. Huang, F. Conradie et al., "Clinical and pharmacogenetic factors affecting neonatal bilirubinemia following atazanavir treatment of mothers during pregnancy," *AIDS Research and Human Retroviruses*, vol. 29, no. 10, pp. 1287–1292, 2013.

[44] A. Vivanti, T. S. Soheili, W. Cuccuini et al., "Comparing genotoxic signatures in cord blood cells from neonates exposed in utero to zidovudine or tenofovir," *AIDS*, vol. 29, no. 11, pp. 1319–1324, 2015.

[45] M. Perry, G. P. Taylor, C. A. Sabin et al., "Lopinavir and atazanavir in pregnancy: comparable infant outcomes, virological efficacies and preterm delivery rates," *HIV Medicine*, vol. 17, no. 1, pp. 28–35, 2016.

19

Management of HIV Infection during Pregnancy in the United States: Updated Evidence-Based Recommendations and Future Potential Practices

Bassam H. Rimawi,[1] Lisa Haddad,[2] Martina L. Badell,[3] and Rana Chakraborty[4]

[1]School of Medicine, Department of Gynecology and Obstetrics, Division of Maternal Fetal Medicine and Reproductive Infectious Diseases, Emory University, 550 Peachtree Street, Atlanta, GA 30308, USA

[2]School of Medicine, Department of Gynecology and Obstetrics, Division of Family Planning, Emory University, 550 Peachtree Street, Atlanta, GA 30308, USA

[3]School of Medicine, Department of Gynecology and Obstetrics, Division of Maternal Fetal Medicine, Emory University, 550 Peachtree Street, Atlanta, GA 30308, USA

[4]School of Medicine, Department of Pediatrics, Division of Infectious Diseases, Emory University, 2015 Uppergate Drive, NE, Atlanta, GA 30322, USA

Correspondence should be addressed to Bassam H. Rimawi; bassamrimawi@yahoo.com

Academic Editor: Bryan Larsen

All HIV-infected women contemplating pregnancy should initiate combination antiretroviral therapy (cART), with a goal to achieve a maternal serum HIV RNA viral load beneath the laboratory level of detection prior to conceiving, as well as throughout their pregnancy. Successfully identifying HIV infection during pregnancy through screening tests is essential in order to prevent *in utero* and intrapartum transmission of HIV. Perinatal HIV transmission can be less than 1% when effective cART, associated with virologic suppression of HIV, is given during the ante-, intra-, and postpartum periods. Perinatal HIV guidelines, developed by organizations such as the World Health Organization, American College of Obstetricians and Gynecologists, and the US Department of Health and Human Services, are constantly evolving, and hence the aim of our review is to provide a useful concise review for medical providers caring for HIV-infected pregnant women, summarizing the latest and current recommendations in the United States.

1. Introduction

Neonatal HIV infections are a result of transmission from a mother to her unborn fetus *in utero*, or during the intrapartum period, or postpartum secondary to breastfeeding [1]. In the US, perinatal transmission has been reduced to less than 1% in many states, reflecting implementation of key interventions during pregnancy, including initiating cART to suppress viral load beneath the level of detection and avoidance of breastfeeding during the postpartum period [1, 2]. Perinatal HIV guidelines in the US are constantly evolving. Here, we present a concise review outlining the latest perinatal recommendations, as well as potential future practices for medical providers caring for HIV-infected pregnant women.

2. Incidence of Perinatal HIV Transmission

Globally, without intervention, the cumulative *in utero*, intrapartum, and postpartum HIV transmission rate is approximately 35–40% [2]. In breastfeeding populations, postpartum HIV transmission through breastfeeding contributes about 40–45% of all mother-to-child transmissions (http://www.unaids.org/en/media/unaids/contentassets/documents/unaidspublication/2011/20110609_JC2137_Global-Plan-Elimination-HIV-Children_en.pdf). Maternal HIV viral load level is by far the most predictive factor for perinatal HIV transmission. Higher HIV viral loads correlate with a greater risk of perinatal transmission, although transmission can occur with any viral load, even when the systemic plasma viral load is beneath the level of detection [3]. Globally, the transmission rates for HIV can be reduced to less than 1% in pregnant women being compliant on their cART with virologic suppression and other perinatal recommendations [4, 5]. Without any intervention, this transmission rate is closer to 25% [2]. Among Hispanic/Latino and Caucasian women, the rates of HIV transmission have remained relatively stable in 2012 (<2% and 1%, resp.) [1, 2].

3. Preconception Counseling

All reproductively aged HIV-infected women should seek counseling prior to contemplating pregnancy, so that a detailed discussion on childbearing can be established. A key focus of discussions should include prevention of mother-to-child transmission (MTCT) of HIV, by initiation or continuation of an appropriately selected cART regimen [6], compliance with these medications during pregnancy and the postpartum period, and identifying potential barriers [7] that may affect postpartum retention in HIV care [8, 9]. The ability to successfully achieve maximal viral suppression before conception and throughout pregnancy is by far the most predictive means of achieving the lowest risk of potential MTCT [6]. Preconception counseling should be aimed at identifying women who may be victims of intimate partner violence, depression, and other psychological or psychiatric illnesses that may serve as barriers to prevention of MTCT and to treat and gain control of these conditions prior to contemplating pregnancy [10]. These strategies will not only result in safer conception and better compliance with cART but also result in better pregnancy outcomes [10].

4. HIV-Concordant and Discordant Couples

Consultation should include an expert in perinatal medicine and/or an experienced specialist who cares for HIV infected individuals [11]. With discordant couples that involve HIV-infected women, conception via timed artificial insemination is the safest option either via self-insemination or via intrauterine insemination [12]. When the discordant couple involves an HIV-infected male, the safest option for pregnancy is via insemination with donor HIV negative sperm. If the couple does not desire donor sperm, semen analysis is recommended prior to attempted pregnancy to avoid unnecessary exposure to genital fluid if semen abnormalities exist. Also sperm preparation techniques followed by intrauterine insemination or *in vitro* fertilization may reduce exposure risks [12].

5. Antepartum Care of HIV-Infected Women

Pitfalls and missed opportunities in healthcare delivery include failure of medical providers to screen pregnant women for HIV, ideally in the first trimester or at their first prenatal visit [7]. Transmission events are often documented in pregnant women who present with limited or no prenatal care, and those who decline HIV screening during pregnancy [13]. Pregnant women who have not previously had HIV

screening and present to a labor and delivery suite in labor urgently require rapid HIV testing at the time of admission [14]. If a positive rapid HIV test is noted, and these patients are deemed to be in active labor or delivery is warranted for other obstetrical indications, then immediately implementing interventions to reduce intrapartum HIV transmission is recommended, which includes a combination of maternal administration of at least 3 hours of intravenous zidovudine therapy prior to a cesarean delivery and postnatal infant prophylaxis with a dual ARV combination regimen of zidovudine and nevirapine [15]. Awaiting laboratory confirmation should not delay these urgent interventions [11].

For known positive mothers, HIV RNA quantitative viral loads should be assessed monthly; however, some medical providers may consider wider interval blood draws to every 2 months, in those pregnant women who have consistently had a suppressed HIV-1 RNA viral load beneath the level of detection while on effective cART [16]. Figure 1 illustrates algorithmic management of HIV during pregnancy.

6. The Diagnosis of HIV during Pregnancy

A positive screening test with traditional HIV testing modalities, either with an HIV 1/2 Antigen/Antibody test or with a Fourth Generation test with reflexes essentially establishes a diagnosis of HIV infection [17]. Newer testing modalities include reflex Multispot rapid HIV testing, which includes a combined HIV-1/HIV-2 rapid test to distinguish between HIV-1 and 2 infection; hence, a positive Multispot test confirms a diagnosis of HIV [17, 18]. However, if the Multispot test is negative, additional reflex testing for establishing a diagnosis of HIV infection includes proceeding with a polymerase chain reaction (PCR) test [18]. The sensitivity and specificity of rapid HIV testing are close to 100%, while the positive predictive value (PPV) depends on the prevalence of the disease in the general population being tested [19, 20]. In populations in which the HIV prevalence is low, a lower PPV is noted [19]. Table 1 demonstrates the different diagnostic tests that are available for establishing a diagnosis of HIV in pregnant women.

7. Coinfection Screening and Vaccination Recommendations

In addition to routine prenatal labs obtained during the first trimester, or at entry into prenatal care, which already includes the assessment of hepatitis B and syphilis, screening for hepatitis C coinfection is recommended for HIV positive women [16]. Those who have a negative hepatitis B surface antibody status should receive hepatitis B vaccine series during pregnancy, regardless of which trimester they are in, as well as screening for immunity to hepatitis A, as a combination vaccine for hepatitis B and hepatitis A exists, formerly known as Twinrex [21]. Patients who are coinfected with these other viral entities should seek consultation with HIV and hepatitis-experienced medical provider(s). For patients with hepatitis B infection, all newborn infants should receive both the hepatitis B vaccine series and hepatitis B immune globulin

TABLE 1: Testing modalities for diagnosing HIV in pregnancy[*].

HIV tests	What they test for	Window period	Available results	Sensitivity	Specificity
ELISA	HIV antibodies	3 Months	2 days–2 weeks	>99%	>98%
Antigen test (p24)	P24 viral proteins	11 days–1 month	2 days–1 week	90%	100%
4th generation tests	Antibodies and p24	11 days–1 month	2 days–2 weeks	>99.7%	>99.3%
PCR/NAAT tests	Genetic material of HIV	12 days	2 days–1 week	>99%	>99%
Rapid test	Antibodies	3 Months	Within 20 minutes	>99%	>98%

[*]AIDSinfo. Recommendations for use of antiretroviral drugs in pregnant HIV-1-infected women for maternal health and interventions to reduce perinatal HIV transmission in the United States. *HHS panel on treatment of HIV-infected pregnant women and prevention of perinatal transmission, a working group of the office of AIDS research advisory council (OARAC)*, 2015, http://aidsinfo.nih.gov/guidelines.

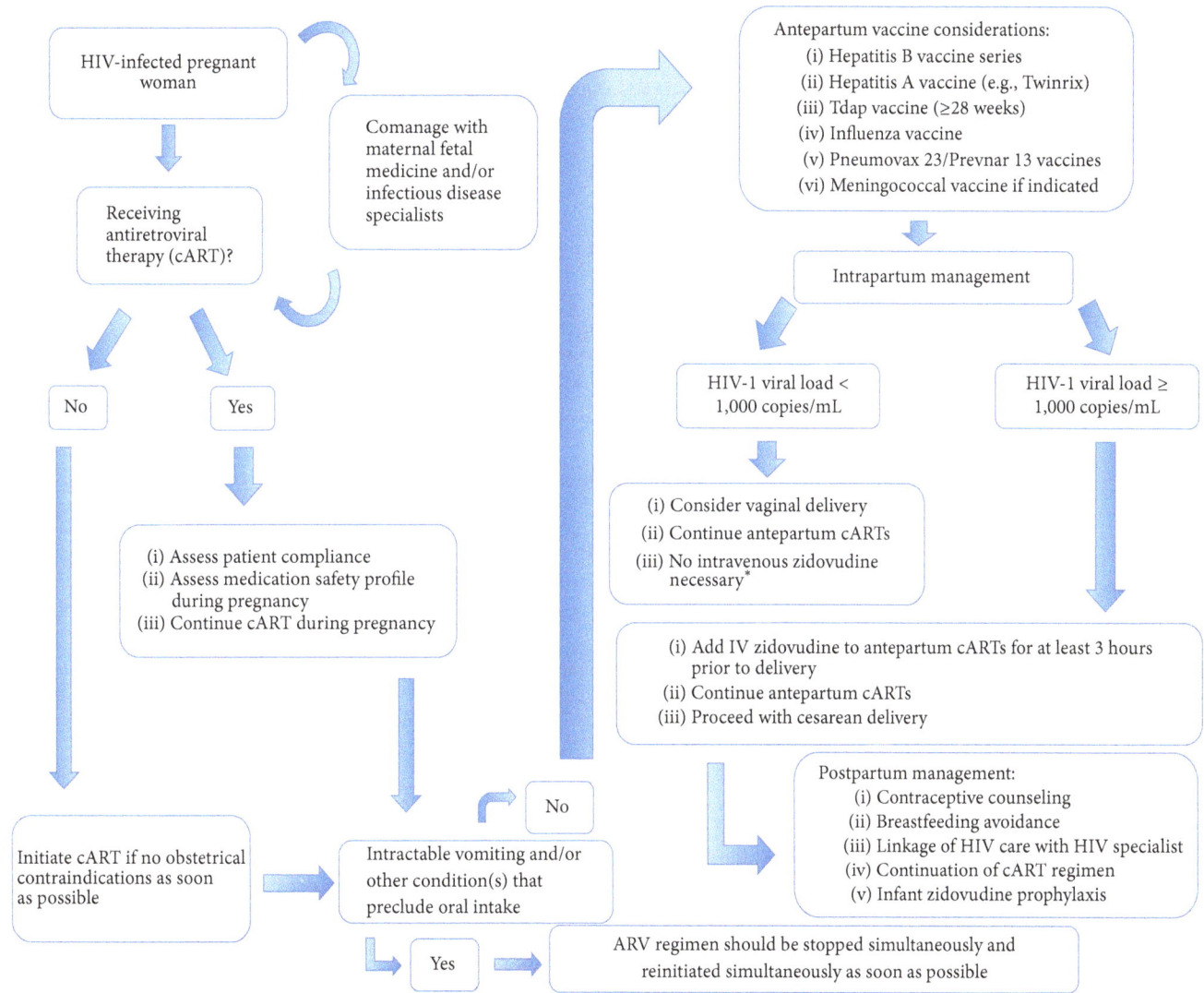

FIGURE 1: Algorithm for management of HIV during pregnancy. [*]Intravenous (IV) zidovudine is not required for HIV-infected women who are compliant with cART and who have an HIV-viral load < 1000 copies/mL at the time of delivery. HIV: human immunodeficiency virus, cART: combination antiretroviral therapy, PO: per os (by mouth), CBC: complete blood count, CMP: complete metabolic panel, CD4: cluster of differentiation 4, and mL: milliliter.

preferably within 12 hours after delivery, regardless of the maternal hepatitis B viral load [22, 23].

In addition to vaccination against hepatitis A and B during pregnancy, additional vaccines to offer HIV-infected women during pregnancy should include the influenza vaccine (inactivated) during the influenza season, which can

be offered to unvaccinated pregnant women during any trimester of pregnancy, as well as combined diphtheria, tetanus, and pertussis (Tdap) vaccine around 28–36 weeks of gestation [23]. Additional vaccines that may be given to HIV-infected pregnant women include Pneumovax 23 (23-valent pneumococcal polysaccharide) vaccine and Prevnar 13

TABLE 2: Treatment regimens for HIV-infected pregnant women.

Brand name	Preparation	Comments
	Preferred regimens	
	Two-NRTI backbone	
Trizivir	ABC/3TC	Patients with an HIV RNA viral load > 100,000 copies/mL should not receive a combination therapy consisting of ABC/3TC with ATV/ritonavir or efavirenz.
Truvada	TDF/FTC or 3TC	TDF-based dual NRTI combinations should be used with caution in patients with renal insufficiency.
Combivir	ZDV/3TC	NRTI combination therapy requires twice daily administration and increases potential for hematologic toxicities.
	Protease inhibitor regimens	
Reyataz	ATV/r plus a two-NRTI backbone	Maternal hyperbilirubinemia.
Prezista	DRV/r plus a two-NRTI backbone	Must be used twice daily in pregnancy.
	NNRTI regimen	
Efavirenz	EFV plus a two-NRTI backbone*	Concern because of birth defects seen in primate study, unclear risk in humans.
	Integrase inhibitor regimen	
Raltegravir	RAL plus a two-NRTI backbone	Rapid viral load reduction. Twice-daily dosing required.
	Alternative regimens	
	Protease inhibitor regimens	
Kaletra	LPV/r	More nausea than preferred regimens. Twice-daily administration in pregnancy.
	NNRTI regimens	
Complera	RPV/TDF/FTC (or RPV plus a two-NRTI backbone)	RPV not recommended with pretreatment HIV RNA > 100,000 copies/mL or CD4 cell count < 200 cells/mm^3. Do not use with PPIs. PK data available in pregnancy but relatively little experience with use in pregnancy. Available in co formulated single-pill once daily regimen.

NRTI: nucleoside or nucleotide reverse transcriptase inhibitor, NNRTI: nonnucleoside or nonnucleotide reverse transcriptase inhibitor, ABC: abacavir, 3TC: lamivudine, TDF: tenofovir disoproxil, FTC: emtricitabine, ZDV: zidovudine, ATV: atazanavir, r: ritonavir (boosted regimen), DRV: darunavir, *EFV: efavirenz, recommended to be started after 8 weeks of gestation, RAL: raltegravir, LPV: lopinavir, and RPV: rilpivirine.

(13-valent pneumococcal conjugate) vaccine [23]. Vaccines that should not be given during pregnancy and postponed until the postpartum period include vaccination against varicella, zoster, human papillomavirus (HPV) and measles, mumps, and rubella (MMR), if testing results are equivocal or nonimmune [23]. At this time, vaccination with serogroup B meningococcal (MenB) vaccine should not be given during pregnancy, as there is not enough information about the potential risks of this vaccine during pregnancy or during the postpartum period for breastfeeding women [24].

8. Safety of Antiretroviral Agents during Pregnancy

The most effective method of identifying adverse fetal/neonatal outcomes is to report all drug exposures to the

Antiretroviral Pregnancy Registry [25]. The information needed to participate in this registry can be readily located online at http://www.apregistry.com/. Table 2 illustrates the different treatment regimens by class for HIV-Infected pregnant women, while Table 3 illustrates the most common reported adverse pregnancy outcomes of certain ARVs.

Small cohort studies have raised the concern that ARVs during pregnancy were associated with low birth weight and preterm birth [26–29], while these concerns may be in fact due to the severity of the disease, rather than the association with ARVs [30]. Other studies have evaluated the use of protease inhibitors and the risk of preterm delivery (PTD) [31–34], as well as the use of zidovudine and the risk of congenital cardiac defects [35], while others have shown favorable pregnancy outcomes [36].

Specific ARV regimens from HIV-pregnant women who gave birth to HIV exposed HIV negative infants have been

TABLE 3: Pregnancy outcomes of individual antiretroviral agents during pregnancy[*].

Brand name	Reported adverse pregnancy outcomes	
	Maternal	Fetal/neonatal
NRTI		
Zidovudine	Potential for hematologic toxicities (anemia and bone marrow suppression) [52], including elevated liver function tests [53], myelotoxicity [54], acute pancreatitis [54], preeclampsia, and other hypertensive disorders [55]	PTD [37], SGA [37], LBW [37], and CHD [35]
Tenofovir disoproxil fumarate	Kidney [56] and bone toxicity [57]	Decreased bone mineral density content [58]
NNRTI		
Efavirenz	Rash and drug interactions [59]	Initial concern of birth defects seen in primate study [60]; however, recent studies have not shown an increased risk of neural tube defects [61]
Abacavir	Abacavir should not be used in patients who test positive for HLA-B[*]5701 because a positive test may increase the risk of a hypersensitivity reaction [56], nausea, vomiting, diarrhea, and abdominal pain [59]	None
Didanosine	Pancreatitis (acute and chronic) [54] and neuropathy	Initial studies concerning for an association with fetal anomalies, specifically head and neck anomalies when exposed during the first trimester [35]; however, recent studies found no adverse outcomes [62]
Nevirapine	10-fold increased risk of hepatotoxicity[¥] [63, 64]	No reported fetal malformations [64]
Emtricitabine	Headache, nausea, vomiting, and diarrhea [59]	None [65]
Protease inhibitors		
Ritonavir	Nausea, vomiting, increased triglycerides, and transaminases [59]	
Atazanavir	Abdominal pain, diarrhea, nausea, and increased liver function tests [59]	PTD [31, 32, 34, 66]
Lopinavir	Nausea, vomiting, diarrhea, and pancreatitis [59]	PTD [21, 31, 34, 66]
Darunavir	Maternal hyperbilirubinemia and nausea [59]	PTD [31, 32, 34, 66]

[*]Table provides a short list of the updated ARV's and their reported safety issues.
[¥]Nevirapine can cause fatal and severe hepatotoxicity among women with CD4 lymphocytes > 250 cells/μL.
NRTI: nucleoside or nucleotide reverse transcriptase inhibitor, NNRTI: nonnucleoside or nonnucleotide reverse transcriptase inhibitor, PTD: preterm delivery (delivery prior to 37 weeks), SGA: small for gestational age (birth weight less than the 10th percentile for their gestational age), LBW: low birth weight (birth weight less than 2500 grams), and CHD: congenital heart defects.

evaluated from a large cohort in sub-Sahara Africa of more than 3000 patients for their association with adverse pregnancy outcomes, specifically for PTD, small for gestational age (SGA), and low birth weight (LBW) [37, 38] in relation to the duration of ARV exposure. The authors noted a 30% increased risk of preterm delivery amongst infants ARV-exposed women, with the highest risk in women who initiated ARVs prior to conception, compared to those who initiated ARVs during pregnancy or received zidovudine monotherapy [37]. Similarly, there was a 20% increased

risk of infants being diagnosed with SGA when exposed to ARVs during pregnancy and before conception; however, when they assessed different ARV exposures, there was no difference in the overall SGA neonates [37].

The highest rates of PTD (25%) and SGA (13%) were those women treated with protease inhibitors during pregnancy [37]. They also found an increased likelihood of LBW amongst women who initiated ARVs prior to conception and those who were exposed to ARVs during pregnancy. Overall, they found that pregnant women exposed to ARVs of longer duration with initiation of ARVs prior to pregnancy had the highest rates of PTD, SGA, and LBW [37]. It is unclear the exact mechanism of why these adverse pregnancy outcomes were seen [39, 40], and further comparative evaluations of different regimens are needed.

Intrapartum, maternal infusion of zidovudine dosing has been investigated and compared to therapeutic exposures in order to assess fetal concentrations [41]. Reducing the maternal infusion dosage from a loading dose of 2 mg/kg to 1 mg/kg over 1 hour, followed by a reduction in the maintenance dosage of 1 mg/kg to 0.5 mg/kg each hour until delivery, reduced fetal exposures [41]. This can also be achieved by taking zidovudine orally every 5 hours, starting at the onset of labor until the time of delivery, followed by neonatal zidovudine prophylaxis as soon as possible after birth [41]. This reduction in zidovudine dosage during the first few days of neonatal life also is important as well.

While treatment of HIV during pregnancy is crucial and the benefits outweigh the risks for the prevention of MTCT, the safety profile of ARVs during pregnancy has shown conflicting evidence. It is ideal that medical providers caring for HIV infected reproductive age women start ARVs prior to pregnancy and continue these throughout pregnancy, or as early as tolerated during pregnancy to achieve the ultimate goal of viral suppression and prevention of MTCT.

9. Postpartum Care

All HIV-infected women should have a routine postpartum follow-up visit with their obstetric provider. After delivery, establishing retention in HIV care is critical, with referral to an infectious disease specialist. Counseling patients regarding adherence to cART, irrespective of CD4 count, is very important, as some HIV-infected women become noncompliant with cART during follow-up after delivery.

Future efforts should be geared towards adapting new strategies in the US to achieve postpartum retention in HIV care settings [42], particularly because there are a limited number of available published reports addressing these strategies during the postpartum period. These strategies include discussion about unintended pregnancy prevention with contraceptive counseling, as well as HIV/STD preventive strategies such as consistent condom use and preexposure prophylaxis. In addition, similar to the preconception-counseling period, postpartum counseling should address intimate partner violence, postpartum depression, and other mental health issues that require treatment, as well as providing linkage to intimate partner violence services [43, 44].

10. Infant Follow-Up and Postnatal Prophylaxis

Regardless of maternal viral load, after birth, all babies born to HIV-infected women should be bathed immediately to remove any potentially infectious maternal secretions [18]. Baseline complete blood counts and HIV diagnostic testing by HIV DNA PCR are to establish or rule out HIV infection, followed by ZDV prophylaxis. Within 12 hours after birth,

and ideally no later than 24 hours, all neonates born to HIV positive mothers should receive a course of ZDV therapy, which will be continued for 6 weeks in the US; however, a 4-week regimen can be considered for full-term infants whose mothers had maintained HIV viral suppression antenatally [45, 46].

A recent study evaluated three postpartum cART regimens for neonates born to mothers infected with HIV who have not received any antepartum cART or had a viral load of >1,000 copies/mL near the time of delivery [47]. Combination prophylaxis with either a 2-drug (zidovudine plus nevirapine) regimen or a 3-drug regimen (zidovudine plus nelfinavir and lamivudine) was found to have superior efficacy, when compared to zidovudine monotherapy alone, with significantly reduced transmission rates of HIV [47]. The Department of Health and Human Services (DHHS) for the US currently recommends that at least 3 doses of nevirapine within the first 7 days of life be administered, in addition to ZDV therapy as prophylaxis during high-risk perinatal exposure when maternal HIV viral load is or is assumed to be more than 1,000 copies/mL.

Premastication of food for infants of HIV-infected mothers should be avoided, as this can potentiate the risk of HIV transmission [48]. Free clinical perinatal HIV consultation, including the care of an HIV-exposed neonate, is available for medical providers at The National Perinatal HIV Hotline at 1-888-448-8765.

Although early-term deliveries can be associated with increased neonatal intensive care unit admissions and higher hospital costs, when compared to those beyond 39 weeks [49], the recommendations currently endorsed by the American College of Obstetricians and Gynecologists (ACOG) is for cesarean deliveries at 38 weeks for pregnant women with HIV-1 RNA viral loads > 1,000 copies/mL [50]. We currently recommend delivery prior to 39 weeks of gestation for other high-risk conditions if the benefit of earlier delivery outweighs the risk of expectant management; therefore, decreasing the risk of spontaneous labor/rupture of membranes between 38 to 39 weeks in women with an HIV-1 RNA viral loads > 1,000 copies/mL outweighs very small increased transient risks of delivery at 38 versus 39 weeks for the neonate [51].

11. Summary of Future Potential Practices

(i) It is ideal that medical providers caring for HIV infected reproductive age women start ARVs prior to pregnancy and continue these throughout pregnancy, or as early as tolerated during pregnancy to achieve the ultimate goal of viral suppression and prevention of MTCT.

(ii) During the preconception counseling and postpartum periods, medical providers should identify women who may be victims of intimate partner violence, depression, and other psychological or psychiatric illnesses that may serve as barriers to prevention of MTCT and to treat and gain control of these conditions prior to contemplating pregnancy.

(iii) These strategies not only will result in safer conception and better compliance with cART but also will result in better pregnancy outcomes and less adverse pregnancy outcomes, as these patients will be more compliant with their prenatal visits and follow recommendations outlined by their obstetrical provider.

(iv) Prevention of pitfalls and missed opportunities in healthcare delivery can be achieved by medical providers screening all pregnant women for HIV, ideally in the first trimester or at their first prenatal visit, establishing an early diagnosis of HIV and initiating cART early in the pregnancy.

(v) Postpartum retention in HIV care settings is critical and can best be achieved through strategies that include a discussion about future unintended pregnancies with contraceptive counseling, as well as preventive strategies such as consistent condom use and preexposure prophylaxis.

Competing Interests

Rana Chakraborty is supported by the NICHD IMPAACT Network (HHSN275701300003C), by the CDC (1U01PS003322-01), by the NIH (5R01AA018096), and by the CDC Grant (5U48DP001909-04). Lisa Haddad is supported by the NICHD (1K23HD078153-01A1). Martina L. Badell NICHD is supported by IMPAACT Network (HHSN275701300003C). Bassam H. Rimawi reports no competing interests.

Acknowledgments

Rana Chakraborty has received research support from Gilead.

References

[1] Center for Disease Control and Prevention (CDC), *HIV among Pregnant Women, Infants, and Children in the United States*, CDC, Atlanta, Ga, USA, 2012.

[2] A. P. Kourtis, F. K. Lee, E. J. Abrams, D. J. Jamieson, and M. Bulterys, "Mother-to-child transmission of HIV-1: timing and implications for prevention," *The Lancet Infectious Diseases*, vol. 6, no. 11, pp. 726–732, 2006.

[3] J. P. A. Ioannidis, E. J. Abrams, A. Ammann et al., "Perinatal transmission of human immunodeficiency virus type 1 by pregnant women with RNA virus loads <1000 copies/mL," *Journal of Infectious Diseases*, vol. 183, no. 4, pp. 539–545, 2001.

[4] L. Mandelbrot, J. Le Chenadec, A. Berrebi et al., "Perinatal HIV-1 transmission: interaction between zidovudine prophylaxis and mode of delivery in the French perinatal cohort," *The Journal of the American Medical Association*, vol. 280, no. 1, pp. 55–60, 1998.

[5] "The mode of delivery and the risk of vertical transmission of human immunodeficiency virus type 1—a meta-analysis of 15 prospective cohort studies. The International Perinatal HIV Group," *The New England Journal of Medicine*, vol. 340, no. 13, pp. 977–987, 1999.

[6] J. Jean, A. Coll, M. Monda, J. Potter, and D. Jones, "Perspectives on safer conception practices and preconception counseling among women living with HIV," *Health Care for Women International*, 2015.

[7] A. F. Camacho-Gonzalez, M.-H. Kingbo, A. Boylan, A. R. Eckard, A. Chahroudi, and R. Chakraborty, "Missed opportunities for prevention of mother-to-child transmission in the United States," *AIDS*, vol. 29, no. 12, pp. 1511–1515, 2015.

[8] S. Nesheim, L. F. Harris, and M. Lampe, "Elimination of perinatal HIV infection in the USA and other high-income countries: achievements and challenges," *Current Opinion in HIV & AIDS*, vol. 8, no. 5, pp. 447–456, 2013.

[9] S. Nesheim, A. Taylor, M. A. Lampe et al., "A framework for elimination of perinatal transmission of HIV in the United States," *Pediatrics*, vol. 130, no. 4, pp. 738–744, 2012.

[10] A. S. Coll, J. E. Potter, N. Chakhtoura, M. L. Alcaide, R. Cook, and D. L. Jones, "Providers' perspectives on preconception counseling and safer conception for HIV-infected women," *AIDS Care*, vol. 28, no. 4, pp. 513–518, 2016.

[11] S. Chaithongwongwatthana, "Conceptive options for people living with HIV," *Journal of the Medical Association of Thailand*, vol. 98, supplement 1, pp. S123–S126, 2015.

[12] M. V. Sauer, "Sperm washing techniques address the fertility needs of HIV-seropositive men: a clinical review," *Reproductive BioMedicine Online*, vol. 10, no. 1, pp. 135–140, 2005.

[13] G. C. Jayaraman, J. K. Preiksaitis, and B. Larke, "Mandatory reporting of HIV infection and opt-out prenatal screening for HIV infection: effect on testing rates," *Canadian Medical Association Journal*, vol. 168, no. 6, pp. 679–682, 2003.

[14] "Committee opinion no: 635: prenatal and perinatal human immunodeficiency virus testing: expanded recommendations," *Obstetrics & Gynecology*, vol. 125, no. 6, pp. 1544–1547, 2015.

[15] M. Bulterys, D. J. Jamieson, M. J. O'Sullivan et al., "Rapid HIV-1 testing during labor: a multicenter study," *The Journal of the American Medical Association*, vol. 292, no. 2, pp. 219–223, 2004.

[16] ACOG Committee on Obstetric Practice, "ACOG committee opinion number 304, November 2004. Prenatal and perinatal human immunodeficiency virus testing: expanded recommendations," *Obstetrics & Gynecology*, vol. 104, no. 5, part 1, pp. 1119–1124, 2004.

[17] B. Weber, R. Thorstensson, S. Tanprasert, U. Schmitt, and W. Melchior, "Reduction of the diagnostic window in three cases of human immunodeficiency-1 subtype E primary infection with fourth-generation HIV screening assays," *Vox Sanguinis*, vol. 85, no. 2, pp. 73–79, 2003.

[18] P. L. Havens, R. Chakraborty, E. Cooper et al., "HIV testing and prophylaxis to prevent mother-to-child transmission in the united states," *Pediatrics*, vol. 122, no. 5, pp. 1127–1134, 2008.

[19] N. M. Doyle, J. E. Levison, and M. O. Gardner, "Rapid HIV versus enzyme-linked immunosorbent assay screening in a low-risk Mexican American population presenting in labor: a cost-effectiveness analysis," *American Journal of Obstetrics and Gynecology*, vol. 193, no. 3, part 2, pp. 1280–1285, 2005.

[20] Centers for Disease Control and Prevention, "Revised classification system for HIV infection and expanded surveillance case definition for AIDS among adolescents and adults," *The Journal of the American Medical Association*, vol. 269, no. 6, pp. 729–730, 1993.

[21] M. W. F. Rac and J. S. Sheffield, "Prevention and management of viral hepatitis in pregnancy," *Obstetrics and Gynecology Clinics of North America*, vol. 41, no. 4, pp. 573–592, 2014.

[22] R. S. Brown Jr., B. J. McMahon, A. S. F. Lok et al., "Antiviral therapy in chronic hepatitis B viral infection during pregnancy: a systematic review and meta-analysis," *Hepatology*, vol. 63, no. 1, pp. 319–333, 2016.

[23] J. Dionne-Odom, A. T. N. Tita, and N. S. Silverman, "Hepatitis B in pregnancy screening, treatment, and prevention of vertical transmission," *American Journal of Obstetrics and Gynecology*, vol. 214, no. 1, pp. 6–14, 2016.

[24] Advisory Committee on Immunization Practices Centers for Disease Control and Prevention, "Guiding principles for development of ACIP recommendations for vaccination during pregnancy and breastfeeding," *Morbidity and Mortality Weekly Report*, vol. 57, no. 21, p. 580, 2008.

[25] A. D. White and E. B. Andrews, "The pregnancy registry program at glaxo wellcome company," *Journal of Allergy and Clinical Immunology*, vol. 103, no. 2, pp. S362–S363, 1999.

[26] J. Y. Chen, H. J. Ribaudo, S. Souda et al., "Highly active antiretroviral therapy and adverse birth outcomes among HIV-infected women in Botswana," *The Journal of Infectious Diseases*, vol. 206, no. 11, pp. 1695–1705, 2012.

[27] L. Yu, W.-Y. Li, R. Y. Chen et al., "Pregnancy outcomes and risk factors for low birth weight and preterm delivery among HIV-infected pregnant women in Guangxi, China," *Chinese Medical Journal*, vol. 125, no. 3, pp. 403–409, 2012.

[28] F. Martin and G. P. Taylor, "Increased rates of preterm delivery are associated with the initiation of highly active antiretrovial therapy during pregnancy: a single-center cohort study," *Journal of Infectious Diseases*, vol. 196, no. 4, pp. 558–561, 2007.

[29] M. Lopez, F. Figueras, S. Hernandez et al., "Association of HIV infection with spontaneous and iatrogenic preterm delivery: effect of HAART," *AIDS*, vol. 26, no. 1, pp. 37–43, 2012.

[30] E. Aaron, A. Bonacquisti, L. Mathew, G. Alleyne, L. P. Bamford, and J. F. Culhane, "Small-for-gestational-age births in pregnant women with HIV, due to severity of HIV disease, not antiretroviral therapy," *Infectious Diseases in Obstetrics and Gynecology*, vol. 2012, Article ID 135030, 9 pages, 2012.

[31] J. Sibiude, J. Warszawski, R. Tubiana et al., "Premature delivery in HIV-infected women starting protease inhibitor therapy during pregnancy: role of the ritonavir boost?" *Clinical Infectious Diseases*, vol. 54, no. 9, pp. 1348–1360, 2012.

[32] H. Minkoff and M. Augenbraun, "Antiretroviral therapy for pregnant women," *American Journal of Obstetrics and Gynecology*, vol. 176, no. 2, pp. 478–489, 1997.

[33] A. B. Morris, A. R. Dobles, S. Cu-Uvin et al., "Protease inhibitor use in 233 pregnancies," *Journal of Acquired Immune Deficiency Syndromes*, vol. 40, no. 1, pp. 30–33, 2005.

[34] A. M. Cotter, A. G. Garcia, M. L. Duthely, B. Luke, and M. J. O'Sullivan, "Is antiretroviral therapy during pregnancy associated with an increased risk of preterm delivery, low birth weight, or stillbirth?" *Journal of Infectious Diseases*, vol. 193, no. 9, pp. 1195–1201, 2006.

[35] J. Sibiude, L. Mandelbrot, S. Blanche et al., "Association between prenatal exposure to antiretroviral therapy and birth defects: an analysis of the French perinatal cohort study (ANRS CO1/CO11)," *PLoS Medicine*, vol. 11, no. 4, Article ID e1001635, 2014.

[36] M. C. Marazzi, L. Palombi, K. Nielsen-Saines et al., "Extended antenatal use of triple antiretroviral therapy for prevention of mother-to-child transmission of HIV-1 correlates with favorable pregnancy outcomes," *AIDS*, vol. 25, no. 13, pp. 1611–1618, 2011.

[37] N. Li, M. M. Sando, D. Spiegelman et al., "Antiretroviral therapy in relation to birth outcomes among HIV-infected Women: a cohort study," *Journal of Infectious Diseases*, vol. 213, no. 7, pp. 1057–1064, 2016.

[38] L. Mofenson, "Antiretroviral therapy and adverse pregnancy outcome: the elephant in the room?" *Journal of Infectious Diseases*, vol. 213, no. 7, pp. 1051–1054, 2016.

[39] K. M. Powis and R. L. Shapiro, "Protease inhibitors and adverse birth outcomes: is progesterone the missing piece to the puzzle?" *The Journal of Infectious Diseases*, vol. 211, no. 1, pp. 4–7, 2015.

[40] S. Fiore, M.-L. Newell, D. Trabattoni et al., "Antiretroviral therapy-associated modulation of Th1 and Th2 immune responses in HIV-infected pregnant women," *Journal of Reproductive Immunology*, vol. 70, no. 1-2, pp. 143–150, 2006.

[41] F. Fauchet, J.-M. Treluyer, E. Valade et al., "Maternal and fetal zidovudine pharmacokinetics during pregnancy and labour: too high dose infused at labour?" *British Journal of Clinical Pharmacology*, vol. 78, no. 6, pp. 1387–1396, 2014.

[42] M. K. Buchberg, F. E. Fletcher, D. J. Vidrine et al., "A mixed-methods approach to understanding barriers to postpartum retention in care among low-income, HIV-infected women," *AIDS Patient Care and STDs*, vol. 29, no. 3, pp. 126–132, 2015.

[43] L. H. Rubin, J. A. Cook, D. D. Grey et al., "Perinatal depressive symptoms in HIV-infected versus HIV-uninfected women: a prospective study from preconception to postpartum," *Journal of Women's Health*, vol. 20, no. 9, pp. 1287–1295, 2011.

[44] J. R. Ickovics, M. E. Hamburger, D. Vlahov et al., "Mortality, CD4 cell count decline, and depressive symptoms among HIV-seropositive women: longitudinal analysis from the HIV epidemiology research study," *The Journal of the American Medical Association*, vol. 285, no. 11, pp. 1466–1474, 2001.

[45] J. Neubert, M. Pfeffer, A. Borkhardt et al., "Risk adapted transmission prophylaxis to prevent vertical HIV-1 transmission: effectiveness and safety of an abbreviated regimen of postnatal oral Zidovudine," *BMC Pregnancy and Childbirth*, vol. 13, article 22, 2013.

[46] W. Ferguson, M. Goode, A. Walsh, P. Gavin, and K. Butler, "Evaluation of 4 weeks' neonatal antiretroviral prophylaxis as a component of a prevention of mother-to-child transmission program in a resource-rich setting," *Pediatric Infectious Disease Journal*, vol. 30, no. 5, pp. 408–412, 2011.

[47] K. Nielsen-Saines, D. H. Watts, V. G. Veloso et al., "Three postpartum antiretroviral regimens to prevent intrapartum HIV infection," *The New England Journal of Medicine*, vol. 366, no. 25, pp. 2368–2379, 2012.

[48] W. E. Ivy III, K. L. Dominguez, N. Y. Rakhmanina et al., "Premastication as a route of pediatric HIV transmission: case-control and cross-sectional investigations," *Journal of Acquired Immune Deficiency Syndromes*, vol. 59, no. 2, pp. 207–212, 2012.

[49] D. M. Ashton, "Elective delivery at less than 39 weeks," *Current Opinion in Obstetrics and Gynecology*, vol. 22, no. 6, pp. 506–510, 2010.

[50] Committee on Obstetric Practice, "ACOG committee opinion-scheduled cesarean delivery and the prevention of vertical transmission of HIV infection," *International Journal of Gynecology & Obstetrics*, vol. 73, no. 3, pp. 279–281, 2001.

[51] A. R. Fleischman, M. Oinuma, and S. L. Clark, "Rethinking the definition of 'term pregnancy'," *Obstetrics and Gynecology*, vol. 116, no. 1, pp. 136–139, 2010.

[52] "Erythropoietin for zidovudine-induced anemia," *The New England Journal of Medicine*, vol. 323, no. 15, pp. 1069–1070, 1990.

[53] T. J. Nagu, M. Kanyangarara, C. Hawkins et al., "Elevated alanine aminotransferase in antiretroviral-naïve HIV-infected African patients: magnitude and risk factors," *HIV Medicine*, vol. 13, no. 9, pp. 541–548, 2012.

[54] N. M. E. Oliveira, F. A. U. Y. Ferreira, R. Y. U. Yonamine, and E. Z. I. Chehter, "Antiretroviral drugs and acute pancreatitis in HIV/AIDS patients: is there any association? A literature review," *Einstein*, vol. 12, no. 1, pp. 112–119, 2014.

[55] R. C. Wimalasundera, N. Larbalestier, J. H. Smith et al., "Pre-eclampsia, antiretroviral therapy, and immune reconstitution," *The Lancet*, vol. 360, no. 9340, pp. 1152–1154, 2002.

[56] M. Mirochnick and E. Capparelli, "Pharmacokinetics of antiretrovirals in pregnant women," *Clinical Pharmacokinetics*, vol. 43, no. 15, pp. 1071–1087, 2004.

[57] E. De Clercq, "Tenofovir alafenamide (TAF) as the successor of tenofovir disoproxil fumarate (TDF)," *Biochemical Pharmacology*, 2016.

[58] G. K. Siberry, D. L. Jacobson, H. J. Kalkwarf et al., "Lower newborn bone mineral content associated with maternal use of tenofovir disoproxil fumarate during pregnancy," *Clinical Infectious Diseases*, vol. 61, no. 6, pp. 996–1003, 2015.

[59] R. A. Murphy, H. Sunpath, D. R. Kuritzkes, F. Venter, and R. T. Gandhi, "Antiretroviral therapy-associated toxicities in the resource-poor world: the challenge of a limited formulary," *Journal of Infectious Diseases*, vol. 196, supplement 3, pp. S449–S456, 2007.

[60] H. Bussmann, C. W. Wester, C. N. Wester et al., "Pregnancy rates and birth outcomes among women on efavirenz-containing highly active antiretroviral therapy in Botswana," *Journal of Acquired Immune Deficiency Syndromes*, vol. 45, no. 3, pp. 269–273, 2007.

[61] N. Ford, L. Mofenson, Z. Shubber et al., "Safety of efavirenz in the first trimester of pregnancy: an updated systematic review and meta-analysis," *AIDS*, vol. 28, supplement 2, pp. S123–S131, 2014.

[62] P. L. Williams, M. J. Crain, C. Yildirim et al., "Congenital anomalies and in utero antiretroviral exposure in human immunodeficiency virus-exposed uninfected infants," *JAMA Pediatrics*, vol. 169, no. 1, pp. 48–55, 2015.

[63] M. S. Baylor and R. Johann-Liang, "Hepatotoxicity associated with nevirapine use," *Journal of Acquired Immune Deficiency Syndromes*, vol. 35, no. 5, pp. 538–539, 2004.

[64] R. Manfredi and L. Calza, "Safety issues about nevirapine administration in HIV-infected pregnant women," *Journal of Acquired Immune Deficiency Syndromes*, vol. 45, no. 3, pp. 365–368, 2007.

[65] Antiretroviral Pregnancy Registry Steering Committee, *Antiretroviral Pregnancy Registry International Interim Report for 1989–2014*, Registry Coordinating Center, Wilmington, NC, USA, 2014, http://www.APRegistry.com/.

[66] K. Morris, "Short course of AZT halves HIV-1 perinatal transmission," *The Lancet*, vol. 351, no. 9103, p. 651, 1998.

20

Perinatal Mortality Associated with Positive Postmortem Cultures for Common Oral Flora

Mai He,[1,2,3] Alison R. Migliori,[1] Patricia Lauro,[1] C. James Sung,[1,2] and Halit Pinar[1,2]

[1]Department of Pathology & Laboratory Medicine, Women & Infants Hospital of Rhode Island, Providence, RI, USA
[2]Department of Pathology & Laboratory Medicine, Warren Alpert Medical School of Brown University, Providence, RI, USA
[3]Department of Pathology and Immunology, Washington University School of Medicine, St Louis, MO, USA

Correspondence should be addressed to Mai He; mikehemd@gmail.com

Academic Editor: Bryan Larsen

Introduction. To investigate whether maternal oral flora might be involved in intrauterine infection and subsequent stillbirth or neonatal death and could therefore be detected in fetal and neonatal postmortem bacterial cultures. *Methods*. This retrospective study of postmortem examinations from 1/1/2000 to 12/31/2010 was searched for bacterial cultures positive for common oral flora from heart blood or lung tissue. Maternal age, gestational age, age at neonatal death, and placental and fetal/neonatal histopathological findings were collected. *Results*. During the study period 1197 postmortem examinations (861 stillbirths and 336 neonatal deaths) were performed in our hospital with gestational ages ranging from 13 to 40+ weeks. Cultures positive for oral flora were identified in 24 autopsies including 20 pure and 8 mixed growths (26/227, 11.5%), found in 16 stillbirths and 8 neonates. Microscopic examinations of these 16 stillbirths revealed 8 with features of infection and inflammation in fetus and placenta. The 7 neonatal deaths within 72 hours after birth grew 6 pure isolates and 1 mixed, and 6 correlated with fetal and placental inflammation. *Conclusions*. Pure isolates of oral flora with histological evidence of inflammation/infection in the placenta and fetus or infant suggest a strong association between maternal periodontal conditions and perinatal death.

1. Introduction

Infection is a leading cause of preterm birth, stillbirth, and neonatal death [1–5]. Both infection and the inflammatory response play significant roles in the pathogenetic processes leading to adverse pregnancy outcomes. Most intrauterine infection is caused by bacteria, most commonly species that are normally part of the genital tract flora. Nongenital tract organisms such as those found in the oral cavity can also populate the intrauterine environment via hematogenous spread or oral-genital contact [3, 5]. Therefore, the potential sources of infection can be both the mother and her partner. Possible associations between maternal periodontal diseases and adverse pregnancy outcomes have attracted considerable attention [3, 6–9].

Intrauterine infection and the inflammatory response can be examined via different approaches. These include culture- and nonculture based detection of microorganisms and the measurement of inflammatory cytokines in amniotic fluid,

placenta, and blood or tissue from the mother or neonate. In the case of autopsy, histological examination for features of infection and/or inflammation can be performed in placental or in fetal tissue. In a simplified way, chorioamnionitis can be regarded as evidence of a maternal inflammatory response. Funisitis, the inflammation of the umbilical cord, and vasculitis of fetal vessels in the fetoplacental unit can be regarded as histological markers for fetal inflammatory response. The infected amniotic fluid can be swallowed by the fetus in utero, depositing inflammatory cells in the lungs and gastrointestinal tract. The presence of maternal and fetal inflammatory responses, inflammatory cells in fetal tissue, and/or positive fetal tissue and blood cultures are sometimes referred to as amniotic fluid infection syndrome (AFIS) [10].

Previous studies have applied these approaches to examine the relationship between maternal periodontal conditions and amniotic fluid or fetal blood cultures from preterm births and stillbirths [9, 11–13]. Goepfert et al. compared maternal oral conditions with placental histological findings and placental/cord blood cultures but found that neither were associated with periodontal disease [13]. However, while periodontal disease has been shown to be a risk factor for stillbirth [14, 15], there are very few studies looking into the presence of common oral flora in postmortem bacterial cultures in cases of stillbirth or neonatal death within 72 hours of birth [9, 12].

We hypothesize that if oral flora is involved in intrauterine infection and subsequent stillbirth or neonatal death, these bacteria might be present in fetal or neonatal tissue or blood. The current study was aimed at exploring the potential association between oral flora and adverse pregnancy outcomes by investigating bacterial culture results from perinatal autopsies. The study was further correlated with histological features of infection and inflammation of the placenta and fetal/neonatal tissue.

2. Materials and Methods

This was a single-institute retrospective study conducted via chart review (IRB approval No. 10-0129). Our hospital is a tertiary care center for pregnant women in which more than 80% of the deliveries statewide take place. Postmortem examinations of stillborns and neonates were performed following the standard division protocol, including the sampling from heart blood cultures and routine lung tissue cultures [16].

2.1. Bacterial Culture and Identification.

Patient bacterial specimens are cultured on the various media using a standardized method. The lung culture is performed on BAP (Blood agar with 5% sheep blood), MacConkey agar, Chocolate agar, reducible BAP, and Thioglycollate broth. All plates are incubated for 18–24 hours at 35°C in 5% CO_2, except for reducible BAP, which is incubated in an anaerobe jar at 35°C. All lung culture plates are incubated for 4 days and examined daily.

Blood cultures consist of a pediatric aerobic bottle and an adult anaerobic bottle. If a scant amount of blood is obtained, only the pediatric aerobic bottle will be inoculated, which is effective with as little as 1 mL of blood. The blood culture bottles are incubated in the BacT/Alert® (BioMerieux) continuous monitoring blood culture system for 5 days. Positive blood cultures are transferred to BAP, Chocolate agar, and MacConkey agar plates. These plates are incubated for 18–24 hours at 35°C in 5% CO_2. A reducible blood agar plate is inoculated and incubated in an anaerobic jar at 35°C.

The Vitek 2® (BioMerieux) automated identification system is used to identify most Gram-negative enteric bacilli, Pseudomonas, and other nonlactose fermenting Gram-negative bacilli and Gram-positive cocci such as Staphylococcus species and Streptococcus species. Yeast isolates are also identified on the Vitek 2 system. The RapID™ System is used for identification of anaerobic bacteria, Gram-positive bacilli, Haemophilus species, and Neisseria species.

2.2. Study Design.

After receiving approval from the Institutional Review Board (IRB), records of postmortem examinations (PMs, autopsies) performed during 1/1/2000 to 12/31/2010 were searched for positive bacterial cultures from fetal heart blood or fetal lung tissue. Relevant clinical information including maternal age, gestational age (GA) at birth, chronological age at neonatal death, and placental and fetal/neonatal histopathology was collected for each of these cases.

Common oral flora, as suggested by Socransky et al. [17], includes known periodontal pathogens such as Aggregatibacter actinomycetemcomitans, Porphyromonas gingivalis, Tannerella forsythia, Treponema denticola, Fusobacterium nucleatum, Prevotella intermedia, Eikenella corrodens, and Eubacterium nodatum; Gram-positive bacteria such as Streptococcus sanguis, mutants, mitis, and salivarius; and other Gram-negative anaerobic bacteria such as Campylobacter rectus.

3. Results

During the study period, 1197 PMs (861 stillbirths and 336 neonatal deaths) were performed in our hospital with GA ranging from 13 to 40+ weeks. Among these, 227 (19%) yielded positive blood and/or lung cultures, including 165 stillbirths and 62 neonates. Positive cultures for oral flora were identified in 24 cases including 18 pure and 8 mixed growths (more than one species isolated; 26/227, 11.5%), found in 16 stillbirths and 8 neonatal deaths in the following summary of bacterial cultures in postmortem examination of stillbirth and neonatal death from 2000 to 2011.

Bacterial Cultures in Perinatal Autopsies. There were 1197 cases of postmortem examinations with gestational age from 13 to 40+ weeks:

 (i) 861 stillbirths (S) and 336 neonatal deaths (N),

 (ii) 227 (19%, 165S and 62N) with positive postmortem bacterial cultures,

 (iii) 24 (10%, 16S and 8N) cases with positive cultures of oral flora (Some autopsy cases yielded more than one positive bacterial culture),

 (iv) 18 cultures growing pure bacterial species,

 (v) 8 cultures growing mixed bacterial species.

Histopathology-Bacterial Cultures Correlations. There were 16 stillbirths (median gestational age 22 weeks):

 (i) 8 AFIS,

 (ii) 5 with placental inflammation only,

 (iii) 3 without histological features of infection or inflammation.

There were also 8 neonatal deaths:

 (i) 7 died within 72 hours of birth,

 (ii) 6 AFIS,

 (iii) 6 with pure bacterial isolates,

 (iv) 1 with mixed culture results.

Among these 24 cases, 19 (79.2%) exhibited histological features of infection and inflammation in fetal and/or placental tissue.

Of the 16 stillbirth autopsies (median GA 22 weeks), 16 postmortem bacterial cultures grew oral flora species. Microscopic examination of fetal and placental tissue in these cases revealed 8 with AFIS, 5 with placental inflammation, and 3 with no histological inflammation. The 7 neonatal deaths within 72 hours after birth (median GA 21 weeks) grew 6 pure isolates and 1 mixed culture, and 6 cases had AFIS. The clinicopathological findings of all 24 cases are summarized in Table 1.

Figures 1 and 2 demonstrate representative microscopic pictures of both placenta and fetal tissue. Acute inflammation is present in the placental membranes and chorionic plate, consistent with acute chorioamnionitis and suggestive of maternal inflammatory response. When fetal blood vessels at the chorionic plate or umbilical cord are involved, fetal inflammatory response is suggested.

The frequencies of isolated microbes and their microbiological-histological correlations are reported in Table 2. S. mitis was isolated from 9 cultures of 6 cases, including 4 stillbirths and 2 neonatal deaths within 4 hours. In 3 cases, there were pure bacterial isolates associated with histological features of infection/inflammation in both fetal and placental tissue (i.e., AFIS). Peptostreptococcus species were isolated from 5 cases with one stillbirth growing a pure culture and showing features of AFIS. One stillbirth and one immediate neonatal death at midgestation exhibited Prevotella-associated AFIS. Three cultures grew S. sanguis including one pure isolate associated with AFIS in a stillbirth. Other microbes were found in single cases.

4. Discussion

During the study period of 11 years, bacterial species considered to be common oral flora were identified in 26 cultures from 24 autopsies, yielding an incidence of 2% (24/1197). Eleven autopsies grew pure oral bacterial species and had histological features of infection or inflammation in both fetal and placental tissue, suggesting an association between cultures positive for oral flora and intrauterine infection in these cases of stillbirth or immediate neonatal death.

The most common species isolated was Streptococcus mitis, which was isolated from nine cultures in 6 cases (Figure 1 and Table 2). Streptococcus mitis is a type of group D Streptococcus and falls under the umbrella of viridans group streptococci. The oral streptococcal group (mitis phylogenetic group) currently consists of nine recognized species, although the group has been traditionally difficult to classify, with frequent changes in nomenclature over the years. There are several reports of severe neonatal infection by this group with resultant demise [18]. Interestingly, these neonatal infections occurred within 72 hours after birth, implying that these bacteria may have had a maternal origin.

S. sanguis is part of the normal oral flora and alters dental plaque to make it less habitable to other strains of Streptococcus that cause tooth decay. S. salivarius was isolated from one stillbirth as a pure isolate from both blood and lung tissue. The diagnosis at autopsy was amniotic fluid infection syndrome (AFIS). S. salivarius colonizes the mouth and upper respiratory tract shortly after birth and is therefore the principle commensal bacterium of the human mouth. It was isolated as a pure culture associated with AFIS. S. anginosus was isolated in a mixed culture from the blood in a case of twin-twin transfusion syndrome. Although it appears that contamination occurred in the current case, this species has previously been seen in autopsy, placental, and fetal tissue bacterial cultures from midgestation abortions [19]. S. mutans is commonly found in the human mouth and is the primary cause of cavities and tooth decay. In the current study, S. mutans was found as a pure isolate from the blood obtained from a 15-week stillborn. The placenta demonstrated features of both maternal and fetal inflammatory response. Although we did not investigate viridans group streptococci in the current study, a previous study claimed it is a cause of neonatal sepsis, second in frequency only to GBS [20]. There is a case series from our institute in which cultures from 18 perinatal autopsies grew S. viridans during a 14-year period [21].

Besides the Streptococcus species, the second most common isolates in our study were Peptostreptococcus species, which were found in five cases (one pure and four mixed). This is a genus of anaerobic, Gram-positive commensal organisms that colonize the mouth, skin, gastrointestinal tract, vagina, and urinary tract. Prevotella species, formerly known as Bacteroides melaninogenicus, are human pathogens associated with periodontal disease and upper respiratory tract infections. In the current study, Prevotella species were isolated from the fetal lung of an AFIS case, from the lung of a 31-week stillbirth in which no placenta was available for examination, and from a placental culture from a 22-week stillbirth exhibiting maternal and fetal inflammatory response in the placenta.

Fusobacterium is a genus of anaerobic, Gram-negative bacilli that is commonly found in the human oropharynx. In our study it was a pure isolate from fetal blood in two cases of AFIS. These species are pathogens that are associated with not only periodontal disease, but also ulcerative colitis and colon cancer. Han et al. identified the same Fusobacterium 16s rDNA in supra- and subgingival plaque samples and in the fetal lung and stomach, thus establishing that the source of fetal infection was this microorganism [9]. Heller et al. reported finding filamentous organisms consistent with Fusobacterium sp. in the placenta using Warthin-Starry stains in three cases of stillbirths during a 2-year period in one hospital. There was no microbiological identification [22]. In another study, Han considered F. nucleatum to be the most prevalent oral species associated with adverse pregnancy outcome [23].

Kostadinov and Pinar, also from our institute, reported a case of neonatal death associated with Eikenella corrodens [12]. Eikenella corrodens is part of the oral flora and often seen in infections involving human bite wounds (Figure 2).

There is increasing evidence to support an interaction between maternal oral flora and the intrauterine environment; pregnancy can lead to an alteration of oral bacterial

TABLE 1: Autopsy diagnosis, placental pathology, and bacterial culture results.

Case	Main autopsy diagnosis	Placental finding of inflammation	Blood culture	Lung culture	Other cultures	Mode of delivery	GA	Fetal gender	Length of survival	Mat Age	Maternal medical or obstetric history
1	AFIS, dysmorphic features, and normal CG	Acute chorioamnionitis. Acute vasculitis of chorionic plate.	*S. sanguis*	None	None	Unk	17	F	0	35	Abnormal Thrombophilia. 3 pregnancy losses: first loss at 22 weeks; Turner's syndrome; this is the 2nd loss. 3rd with normal CG.
2	Extreme prematurity, AFIS	Acute chorioamnionitis. Gram-positive cocci seen on Gram stain.	*S. mitis*	No growth	None	VD	20	M	15 min	35	Gestational diabetes mellitus
3	AFIS	Necrotizing acute chorioamnionitis. 3-vessel acute vasculitis and funisitis of the umbilical cord.	*S. salivarius*	*S. salivarius*	None	VD	19	F	0	29	
4	IUFD cause cannot be determined	None	No growth	*Enterococcus species, Peptostreptococcus*	None	Unk	16	F	0	34	Maternal obesity
5	AFIS	Acute chorioamnionitis. 3-vessel acute vasculitis and funisitis of the umbilical cord. Acute vasculitis of chorionic plate.	*S. mitis*	*S. mitis*	None	VD	35	F	0	21	
6	AFIS, extreme prematurity	Acute chorioamnionitis. Necrotizing acute chorioamnionitis. 3-vessel acute vasculitis and funisitis of the umbilical cord. Acute vasculitis of chorionic plate.	*Prevotella species*	No growth	None	VD	22	M	15 min	19	
7	Dysmorphic features, AFIS	Acute chorioamnionitis. Acute vasculitis of the umbilical cord.	Not taken	*S. sanguis, S. viridans group, P. anaerobius*	None	VD	19	F	0	37	
8	Intrauterine infection	Acute chorioamnionitis. Acute vasculitis and funisitis of the umbilical cord.	*Peptostreptococcus species*	No growth	*Prevotella* from placenta	VD	22	M	0	20	
9	Undetermined	None	*S. mitis*	No growth	None	VD	21	F	0	30	
10	AFIS	Evidence of amniotic fluid infection with fetal inflammatory response.	*Fusobacterium species*	No growth	None	VD	22	M	0	24	
11	Trisomy 18	No placenta submitted	*S. epidermidis*	*S. epidermidis, S. mitis*	None	C/S	36	F	22 days	31	
12	Extreme prematurity, AFIS	Severe necrotizing acute chorioamnionitis. Acute vasculitis and funisitis of the umbilical cord.	*Fusobacterium*	None	None	VD	22	F	5 hours	22	

TABLE 1: Continued.

Case	Main autopsy diagnosis	Placental finding of inflammation	Blood culture	Lung culture	Other cultures	Mode of delivery	GA	Fetal gender	Length of survival	Mat Age	Maternal medical or obstetric history
13	AFIS	Necrotizing acute chorioamnionitis. 3-vessel acute vasculitis and funisitis of umbilical cord. Acute vasculitis of chorionic plate.	Not taken	1+Staphylococcus coagulase negative. 3+ Peptostreptococcus species and 4+ Lactobacillus species	None	VD	40+	F	0	20	No prenatal care (unaware of pregnancy). Renal failure and DVT. On weight loss medication.
14	AFIS	Acute chorioamnionitis. 3-vessel acute vasculitis and funisitis of the umbilical cord. Acute vasculitis of chorionic plate.	Anaerobic Gram(−) bacteria, fusiform type, fastidious	No growth	None	VD	38	F	0	30	
15	Twin-twin transfusion syndrome IUGR, abruption,	None	S. anginosus and Peptostreptococcus	Staphylococcus coagulase negative	None	C/S	30	Unk	0	24	
16	intrauterine infection, and no inflammation seen in fetal tissue	Evidence of intrauterine infection with fetal inflammatory response.	S. mitis and E. faecalis	None	None	VD	28	M	0	33	Previous pregnancy loss at 23 weeks of GA. Antiphospholipid syndrome, prophylactic heparin, and aspirin.
17	Intrauterine infection with fetal inflammatory response, no inflammation seen in fetal tissue	Acute chorioamnionitis. 1-vessel acute vasculitis of umbilical cord.	E. faecalis and S. mitis	None	GBS in urine	VD	27	F	0	35	Ampicillin for GBS in urine. Prior pregnancy-induced hypertension with full term delivery. Hypothyroidism, on levoxyl daily.
18	Intrauterine infection with fetal inflammatory response, no inflammation seen in fetal tissue	Acute chorioamnionitis. 1-vessel acute vasculitis of umbilical cord. Acute vasculitis of chorionic plate.	S. mutans	None	None	VD	15	F	0	23	G3P0. Cervical cerclage. Two previous second trimester losses
19	Extreme prematurity, no inflammation seen in fetal tissue	Acute chorioamnionitis. 1-vessel acute vasculitis and funisitis of umbilical cord. Acute vasculitis of chorionic plate.	S. mitis	None	None	VD	19+	M	3 hours 40 minutes	33	
20	AFIS	Acute necrotizing chorioamnionitis of twin A	E. corrodens	E. corrodens	None	Unk	23	F	>10 minutes	14	Bleeding gums
21	AFIS	Acute chorioamnionitis. 3-vessel acute vasculitis and funisitis of umbilical cord. Acute vasculitis of chorionic plate.	S. mitis	S. mitis		Unk	36+	M	0	32	
22	AFIS	Acute chorioamnionitis. 2-vessel acute vasculitis and funisitis of umbilical cord.		S. mitis, S. sanguis	None	VD	19+	F	2 hours	30	G4P0. Cervical cerclage. Prophylactic antibiotics
23	AFIS	Acute chorioamnionitis.	None	Prevotella bivia	None	Unk	21	M	2 hours	15	
24	Fetal hypoxia	No placenta submitted	None	Prevotella bivia	None	C/S	31	M	0	20	Pregnancy-induced hypertension, treated with Labetalol

AFIS, amniotic fluid infection syndrome; CG, cytogenetics; C/S, cesarean section; F, female; GA, gestational age; GBS, group B streptococcus; IUFD, intrauterine fetal demise; M, male; Mat, maternal; Unk, unknown; VD, vaginal delivery.

TABLE 2: Microbiological and histological correlation in autopsies with positive cultures for oral flora.

Microbe	Number of cases with positive cultures	Pure culture	Mixed culture	Cases with AFIS	Cases with pure cultures and AFIS	Cases with placental finding of inflammation only	Cases with no histological evidence of inflammation	Note
S. mitis	9	5	4	4	3	3	1	Case 11 had no placenta submitted
Peptostreptococcus	5	1	4	2	1	1	2	
Prevotella	4	4	0	2	2	1	0	Case 24 had no placenta submitted
S. sanguis	3	1	2	3	1	1	0	
Fusobacterium	2	2	0	2	2	0	0	
S. salivarius	1	1	0	1	1	0	0	
S. anginosus	1	0	1	0	0	0	0	Case 15 had no placenta submitted
S. mutans	1	1	0	0	0	1	0	
E. corrodens	1	1	0	1	1	0	0	

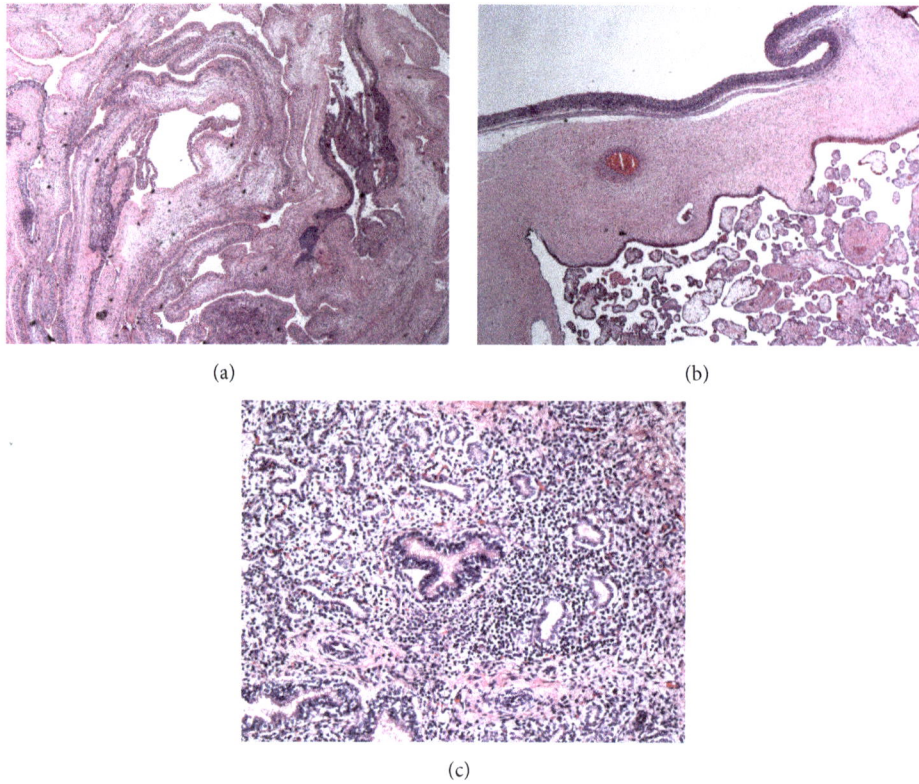

(a)

(b)

(c)

FIGURE 1: Histopathology of a neonatal death born at 20 weeks with postmortem blood cultures growing *Streptococcus mitis*. (a), (b) Acute necrotizing chorioamnionitis (H&E, 40x). (c) Bronchopneumonia (H&E, 200x).

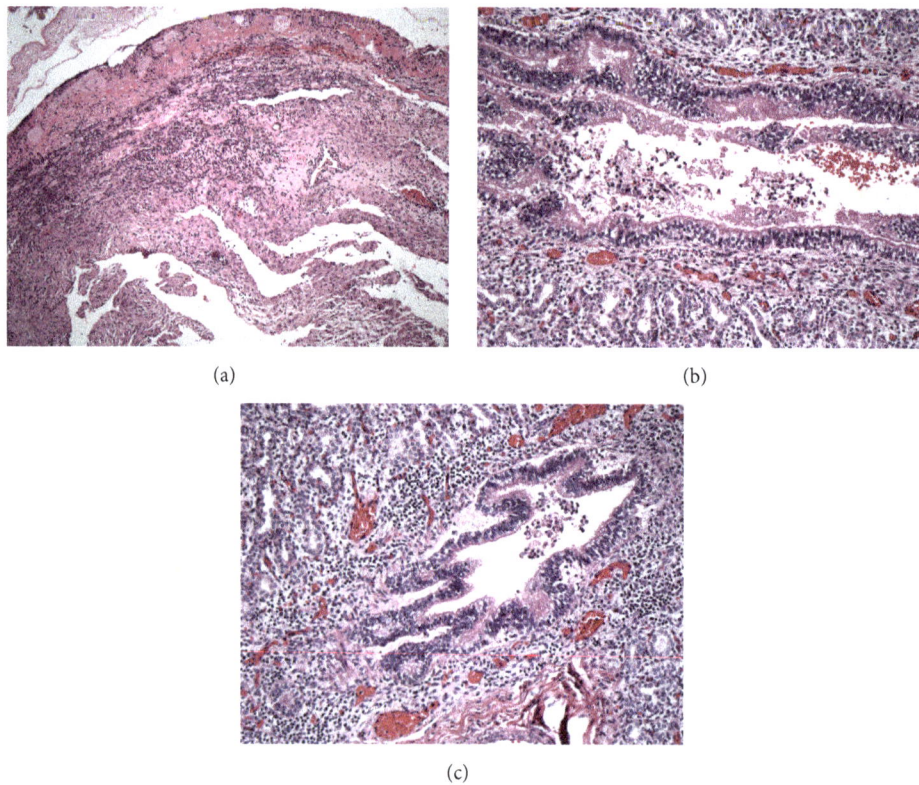

(a)

(b)

(c)

FIGURE 2: Histopathology of a neonatal death born at 23 weeks to a 14-year-old mother with bleeding gums, postmortem blood, and lung cultures growing *Eikenella corrodens*. (a) Acute necrotizing chorioamnionitis (H&E, 40x). (b), (c) Bronchopneumonia (H&E, 200x).

conditions, and oral flora may affect the outcome of pregnancy [24, 25]. Oral-genital contact further complicates the situation. Previous studies revealed that common oral bacteria have been isolated from amniotic fluid [26] and placenta [27], and there are several case reports of stillbirths whose postmortem cultures grew oral flora [9, 12]. Microbiological-histological correlation analysis is necessary to establish the causal relationship between oral bacterial infection and stillbirth. This study demonstrated that common oral flora species can be isolated from postmortem bacterial cultures in cases of stillbirth or neonatal death. These isolates in addition to histological evidence of inflammation in both placenta and fetal/neonatal tissue suggest a strong association between the presence of oral flora in the intrauterine environment and perinatal death.

Since oral health and dental charts are not included in the practice of prenatal care, one of the limitations of this study was the lack of data on the maternal periodontal conditions. Given the probable association between maternal oral flora and fetal/neonatal demise, it may be advisable to include oral and dental assessments as part of prenatal management.

The most significant limitation to the current study was the reliance on bacterial cultures; thus we were not being able to elucidate the occurrence of fastidious bacteria in our cases (i.e., species that cannot be cultured using standard laboratory methods). Han et al. reported an uncultivated oral *Bergeyella* strain in the amniotic fluid in a case of preterm birth [28]. DiGiulio et al. used a combination of ribosomal DNA identification techniques and conventional cultures to report a greater prevalence and diversity of microbes in amniotic fluid compared to those identified by culture alone. They were able to establish an association between positive PCR results and histological chorioamnionitis and funisitis, as well as a causal relationship between amniotic fluid microbes and preterm labor [29]. Molecular detection of microbes may also be used to reveal similar associations by testing samples from both the oral cavity and amniotic fluid [30, 31]. Histological detection of microorganisms can be used for molecular identification as well [32].

Thus, a future prospective study combining molecular detection techniques and conventional cultures to identify bacteria in the maternal oral cavity, amniotic fluid, and fetal tissue, correlated with histological studies of placenta (and the fetus in cases of stillbirth), could provide more convincing evidence of a causal relationship between intrauterine infection by oral bacteria and stillbirth. This knowledge probably could further contribute to the improvement of pregnancy care.

Disclosure

Part of this study was presented as a poster at the Society for Pediatric Pathology Annual Meeting, Vancouver, CA, March 17-18, 2012.

Competing Interests

The authors report no conflict of interests.

References

[1] Stillbirth Collaborative Research Network Writing Group, "Causes of death among stillbirths," *The Journal of the American Medical Association*, vol. 306, no. 22, pp. 2459–2468, 2011.

[2] R. N. Anderson, B. Smith, and National Vital Statistics System, "Deaths: leading causes for 2002," National Vital Statistics Reports 53(17), 2002, http://www.cdc.gov/mmwr/preview/mmwrhtml/mm5438a8.htm.

[3] R. L. Goldenberg, J. C. Hauth, and W. W. Andrews, "Intrauterine infection and preterm delivery," *New England Journal of Medicine*, vol. 342, no. 20, pp. 1500–1507, 2000.

[4] X. Zhou, R. M. Brotman, P. Gajer et al., "Recent advances in understanding the microbiology of the female reproductive tract and the causes of premature birth," *Infectious Diseases in Obstetrics and Gynecology*, vol. 2010, Article ID 737425, 10 pages, 2010.

[5] V. Agrawal and E. Hirsch, "Intrauterine infection and preterm labor," *Seminars in Fetal and Neonatal Medicine*, vol. 17, no. 1, pp. 12–19, 2012.

[6] X. Xiong, P. Buekens, W. D. Fraser, J. Beck, and S. Offenbacher, "Periodontal disease and adverse pregnancy outcomes: a systematic review," *BJOG: An International Journal of Obstetrics and Gynaecology*, vol. 113, no. 2, pp. 135–143, 2006.

[7] M. Straka, "Pregnancy and periodontal tissues," *Neuroendocrinology Letters*, vol. 32, no. 1, pp. 34–38, 2011.

[8] N. R. Matevosyan, "Periodontal disease and perinatal outcomes," *Archives of Gynecology and Obstetrics*, vol. 283, no. 4, pp. 675–686, 2011.

[9] Y. W. Han, Y. Fardini, C. Chen et al., "Term stillbirth caused by oral fusobacterium nucleatum," *Obstetrics and Gynecology*, vol. 115, no. 2, pp. 442–445, 2010.

[10] S. M. Ross, "Amniotic fluid infection syndrome," *South African Medical Journal*, vol. 58, no. 9, pp. 379–380, 1980.

[11] K. A. Boggess, "Maternal oral health in pregnancy," *Obstetrics & Gynecology*, vol. 111, no. 4, pp. 976–986, 2008.

[12] S. Kostadinov and H. Pinar, "Amniotic fluid infection syndrome and neonatal mortality caused by *Eikenella corrodens*," *Pediatric and Developmental Pathology*, vol. 8, no. 4, pp. 489–492, 2005.

[13] A. R. Goepfert, M. K. Jeffcoat, W. W. Andrews et al., "Periodontal disease and upper genital tract inflammation in early spontaneous preterm birth," *Obstetrics and Gynecology*, vol. 104, no. 4, pp. 777–783, 2004.

[14] E. V. Menezes, M. Y. Yakoob, T. Soomro, R. A. Haws, G. L. Darmstadt, and Z. A. Bhutta, "Reducing stillbirths: prevention and management of medical disorders and infections during pregnancy," *BMC Pregnancy and Childbirth*, vol. 9, no. 1, article no. S4, 2009.

[15] A. Shub, C. Wong, B. Jennings, J. R. Swain, and J. P. Newnham, "Maternal periodontal disease and perinatal mortality," *Australian and New Zealand Journal of Obstetrics and Gynaecology*, vol. 49, no. 2, pp. 130–136, 2009.

[16] H. Pinar, M. Koch, H. Hawkins et al., "The stillbirth collaborative research network postmortem examination protocol," *American Journal of Perinatology*, vol. 29, no. 3, pp. 187–202, 2012.

[17] S. S. Socransky, A. D. Haffajee, M. A. Cugini, C. Smith, and R. L. Kent Jr., "Microbial complexes in subgingival plaque," *Journal of Clinical Periodontology*, vol. 25, no. 2, pp. 134–144, 1998.

[18] J. T. Adams and R. G. Faix, "Streptococcus mitis infection in newborns," *Journal of Perinatology*, vol. 14, no. 6, pp. 473–478, 1994.

[19] H. M. McDonald and H. M. Chambers, "Intrauterine infection and spontaneous midgestation abortion: is the spectrum of microorganisms similar to that in preterm labor?" *Infectious Diseases in Obstetrics and Gynecology*, vol. 8, no. 5-6, pp. 220–227, 2000.

[20] A. Rønnestad, T. G. Abrahamsen, P. Gaustad, and P. H. Finne, "Blood culture isolates during 6 years in a tertiary neonatal intensive care unit," *Scandinavian Journal of Infectious Diseases*, vol. 30, no. 3, pp. 245–251, 1998.

[21] I. Ariel and D. B. Singer, "Streptococcus viridans infections in midgestation," *Pediatric Pathology*, vol. 11, no. 1, pp. 75–83, 1991.

[22] D. S. Heller, C. Moorehouse-Moore, J. Skurnick, and R. N. Baergen, "Second-trimester pregnancy loss at an urban hospital," *Infectious Disease in Obstetrics and Gynecology*, vol. 11, no. 2, pp. 117–122, 2003.

[23] Y. W. Han, "Fusobacterium nucleatum: a commensal-turned pathogen," *Current Opinion in Microbiology*, vol. 23, pp. 141–147, 2015.

[24] A. Basavaraju, S. V. Durga, and B. Vanitha, "Variations in the oral anaerobic microbial flora in relation to pregnancy," *Journal of Clinical and Diagnostic Research*, vol. 6, no. 9, pp. 1489–1491, 2012.

[25] L. M. Adriaens, R. Alessandri, S. Spörri, N. P. Lang, and G. R. Persson, "Does pregnancy have an impact on the subgingival microbiota?" *Journal of Periodontology*, vol. 80, no. 1, pp. 72–81, 2009.

[26] G. B. Hill, "Preterm birth: associations with genital and possibly oral microflora," *Annals of Periodontology*, vol. 3, no. 1, pp. 222–232, 1998.

[27] K. Aagaard, J. Ma, K. M. Antony, R. Ganu, J. Petrosino, and J. Versalovic, "The placenta harbors a unique microbiome," *Science Translational Medicine*, vol. 6, no. 237, Article ID 237ra65, 2014.

[28] Y. W. Han, A. Ikegami, N. F. Bissada, M. Herbst, R. W. Redline, and G. G. Ashmead, "Transmission of an uncultivated *Bergeyella* strain from the oral cavity to amniotic fluid in a case of preterm birth," *Journal of Clinical Microbiology*, vol. 44, no. 4, pp. 1475–1483, 2006.

[29] D. B. DiGiulio, R. Romero, H. P. Amogan et al., "Microbial prevalence, diversity and abundance in amniotic fluid during preterm labor: a molecular and culture-based investigation," *PLoS ONE*, vol. 3, no. 8, Article ID e3056, 2008.

[30] Y. W. Han, T. Shen, P. Chung, I. A. Buhimschi, and C. S. Buhimschi, "Uncultivated bacteria as etiologic agents of intra-amniotic inflammation leading to preterm birth," *Journal of Clinical Microbiology*, vol. 47, no. 1, pp. 38–47, 2009.

[31] Y. W. Han, "Can oral bacteria cause pregnancy complications?" *Women's Health*, vol. 7, no. 4, pp. 401–404, 2011.

[32] M. He, T. Hong, P. Lauro, and H. Pinar, "Identification of bacteria in paraffin-embedded tissues using 16S rDNA sequencing from a neonate with necrotizing enterocolitis," *Pediatric and Developmental Pathology*, vol. 14, no. 2, pp. 149–152, 2011.

21

Cervicovaginal Bacteriology and Antibiotic Sensitivity Patterns among Women with Premature Rupture of Membranes in Mulago Hospital, Kampala, Uganda

Milton W. Musaba,[1] **Mike N. Kagawa,**[2] **Charles Kiggundu,**[3] **Paul Kiondo,**[2] **and Julius Wandabwa**[4]

[1] Mbale Regional Referral & Teaching Hospital, P.O. Box 921, Mbale, Uganda
[2] School of Medicine, College of Health Sciences, Makerere University, P.O. Box 7072, Kampala, Uganda
[3] Mulago National Referral & Teaching Hospital, P.O. Box 7051, Kampala, Uganda
[4] Faculty of Health Sciences, Busitema University, P.O. Box 1460, Mbale, Uganda

Correspondence should be addressed to Milton W. Musaba; miltonmusaba@gmail.com

Academic Editor: David Baker

Background. A 2013 Cochrane review concluded that the choice of antibiotics for prophylaxis in PROM is not clear. In Uganda, a combination of oral erythromycin and amoxicillin is the 1st line for prophylaxis against ascending infection. Our aim was to establish the current cervicovaginal bacteriology and antibiotic sensitivity patterns. *Methods.* Liquor was collected aseptically from the endocervical canal and pool in the posterior fornix of the vagina using a pipette. Aerobic cultures were performed on blood, chocolate, and MacConkey agar and incubated at 35–37°C for 24–48 hrs. Enrichment media were utilized to culture for GBS and facultative anaerobes. Isolates were identified using colonial morphology, gram staining, and biochemical analysis. Sensitivity testing was performed via Kirby-Bauer disk diffusion and dilution method. Pearson's chi-squared (χ^2) test and the paired t-test were applied, at a P value of 0.05. *Results.* Thirty percent of the cultures were positive and over 90% were aerobic microorganisms. Resistance to erythromycin, ampicillin, cotrimoxazole, and ceftriaxone was 44%, 95%, 96%, and 24%, respectively. Rupture of membranes (>12 hrs), late preterm, and term PROM were associated with more positive cultures. *Conclusion.* The spectrum of bacteria associated with PROM has not changed, but resistance to erythromycin and ampicillin has increased.

1. Background

Prelabour rupture of membranes is the commonest antecedent to preterm and term labour [1]. The aetiology of preterm delivery has been attributed to a number of causes such as decidual hemorrhage, inflammation of the fetal membranes, activation of the maternal-fetal hypothalamic pituitary axis, structural abnormalities like cervical incompetence, pathologic distension of the uterus, and uterine abnormalities [2]. However, there is strong epidemiological and biochemical evidence which links preterm and term delivery to ascending infection of the female genital tract [3].

The incidence of maternal and neonatal sepsis ranges from 1 to 25% depending on the duration of rupture of membranes and gestation age [4] or even higher in low resource settings [5]. In Uganda, 22% of the maternal deaths are due to sepsis [6] and sepsis is the 2nd major cause of neonatal mortality [7]. Premature rupture of membranes at or near term complicates 3% of all pregnancies in Mulago Hospital [8]. Anecdotal evidence suggests that most of these patients suffer adverse obstetric outcomes due to sepsis.

Several organisms have been variably associated with PROM in different parts of the world [1]. Previous culture and sensitivity studies in this settings have involved sick neonates and patients with surgical site infections [9, 10]. Only one found that 13.3% of 180 women with PROM in Mulago Hospital had positive amniotic fluid cultures with descending order isolates of *Escherichia coli*, beta hemolytic *Streptococcus*,

Proteus species, and *Peptostreptococcus*, although the antibiotic sensitivity patterns were not done [8].

The choice of antibiotics for prophylaxis should be based on culture and sensitivity patterns as well as epidemiological patterns, but because of limited access to reliable laboratory services in Uganda, broad spectrum antibiotics are given empirically. A combination of oral erythromycin (250 mg) and amoxicillin (500 mg) for 7 days is the 1st line for prophylaxis against ascending genital tract infection following PROM (MOH 2012). It is not clear if this recommendation is based on current culture and sensitivity patterns. In Africa, resistance to commonly used antibiotics has greatly increased over the last 20 years [9]; so we are no longer sure if this recommendation is still relevant. A recent Cochrane review which included 22 studies from high resource settings concluded that the antibiotic of choice for prophylaxis in PROM is not clear [11]. Probably the associated organisms have changed or developed resistance, hence the need to establish the current bacterial culture and sensitivity patterns in this population of patients. This information may inform our choice of antibiotics for prophylaxis against ascending infection following PROM and probably contribute to the body of evidence needed to either revise or maintain the current guideline for management of PROM.

The aim of this study was to establish the current cervicovaginal bacteriology and antibiotic sensitivity patterns.

2. Materials and Methods

2.1. Study Design. A cross-sectional study was conducted on the labour suite at Mulago National Referral and Teaching Hospital Uganda between January and May, 2013.

2.2. Study Setting. Mulago Hospital is the national referral hospital for Uganda and a teaching hospital for Makerere University. The hospital averages 30,000 births per year. In 2011, 868 patients with PROM were admitted in Mulago Hospital, none of them had culture and sensitivity patterns done and the pregnancy outcomes related to sepsis were not easy to ascertain because of poor documentation.

2.3. Sample Size Calculation. The Leslie Kish (1965) formula for determining single proportions was used. *P* was the percentage of positive amniotic fluid cultures among patients with PROM in Mulago National hospital, using 13.3% [8].

2.4. Sampling. We consecutively enrolled 196 women with a diagnosis of PROM and a viable foetus at or after 28 weeks of gestation, over a 5 months' period. Ethical approval was obtained from the School of Medicine Research and Ethics Committee, Makerere University College of Health Sciences, and the Uganda National Council for Science and Technology. Each participant was requested to give written informed consent. An interviewer administered questionnaire was used to collect data on patient demographics and clinical features [12].

Using an aseptic technique, 5 mLs of amniotic fluid was collected from both the endocervical canal and the pool in the posterior fornix of the vagina using a pipette

TABLE 1: Sociodemographic and clinical characteristics (*n* = 196).

Characteristic	Frequency (%)
Mean age	25 (16–47) years
Referral status	
Yes	54 (27.6)
No	142 (72.4)
Gestation age	
Extreme preterm (28–31 weeks)	19 (10)
Late preterm (32–36 weeks)	52 (27)
Term (>37 weeks)	125 (64)
Gravidity	
Primigravida	80 (40)
2-3	60 (31)
>3	56 (29)
Prior antibiotic use	
Yes	46 (23.5)
No	150 (76.5)
Duration of ROM	
<12 hrs	77 (39)
12–24 hrs	20 (10)
>24 hrs	99 (51)

TABLE 2: Isolates from the positive cervicovaginal cultures.

	Number
Gram negative organism	
Bacteroides species*	3
*Citrobacterfreundii***	2
Enterobacterspecies	1
Escherichiacoli	12
KlebsiellaPneumoniae	7
Gram positive organisms	
*Clostridiumtetani**	1
Coagulase-negative *Staphylococcus*	9
Coryneform bacteria	1
Enterococcus species	3
Staphylococcus aureus	13
Streptococcus pyogenes	8
Streptococcuspneumoniae	1
Streptococcusspecies	1
*Viridiansstreptococcus***	3
Listeriamonocytogenes	1
Positive rods isolated*	1
Total	67

*Anaerobe. **Facultative anaerobe.

and transported to the microbiology laboratory within 30 minutes for analysis. Specimen was transported in 3 separate containers: 1 mL inoculated into a selective Todd-Hewitt enrichment media to culture for GBS in a glass bottle; 1 mL inoculated into thioglycolate enrichment media to culture for facultative anaerobes in a glass bottle; 3 mL in a sterile plastic container. The aerobic culture was performed on blood,

TABLE 3: Antibiotic sensitivity profile of positive cervicovaginal cultures.

Antibiotic	Sensitive (%)	Resistant (%)	Intermediate (%)	Total
Ceftriaxone/cefotaxime	16 (76)	5 (24)	0	21
Cotrimoxazole	1 (4)	26 (96)	0	27
Erythromycin	15 (56)	10 (37)	2 (7)	27
Vancomycin	20 (95)	1 (5)	0	21
Chloramphenicol	23 (62)	14 (38)	0	37
Clindamycin	6 (40)	7 (47)	2 (13)	15
Ampicillin	1 (5)	20 (95)	0	21
Penicillin G	9 (38)	15 (63)	0	24
Co-amoxiclav	3 (17)	15 (83)	0	18
Tetracycline	6 (21)	22 (79)	0	28
Meropenem	6 (100)	0	0	6
Ciprofloxacin	21 (66)	11 (34)	0	32
Oxacillin	1 (7)	14 (93)	0	15
Ofloxacin	4 (80)	1 (20)	0	5
Cefazolin	3 (23)	9 (69)	1 (8)	13
Cefuroxime	3 (19)	13 (81)	0	16
Gentamicin	12 (46)	12 (46)	2 (8)	26
Ceftazidime	2 (100)	0	0	2
Nitrofurantoin	1 (100)	0	0	1
Cefotaxime-clavulanic acid	1 (100)	0	0	1

chocolate, and MacConkey agar incubated at 35–37° for 24–48 hours [12]. Colonial morphology, gram staining, and biochemical analysis were used to identify the isolates. The Kirby-Bauer disk diffusion and dilution methods were used to test for sensitivity of the isolates against nitroimidazoles, penicillins, cephalosporins, sulfonamides, aminoglycosides, quinolones/fluoroquinolones, macrolides, and tetracyclines, as specified in the manual of clinical microbiology (Jorgensen, Pfaller et al. 2015). Ten percent of the samples were taken to 2 laboratories (Medical School Laboratory and MBN diagnostic laboratories) for quality control purposes [12].

Data was entered into Epidata version 3.1 and then exported into Stata version 12 for analysis. The proportion of positive amniotic fluid cultures was computed; statistical significance was tested via the chi (χ^2) test [12]. The paired t-test was applied to measure the significance of the factors associated with positive cultures ($P = 0.05$).

3. Results

Fifty-eight (30%) of the 196 cervicovaginal cultures were positive. A quarter of the participants had received an antibiotic prior to admission and the most commonly used antibiotics were ceftriaxone (29), ampicillin (13), erythromycin (9), and metronidazole (9) (Table 1).

Sixty-seven isolates were identified from the 58 positive cultures, 63% were gram positive aerobic bacteria, and only 5 (7.5%) were anaerobes (Table 2).

Resistance to most commonly used broad spectrum antibiotics (ceftriaxone, ampicillin, cotrimoxazole, and erythromycin) was notably high. It is only the less commonly used and more expensive antibiotics like vancomycin and

meropenem that showed the highest levels of sensitivity to the isolated antibiotics (Table 3).

Rupture of membranes for >12 hrs and late preterm and term PROM mothers were associated with a higher percentage of positive cultures. On the other hand prior use of any antibiotic following rupture of membranes and a positive HIV status were associated with fewer positive cultures (Table 4).

4. Discussion

In the current study, we found that the proportion of positive cervicovaginal cultures has doubled since 1996 [8]. This could be attributed to the use of enrichment broths to increase the yield of specific bacterial isolates. A review of 18 published studies involving 1,727 women with PROM in which amniotic fluid was obtained by amniocentesis; a 32.4% rate of positive cultures was reported for women not in labour and 75% for those admitted in labour [13]. Despite the differences in setting and techniques employed, the rate of positive cultures is similar.

The spectrum of bacteria associated with PROM has not changed much over time [8] and it is similar to those isolated from neonates with sepsis in this hospital [7].

We did not isolate any GBS despite the fact that an enrichment medium was used to favour its growth. It has been strongly associated with neonatal sepsis following vertical transmission. This could be so because either we used an antiseptic before introducing a speculum into the vagina or the site, or timing and nature of specimen collected were not ideal [14]

TABLE 4: Factors associated with cervicovaginal culture and sensitivity patterns.

Characteristic	Positive cultures	Negative cultures	Odds ratio (CI)	P values
Referral status				
Yes	14 (26%)	40 (74%)	0.78 (CI 0.49–1.38)	
No	44 (31%)	98 (69%)		0.488
Mean maternal BP	119/74	116/75	Mean = 117/75	
Mean radial pulse	83	85	Mean = 85	
Mean axillary temp.	37	37	Mean = 37	
Gestation age (weeks)				
Extreme preterm (28–31)	8 (42%)	11 (58%)		
Late preterm (32–36)	16 (31%)	36 (39%)	1.4 (CI 1.3–1.6)	0.000
Term (>37)	34 (27%)	91 (73%)		
Gravidity				
Primigravida	24 (30%)	56 (70%)		
2-3	14 (23%)	46 (77%)	1.12 (CI 0.77–1.62)	0.343
>3	20 (36%)	36 (64%)		
Duration of ROM				
<12	16 (21%)	61 (79%)		
12–24	9 (45%)	11 (55%)	1.33 (CI 0.96–1.85)	0.055
>24	33 (33%)	66 (67%)		
HIV serology				
Negative	50 (29%)	123 (71%)	0.76 (CI 0.30–1.92)	0.562
Positive	8 (35%)	15 (65%)		
Prior antibiotic use				
Yes	9 (20%)	37 (80%)	0.50 (CI 0.22–1.13)	0.089
No	49 (33%)	101 (67%)		
Prior steroid use				
Yes	7 (41%)	10 (59%)	1.76 (CI 0.63–4.90)	0.274
No	51 (28%)	128 (72%)		
Regular medication use (ART)				
Yes	6 (35%)	11 (65%)	1.33 (CI 0.47–3.80)	0.59
No	52 (29%)	127 (71%)		
Mean FHR				
<120	0 (0%)	2 (100%)		
120–160	55 (30%)	129 (70%)	1.30 (CI 0.37–4.54)	0.654
>160	3 (30%)	7 (70%)		
Gram stain result				
Positive	38 (50%)	38 (50%)	0.2 (CI 0.10–0.40)	< 0.001
Negative	20 (17%)	100 (83%)		

The yield of anaerobic bacteria was very poor, even though specific measures like the use of enrichment media for transportation of cervicovaginal samples were employed in this study. Several studies from high income settings have strongly associated them with PROM [4], so it would be interesting to study the whole picture in a better resourced laboratory before drawing conclusions [12].

Resistance to commonly used antibiotics is high which is consistent with reports of increasing antibiotic resistance in resource limited setting due to irrational use of antibiotics [9]. Due to limitations in accessing laboratory services in Uganda and other similar settings, there is a recourse to empirical use of broad spectrum antibiotics for prophylaxis against ascending genital tract infections following PROM [12]. The findings of high resistance to erythromycin and ampicillin, the 2 antibiotics recommended by MOH in Uganda, raise concerns regarding their usefulness as 1st choice prophylactic antibiotics. It is possible that either the organisms have developed resistance over time or the associated organisms have changed. Moving forward, trials need to be undertaken to identify the most appropriate antibiotic for prophylaxis following PROM in Uganda.

Although this study was not powered to determine associated factors, it was noted that there were more positive cultures when the duration of rupture of membranes was longer than 24 hrs but this result was not statistically significant;

TABLE 5: Gestation age and cervicovaginal cultures of mothers with PROM.

	Odds ratio	*P* value	95% CI	
Extreme preterm (28–31) R	1.0			
Late preterm (32–36) versus extreme preterm (28–31)	2.3	0.007	1.2	4.1
Term (>37) versus extreme preterm (28–31)	2.7	0.000	1.8	4.0

$P = 0.055$. It is also important to note that as early as 12 hrs after ROM 21% of 77 cultures were positive (Table 4). In this setting, we probably need to initiate prophylaxis early even before the recommended 18 hrs for prolonged ROM. A similar trend was also noted with the gestation age; there were more positive cultures seen with decreasing gestation age. This is consistent with other studies that have identified these two factors as important risk factors for ascending genital tract infection following PROM [15]. Further analysis revealed that mothers with late preterm and term PROM were more likely to have positive cultures compared to mothers with extreme preterm PROM. Both of them were statistically significant $P = 0.007$ and $P = 0.000$, respectively (Table 5).

Prior use of antibiotics following PROM was associated with fewer positive cervicovaginal cultures, which is expected. Although in this current study, only 23.5% of the participants reported use of antibiotics prior to admission following PROM.

5. Conclusions

The proportion of positive cervicovaginal cultures in Mulago National Referral and Teaching Hospital has more than doubled, but the spectrum of associated bacteria isolated has not changed since 1996. Resistance to the most commonly used antibiotics in our setting is high. There is a need for clinical trials to identify the most appropriate antibiotic for prophylaxis in PROM.

Abbreviations

PROM: Premature rupture of membranes
C & S: Culture and sensitivity patterns
GBS: Group B *Streptococcus*
MOH: Ministry of Health.

Competing Interests

The authors declare that they have no competing interests.

Authors' Contributions

Milton W. Musaba participated in conception and design of the proposal, collection of the data and analysis, and drafting the manuscript. Julius Wandabwa and Paul Kiondo were involved in drafting and reviewing the manuscript for accuracy and intellectual content. Mike N. Kagawa and Charles Kiggundu made substantial contribution to the conception and design of the proposal as well as interpretation of the data. All the author's read and approved the final manuscript.

Acknowledgments

Thanks are due to the Staff of Medical School Microbiology Laboratory and MBN Clinical Laboratories for working tirelessly and Javis Tumuhe for helping with the statistical work.

References

[1] S. L. Kenyon, D. J. Taylor, and W. Tarnow-Mordi, "Broad-spectrum antibiotics for preterm, prelabour rupture of fetal membranes: the ORACLE I randomised trial," *Lancet*, vol. 357, no. 9261, pp. 979–988, 2001.

[2] E. R. Newton, "Preterm labor, preterm premature rupture of membranes, and chorioamnionitis," *Clinics in Perinatology*, vol. 32, no. 3, pp. 571–600, 2005.

[3] G. G. G. Donders and G. Bellen, "Management of abnormal vaginal flora as a risk factor for preterm birth," in *Preterm Birth—Mother and Child*, InTech, 2011.

[4] A. T. N. Tita and W. W. Andrews, "Diagnosis and management of clinical chorioamnionitis," *Clinics in Perinatology*, vol. 37, no. 2, pp. 339–354, 2010.

[5] A. C. Seale, M. Mwaniki, C. R. Newton, and J. A. Berkley, "Maternal and early onset neonatal bacterial sepsis: burden and strategies for prevention in sub-Saharan Africa," *The Lancet Infectious Diseases*, vol. 9, no. 7, pp. 428–438, 2009.

[6] MOH, Uganda Clinical Guidelines, 2012.

[7] J. Mugalu, M. K. Nakakeeto, S. Kiguli, and D. H. Kaddu-Mulindwa, "Aetiology, risk factors and immediate outcome of bacteriologically confirmed neonatal septicaemia in Mulago hospital, Uganda," *African Health Sciences*, vol. 6, no. 2, pp. 120–126, 2006.

[8] D. Kaye, "Risk factors for preterm premature rupture of membranes at Mulago Hospital, Kampala," *East African Medical Journal*, vol. 78, no. 2, pp. 65–69, 2001.

[9] A. N. Kimang'a, "A situational analysis of antimicrobial drug resistance in Africa: are we losing the battle?" *Ethiopian Journal of Health Sciences, Jimma, Ethiopia*, vol. 22, pp. 135–143, 2012.

[10] Y. Mpairwe and S. Wamala, *Antibiotic Resistance in Uganda: Situation Analysis and Recommendations*, Uganda National Academy of Sciences, Kampala, Uganda, 2015.

[11] S. Kenyon, M. Boulvain, and J. Neilson, "Antibiotics for preterm rupture of membranes (Review)," *The Cochrane Database of Systematic Reviews*, no. 12, Article ID CD001058, 2010.

[12] L. Mubangizi, F. Namusoke, and T. Mutyaba, "Aerobic cervical bacteriology and antibiotic sensitivity patterns in patients with advanced cervical cancer before and after radiotherapy at a national referral hospital in Uganda," *International Journal of Gynecology and Obstetrics*, vol. 126, no. 1, pp. 37–40, 2014.

[13] R. Romero, R. Gómez, T. Chaiworapongsa, G. Conoscenti, J. C. Kim, and Y. M. Kim, "The role of infection in preterm labour and delivery," *Paediatric and Perinatal Epidemiology*, vol. 15, no. 2, pp. 41–56, 2001.

[14] A. Joachim, M. I. Matee, F. A. Massawe, and E. F. Lyamuya, "Maternal and neonatal colonisation of group B streptococcus at Muhimbili National Hospital in Dar es Salaam, Tanzania: prevalence, risk factors and antimicrobial resistance," *BMC Public Health*, vol. 9, article no. 437, 2009.

[15] M. E. Hannah, A. Ohlsson, D. Farine et al., "Induction of labor compared with expectant management for prelabor rupture of the membranes at term," *New England Journal of Medicine*, vol. 334, no. 16, pp. 1005–1010, 1996.

22

Effect of Genital Sampling Site on the Detection and Quantification of *Ureaplasma* Species with Quantitative Polymerase Chain Reaction during Pregnancy

Gilles Faron,[1] **Ellen Vancutsem,**[2] **Anne Naessens,**[2] **Ronald Buyl,**[3]
Leonardo Gucciardo,[1] **and Walter Foulon**[1]

[1]*Department of Obstetrics and Prenatal Medicine, Universitair Ziekenhuis Brussel, 101 Laarbeeklaan, Jette, 1090 Brussels, Belgium*
[2]*Department of Microbiology, UZ Brussel, 101 Laarbeeklaan, Jette, 1090 Brussels, Belgium*
[3]*Department of Biostatistics and Medical Informatics, Faculty of Medicine and Pharmacy, Vrije Universiteit Brussel,*
 101 Laarbeeklaan, Jette, 1090 Brussels, Belgium

Correspondence should be addressed to Gilles Faron; gilles.faron@uzbrussel.be

Academic Editor: Diane M. Harper

Objective. This study aimed to compare the qualitative and quantitative reproducibility of quantitative PCR (qPCR) for *Ureaplasma* species (*Ureaplasma* spp.) throughout pregnancy and according to the genital sampling site. *Study Design.* Between 5 and 14 weeks of gestation (T1), vaginal, fornix, and two cervical samples were taken. Sampling was repeated during the 2nd (T2) and 3rd (T3) trimester in randomly selected T1 positive and negative women. Qualitative and quantitative reproducibility were evaluated using, respectively, Cohen's kappa (κ) and interclass correlation coefficients (ICC) and repeated measures ANOVA on the log-transformed mean number of DNA copies for each sampling site. *Results.* During T1, 51/127 women were positive for *U. parvum* and 8 for *U. urealyticum* (4 patients for both). Sampling was repeated for 44/55 women at T2 and/or T3; 43 (97.7%) remained positive at the three timepoints. κ ranged between 0.83 and 0.95 and the ICC for cervical samples was 0.86. *Conclusions.* Colonization by *Ureaplasma* spp. seems to be very constant during pregnancy and vaginal samples have the highest detection rate.

1. Introduction

Preterm delivery, defined as birth before 37 weeks, is responsible for 75% of perinatal mortality and for more than 50% of the long-term morbidity among survivors [1]. Spontaneous premature labor or premature preterm rupture of the membranes is involved in 60–65% of premature births [2]. These outcomes could be improved with development of specific care and with more accurate identification of pregnant women with obviously increased risks of premature delivery among the heterogeneous population of more or less symptomatic patients.

Evaluation of the vaginal flora during pregnancy has been pointed out as a potentially interesting screening tool in this context [3, 4]. Although considered to be commensal in the female genital tract, the presence of *Ureaplasma* species (*Ureaplasma* spp.) during pregnancy is independently associated with an increased likelihood of clinical chorioamnionitis, preterm premature rupture of membranes (PPROM), and preterm delivery [5, 6]. *Ureaplasma* spp. induce inflammatory response in chorion and amnion cells [7] and contribute to collagen fragmentation which weakens amniotic membranes [8].

Two methods have been described to screen for *Ureaplasma* spp.: culture is the gold standard, but this method gives no information about the different species (*Ureaplasma urealyticum* (*U. urealyticum*) or *Ureaplasma parvum* (*U. parvum*)) and gives few indications of their quantity. The second method, quantitative polymerase chain reaction (qPCR), has the huge advantage over culture of being able to differentiate *U. urealyticum* and *U. parvum*. Studies on the pathogenicity of *Ureaplasma* spp. in pregnancy have addressed the possibility that there may be a difference in pathogenic potential among species [9]. Moreover, bacterial load could also be a factor which enhances the invasive potential of the microorganism [5]. Culture based studies have reported that women harbor different bacterial populations in the cervix than in the vagina and that the vaginal flora was a dynamic ecosystem [10]. One study has investigated the constancy of the burden of *Ureaplasma* spp. in genital secretions [11] throughout pregnancy, but none has reported the distribution of *U. urealyticum* and *U. parvum* during pregnancy. The influence of the sampling location on the detection and quantification of *Ureaplasma* spp. has also not been studied previously. Therefore, the aim of this study was to compare the qualitative and quantitative reproducibility of a qPCR technique used to identify the presence of both *Ureaplasma* spp. according to the sampling site, within the same woman, throughout pregnancy. As a secondary outcome, we studied the epidemiology of *Ureaplasma* species (*parvum* or *urealyticum*) during pregnancy and the evolution of the colonization of the women, using three timepoints.

2. Material and Methods

This was a prospective study conducted in the antenatal outpatient clinic of the Universitair Ziekenhuis Brussel (UZ Brussel) from February 2011 to January 2015. Healthy women with uncomplicated pregnancies were invited to participate. During the first prenatal visit that was scheduled before 14 weeks of gestation, we gave oral information about the study. Written informed consent was obtained from those agreeing to participate. This study was approved by the hospital's ethics committee. Gestational age was ascertained from the last menstruation date and a first trimester ultrasound examination. The participants were tested between 5 and 14 weeks of gestation. The exclusion criteria included patients under 18 years old, clinical vaginal infection, or documented recent intake of antibiotics (whatever the reason).

After exposing the cervix with a sterile speculum, four samples were taken for PCR quantification of *U. parvum* and *U. urealyticum*, in the following order: vaginal, fornix, and two from the (exo)cervix (cx1 and cx2). Sampling was performed gently to avoid (cervical) bleeding. The samples were transported in the "Universal Transport Medium System" (UTM) (Copan Italia, Italy, containing 3 ml liquid medium) and processed using a qPCR method that was described in a previous publication [12].

We recruited women during the first trimester and they were considered positive if any of the four genital tract samples tested was reactive in qPCR. We intended to repeat the same sampling during the second trimester (between 18 and 27 completed weeks, T2) and during the third trimester (between 28 and 39 weeks, T3) for these positive women. The lack of available publications about this specific research topic made the required sample size impossible to calculate accurately.

For those who were negative at the first sampling we decided to test some of them again, at random, during the second and the third trimester to confirm that the absence of *Ureaplasma* spp. was maintained throughout the pregnancy.

Qualitative reproducibility was assessed by comparing the proportions of qPCR positive tests for each sampling site with a Fisher's exact test, both at the first trimester and in a second analysis for all samples (T1, T2, and T3). Cohen's kappa coefficient (κ) was used to assess the degree of inter-rater agreement between the different sampling sites. The agreement between two observations is generally considered excellent when $\kappa > 0.75$ [13].

The quantitative reproducibility of the test was assessed at two levels among the patients who were found positive:

(1) We calculated the mean number of DNA copies for each sampling site. In order to normalize our results and minimize the outlier effect we used (base 10) logarithmically transformed data. The computed mean log of the two cervical samples was used to compare with those from other sampling sites, except if one of them was negative; in that case we took into account only the value of the positive result. A repeated measures ANOVA, with pairwise comparisons (Bonferroni corrections), was used to analyze the quantitative differences among locations as well as potential differences in carriage among T1, T2, and T3.

(2) To test the degree of quantitative agreement between two samples taken simultaneously from the same location, we considered the two repeated samples taken from the cervix during all trimesters (when both of them were positive) and computed the interclass correlation coefficient (ICC) and its 95% confidence interval (95% CI).

All calculations were carried out using IBM SPSS version 22.0. Baseline data were summarized for each group and compared (comparison of two proportions or two means, with 95% CI). Unpaired t-tests, the two-sided Fisher's exact test, and 95% CI were used when appropriate. A P value < 0.05 was considered to be statistically significant.

3. Results

We recruited 139 women, who were tested between 5 and 14 weeks of pregnancy. Three were lost to follow-up and were excluded from our analysis (Figure 1). Nine women had a miscarriage between 6 and 13 weeks: among them, six were positive for *U. parvum* for all sites, including one patient with associated positivity for *U. urealyticum* in the fornix and the vagina. The three other women had negative results for all sampling sites.

Of the remaining 127 women, 72 (56.7%) had negative qPCR results for all sites and 55 (43.3%) were positive for at least one location during the first trimester. Follow-up samples were taken from the three different locations for 23 of the 72 negative women; 15 were tested in the second trimester and 8 other patients were sampled in both the second and the third trimester. All these women remained negative at all sampling timepoints.

Among the 55 women with +qPCR, 51 (92.7%) were positive for *U. parvum* and 8 (14.5%) were positive for *U. urealyticum*; 4 (7.2%) of these women were positive for both species.

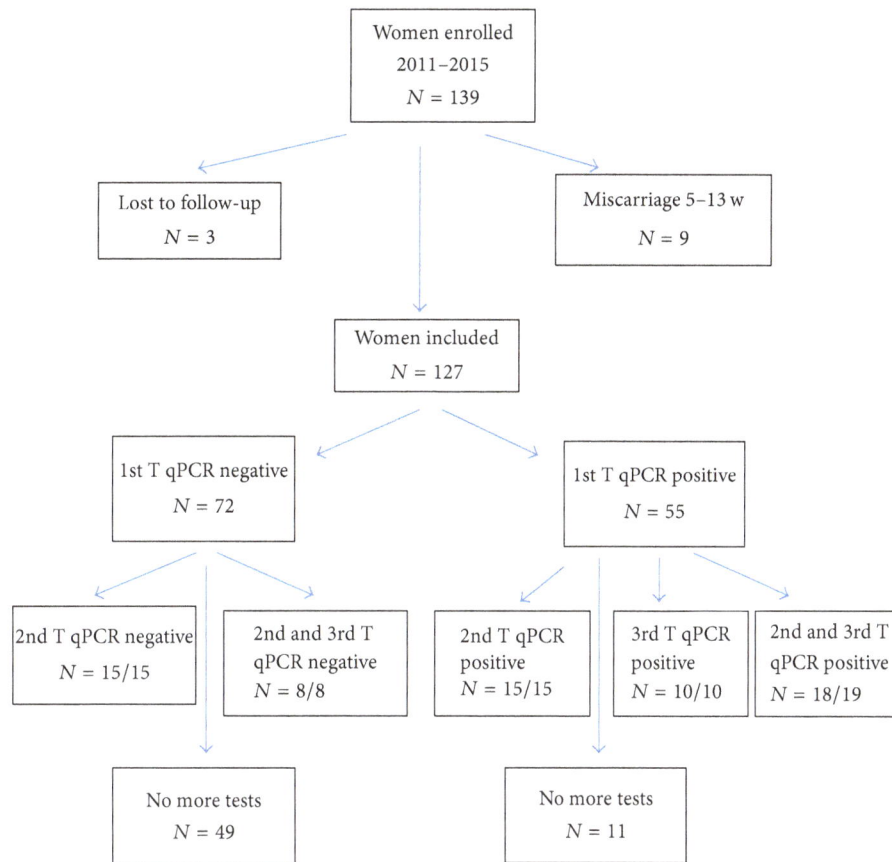

FIGURE 1: Enrolments of participants.

TABLE 1: Number (N, %) of positive samples per location and per trimester in qPCR+ patients.

Sampling location	qPCR + T1 ($N = 55$)	qPCR + T2 ($N = 32$)	qPCR + T3 ($N = 29$)	Total number of tests ($N = 116$)
Vagina (vg)	55 (100%)	32 (100%)	28 (96.6%)	115 (99.1%)
Fornix (fx)	52 (97.5%)	30 (93.8%)	27 (93.1%)	109 (94.0%)
Cervical 1 (cx1)	47 (85.5%)	30 (88.2%)	27 (93.1%)	104 (89.7%)
Cervical 2 (cx2)	44 (80.0%)	27 (84.4%)	26 (87.7%)	97 (83.6%)

Among the 51 women positive for *U. parvum*, 43 were positive at all locations, two were positive only in the vagina, four were positive in the vagina and the fornix (but negative for both cervical samples), and two had discordant results in the cervix. There was a statistically significant lower mean bacterial load (5.08 log copies/mL (95% CI: 4.58–5.59)) in the group of eight women not positive for all locations, in comparison with the mean bacterial load of the 43 women for whom all four samples were positive (5.95 log copies/mL (95% CI: 5.70–6.20)) ($P = 0.008$).

Among the eight women positive for *U. urealyticum*, one was positive only in the vagina and three had discordant results in the cervix; the other four were positive in all locations. The same trend for a lower *U. urealyticum* load in the vagina was noticed in the four women with discordant results (as observed for *U. parvum*) but the difference did not

reach the statistical significance probably due to the small groups (4.58 log copies/mL (3.87–5.30) versus 5.43 (4.08–6.79)), $P = 0.32$.

Among the 55 women who showed +qPCR in the first trimester, 44 were retested later in pregnancy, either in the second trimester (15 women) or during the third trimester (10 women) or during both second and third trimesters (19 women). Among all these positive women, only one woman with an uneventful pregnancy showed discordant qualitative tests results during her pregnancy. This patient had a +qPCR at T1 and T2 (with mean log-transformed values that were not statistically different from those of the other patients) but negative qPCR at T3, with no history of antibiotic treatment in the meantime.

The distribution of the positive samples according to the sample location and the sampling timepoint during pregnancy is detailed in Table 1.

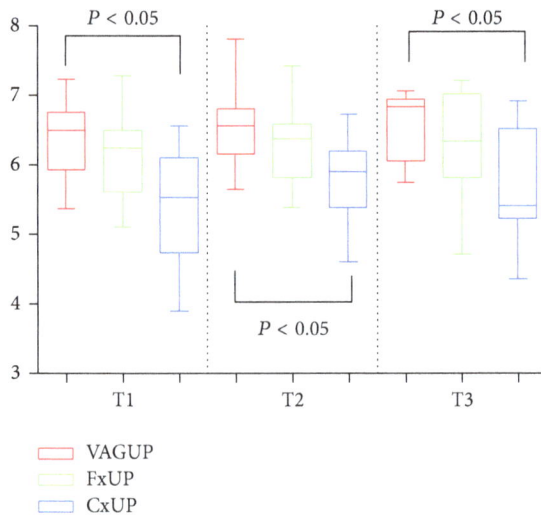

FIGURE 2: Mean log values (with 95% CI) of *U. parvum* (UP) during pregnancy for the three sample sites. VAG UP: vaginal *Ureaplasma parvum*. Fx UP: fornix *Ureaplasma parvum*. Cx UP: cervical *Ureaplasma parvum*. T1: first trimester. T2: second trimester. T3: third trimester.

TABLE 2: Qualitative reproducibility during first trimester.

	κ coefficient
vg/fx	0.95
vg/cx1	0.87
vg/cx2	0.84
fx/cx1	0.87
fx/cx2	0.83
cx1/cx2	0.93

vg: vaginal; fx: fornix; cx: cervical.

The qualitative analysis of the qPCR results with comparison between locations using Cohen's kappa coefficients (κ) revealed high agreement, with κ values between 0.83 and 0.95 (Table 2). The results for vaginal and fornix samples showed the highest agreement.

Eighty-four positive repetitive cervical samplings (T1: $n = 42$; T2: $n = 25$; T3: $n = 17$) were used to test the quantitative agreement between the two cervical sampling locations. The ICC value was 0.86 (95% CI: 0.73–0.92) which should be considered to show good agreement, according to the literature [13].

The evolution of the quantitative qPCR results during pregnancy is summarized in Figure 2 using mean log-transformed values for each sampling site for *U. parvum* at T1, T2, and T3. This analysis was not done for *U. urealyticum* because there were too few positive results.

For each trimester, the mean number of DNA copies for *U. parvum* was highest for vaginal sampling; the lowest numbers were observed for cervical sampling. The fornix burden showed intermediate results. This statistically significant trend was still observed after exclusion of women with negative qPCR results in the cervix, confirming the lower values for cervical microbial load. A trend was observed, showing increasing log-transformed values for *U. parvum* with time during pregnancy. This was seen for all sample locations but did not reach statistical significance.

4. Discussion

Colonization with *Ureaplasma* spp. was found in 43.3% of the women. Colonization with *U. parvum* was far more frequent than with *U. urealyticum* (40.2% versus 6.3%) and this correlates very well with previous studies [12, 14, 15]. Using a different methodology, Knox and Timms concluded that *Ureaplasma* spp. (formerly named *Ureaplasma urealyticum* subdivided into different serovars) were often persistent colonizers of the lower genital tract from mid-pregnancy until the third trimester of pregnancy [11]. Our study, using a more recently developed qPCR technique, confirms this and gives more information about the constancy and the density of *Ureaplasma* spp. in genital secretions from an early gestational age to the end of pregnancy and at different sampling sites.

In our study, positivity as well as negativity for *Ureaplasma* spp. carriage was almost constant during pregnancy, without any intervention. All negative women remained negative throughout the pregnancy, and 98% of the women with a +qPCR result in the first trimester were confirmed with positive samples at T2 and/or T3. These findings are essential for clinicians, because it implies that, in order to study the pathogenicity of *Ureaplasma* spp. during pregnancy, there is no need to use a standardized screening timepoint at a certain gestational age. Therefore one can presume that patients who are positive at a certain time during pregnancy were or will be positive throughout the current pregnancy in the absence of antibiotic intake. Our study was underpowered to be able to analyze outcomes like preterm birth or neonatal complications but to avoid bias we have only tested low-risk pregnant women.

The real-time qPCR for *Ureaplasma* spp. demonstrated excellent qualitative agreement whatever the site of sampling (κ values between 0.81 and 0.95). Nevertheless the probability of a positive qPCR result is significantly greater for a vaginal sample when compared with other sampling sites. This particular trend was observed during all three trimesters for *U. parvum* and at least during the first trimester for *U. urealyticum*. A group of eight women (14.5%) had a positive vaginal qPCR result but negative cervical qPCR. Analyzing the bacterial load in these discordant samples, we found a lower mean vaginal bacterial load when compared with women with positivity at all locations. Remarkably, among the 4/8 women retested later (T2 and/or T3), 3/4 showed the same profile: +qPCR in the vagina and fornix, but still negative in the cervix. We can conclude that the vaginal burden has an impact on the colonization of the cervix: the higher the vaginal bacterial load, the higher the risk of positive cervical colonization. The vaginal colonization should be considered as a "reservoir" allowing secondary colonization of the cervix and further ascending infection in function of different local conditions like change of pH during pregnancy or decline in maternal immunity.

Quantitative analysis of *Ureaplasma* spp. colonization performed at T1, T2, and T3 did not identify significant patterns of variation: the observed trend for augmentation during pregnancy remained lower than 1 log for *U. parvum*. The small number of positive cases for *U. urealyticum* prevented any definitive conclusions for this species.

Overall, the colonization by *U. parvum* was quantitatively greater in the vagina than in cervical samples (Figure 2). These differences reached 1 log (or were very close to 1 log) in almost all the cases, and this may explain why in some cases the qPCR was positive in the vagina and negative in the cervix. These challenging findings may have clinical implications, especially if we wish to optimize the identification of pregnant women with a high risk of late miscarriage or preterm labor using this qPCR technique.

Therefore, several questions deserve to be asked: Do we need to sample the vagina, the cervix, or both? How should we interpret a positive vaginal sample associated with a negative cervical one? The fact that the cervix is not colonized despite a positive vaginal sample could reflect a better immune response with a decreased associated risk of adverse outcomes due to *Ureaplasma* colonization. This is an interesting hypothesis to be tested using a population of pregnant women with negative cervical qPCR combined with a positive vaginal sample. Our study was not powered to answer this clinical question, but we intend to develop a new experimental design based on these findings. Depending on these future results, two screening options could be assessed: a vaginal screening method (easier, no speculum needed) recruiting more positive women and a cervical screening procedure, technically more difficult to perform but recruiting patients at potentially higher risk.

We believe that screening for *Ureaplasma* during pregnancy combined with species identification and quantification should be a new direction of investigation to better understand preterm labor process. Our study has demonstrated that the sampling is easy to perform and is highly reliable and reproducible. The combination of effective screening with an efficient intervention may open new perspectives for prevention of pregnancy complications, including preterm birth.

Additional Points

Condensation. Effect of genital sampling site on *Ureaplasma* spp. qPCR results.

Competing Interests

All authors declare no competing interests (financial or personal) in this article.

References

[1] R. L. Goldenberg, J. F. Culhane, J. D. Iams, and R. Romero, "Epidemiology and causes of preterm birth," *The Lancet*, vol. 371, no. 9606, pp. 75–84, 2008.

[2] J. D. Iams, R. Romero, J. F. Culhane, and R. L. Goldenberg, "Primary, secondary, and tertiary interventions to reduce the morbidity and mortality of preterm birth," *The Lancet*, vol. 371, no. 9607, pp. 164–175, 2008.

[3] R. L. Goldenberg, J. D. Iams, B. M. Mercer et al., "The preterm prediction study: the value of new vs standard risk factors in predicting early and all spontaneous preterm births," *American Journal of Public Health*, vol. 88, no. 2, pp. 233–238, 1998.

[4] P. J. Meis, R. L. Goldenberg, B. Mercer et al., "The preterm prediction study: significance of vaginal infections," *American Journal of Obstetrics and Gynecology*, vol. 173, no. 4, pp. 1231–1235, 1995.

[5] M. Abele-Horn, M. Scholz, C. Wolff, and M. Kolben, "High-density vaginal *Ureaplasma urealyticum* colonization as a risk factor for chorioamnionitis and preterm delivery," *Acta Obstetricia et Gynecologica Scandinavica*, vol. 79, no. 11, pp. 973–978, 2000.

[6] J. Kikhney, D. von Schöning, I. Steding et al., "Is *Ureaplasma* spp. the leading causative agent of acute chorioamnionitis in women with preterm birth?" *Clinical Microbiology and Infection*, 2016.

[7] L. Feng, C. E. Ransom, M. K. Nazzal et al., "The role of progesterone and a novel progesterone receptor, progesterone receptor membrane component 1, in the inflammatory response of fetal membranes to ureaplasma parvum infection," *PLOS ONE*, vol. 11, no. 12, Article ID e0168102, 2016.

[8] C. V. Lal, X. Xu, P. Jackson et al., "Ureaplasma infection-mediated release of matrix metalloproteinase-9 and PGP: a novel mechanism of preterm rupture of membranes and chorioamnionitis," *Pediatric Research*, vol. 81, no. 1, pp. 75–79, 2016.

[9] R. M. Viscardi, "*Ureaplasma* species: role in diseases of prematurity," *Clinics in Perinatology*, vol. 37, no. 2, pp. 393–409, 2010.

[10] T. K. Kim, S. M. Thomas, M. Ho et al., "Heterogeneity of vaginal microbial communities within individuals," *Journal of Clinical Microbiology*, vol. 47, no. 4, pp. 1181–1189, 2009.

[11] C. L. Knox and P. Timms, "Comparison of PCR, nested PCR, and random amplified polymorphic DNA PCR for detection and typing of *Ureaplasma urealyticum* in specimens from pregnant women," *Journal of Clinical Microbiology*, vol. 36, no. 10, pp. 3032–3039, 1998.

[12] E. Vancutsem, O. Soetens, M. Breugelmans, W. Foulon, and A. Naessens, "Modified real-time PCR for detecting, differentiating, and quantifying *Ureaplasma urealyticum* and *Ureaplasma parvum*," *Journal of Molecular Diagnostics*, vol. 13, no. 2, pp. 206–212, 2011.

[13] P. M. Bernard and C. Lapointe, "Mesures composées," in *Mesures Statistiques en Épidémiologie*, P. M. Bernard and C. Lapointe, Eds., pp. 131–143, Presse Universitaire du Québec, Quebec City, Canada, 1st edition, 1991.

[14] F. Kong, Z. Ma, G. James, S. Gordon, and G. L. Gilbert, "Species identification and subtyping of *Ureaplasma parvum* and *Ureaplasma urealyticum* using PCR-based assays," *Journal of Clinical Microbiology*, vol. 38, no. 3, pp. 1175–1179, 2000.

[15] M. Marovt, D. Keše, T. Kotar et al., "*Ureaplasma parvum* and *Ureaplasma urealyticum* detected with the same frequency among women with and without symptoms of urogenital tract infection," *European Journal of Clinical Microbiology and Infectious Diseases*, vol. 34, no. 6, pp. 1237–1245, 2015.

23

Risk of Adverse Infant Outcomes Associated with Maternal Tuberculosis in a Low Burden Setting: A Population-Based Retrospective Cohort Study

Sylvia M. LaCourse,[1] Sharon A. Greene,[2]
Elizabeth E. Dawson-Hahn,[3] and Stephen E. Hawes[2]

[1]*Department of Medicine, Division of Allergy and Infectious Diseases, University of Washington, Seattle, WA 98104, USA*
[2]*Department of Epidemiology, University of Washington, Seattle, WA 98195, USA*
[3]*Department of Pediatrics, University of Washington, Seattle, WA 98121, USA*

Correspondence should be addressed to Sylvia M. LaCourse; sylvial2@uw.edu

Academic Editor: Faustino R. Perez-Lopez

Background. Maternal tuberculosis (TB) may be associated with increased risk of adverse infant outcomes. *Study Design.* We examined the risk of low birth weight (LBW), small for gestational age (SGA), and preterm birth (<37 weeks) associated with maternal TB in a retrospective population-based Washington State cohort using linked infant birth certificate and maternal delivery hospitalization discharge records. We identified 134 women with births between 1987 and 2012 with TB-associated ICD-9 diagnosis codes at hospital delivery discharge and 536 randomly selected women without TB, frequency matched 4 : 1 on delivery year. Multinomial logistic regression analyses were performed to compare the risk of LBW, SGA, and preterm birth between infants born to mothers with and without TB. *Results.* Infants born to women with TB were 3.74 (aRR 95% CI 1.40–10.00) times as likely to be LBW and 1.96 (aRR 95% CI 0.91–4.22) as likely to be SGA compared to infants born to mothers without TB. Risk of prematurity was similar (aRR 1.01 95% CI 0.39–2.58). *Conclusion.* Maternal TB is associated with poor infant outcomes even in a low burden setting. A better understanding of the adverse infant outcomes associated with maternal TB, reflecting recent trends in US TB epidemiology, may inform potential targeted interventions in other low prevalence settings.

1. Introduction

Globally, tuberculosis (TB) is one of leading infectious causes of morbidity and mortality among women of childbearing age [1, 2]. Despite decreasing incidence of TB in the US since the 1990s, TB continues to disproportionately affect specific populations including immigrants [3]. In Washington State, the incidence of TB is similar to the US national average of 3.0 per 100,000; however, the proportion of TB cases occurring among foreign-born residents is greater (72.8% in Washington versus 60.0% in the US) [3, 4]. In 2013, women accounted for 41% of incident TB in Washington [4].

Pregnant and postpartum women may be at increased risk for TB potentially due to the physiologic, hormonal, and immunologic changes associated with pregnancy [5–7].

Additionally, pregnant women may not present with typical symptoms, which may delay diagnosis and lead to poor maternal outcomes [7–12]. Recent modelling estimates suggest that more than 200,000 TB cases occurred among pregnant women worldwide in 2011 [13]. Data regarding infant outcomes associated with maternal TB is conflicting, with some reporting increased adverse outcomes, intrauterine growth retardation, prematurity, small for gestational age, low birth weight, and death [14–19], while others show no increase in adverse outcomes [20].

The majority of studies evaluating adverse infant outcomes associated with maternal TB are case control studies within single facilities or small groups of hospitals, with very few population-based estimates conducted in low prevalence settings [10, 14, 18, 21–23]. A better understanding of

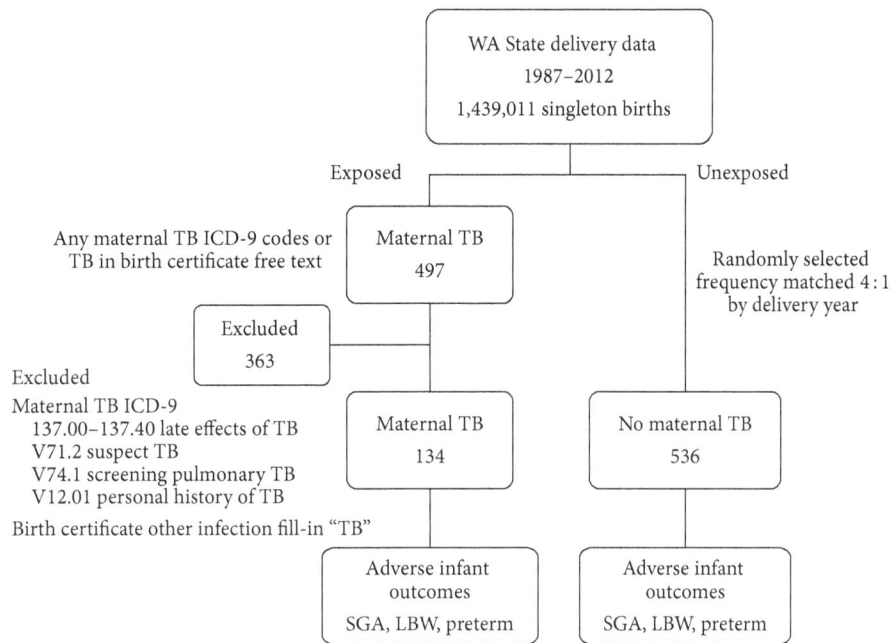

FIGURE 1: Study flow.

the adverse infant outcomes associated with maternal TB reflecting recent trends in US TB epidemiology may inform potential targeted interventions in the US and other low prevalence settings. We conducted a population-based, retrospective cohort study to estimate the risk of low birth weight (LBW), small for gestational age (SGA), and prematurity among infants born to women with TB-associated hospital delivery discharge diagnoses in Washington State.

2. Materials and Methods

Women with singleton births in Washington State from 1987 to 2012 and their infants were identified using the Birth Events Records Database (BERD). The BERD database links more than 95% of Washington State birth certificate data to maternal and infant delivery hospitalization data from the statewide Comprehensive Hospital Abstract Reporting System (CHARS), including hospital discharge diagnosis codes by the International Classification of Diseases ninth revision (ICD-9) [24].

We initially identified all women delivering in Washington State between 1987 and 2012 with any TB-associated delivery diagnosis (ICD-9 codes 10.0–18.96, 647.30–647.34, V71.2, V74.1, and V12.01) or with TB noted on the birth certificate under "maternal infection other," an open-ended data element on the birth certificate (Figure 1). We then excluded women with diagnoses that likely reflected a history of TB (as opposed to current TB), as well as TB suspect/screening (ICD-9 codes V71.2, V74.1, and V12.01), since we were specifically interested in the relationship between active maternal TB during pregnancy and delivery and its relationship to neonatal outcomes. Additionally, we excluded women identified through the open-ended "maternal infection other" on the birth certificate, as we were unable to discern whether

it indicated the mother had latent TB infection or active TB from this data source. After these exclusions, there were 134 women in the final exposed maternal TB cohort (Figure 1). Supplemental Table 1 in Supplementary Material available online at http://dx.doi.org/10.1155/2016/6413713 shows the distribution of TB diagnoses identified from ICD-9 codes. The unexposed cohort was comprised of 536 randomly selected women without TB-associated diagnoses who delivered in Washington, frequency matched (4:1) on year of delivery (Figure 1).

The primary neonatal outcomes of SGA (weight < 10th percentile for age), LBW (<2,500 grams), and preterm birth (<37 weeks) were identified from information recorded on the birth certificate. Gestational age was coded as a composite variable using clinical estimate of gestational age or estimated using the last menstrual period (LMP) if the clinical estimate was missing. Weight for gestational age categories were derived from a population-based reference for Washington State [25]. We also evaluated secondary outcomes of infant mortality and congenital/infant TB from both birth and readmission data within the first two years of life from the BERD and CHARS databases.

Factors identified *a priori* as potential confounders in the relationship between maternal TB and poor neonatal outcomes included maternal age, education, race/ethnicity, parity, prenatal smoking, gestational diabetes, income (USD based on median census tract income), marital status, prenatal care (using the Adequacy of Prenatal Care Utilization index which classifies prenatal care based on date prenatal care was initiated and number of prenatal visits [26]), and maternal country of origin (grouped by World Bank gross national income index categories [27]). Maternal body mass index (BMI) was not available on the birth certificate before 2003. Weight gain during pregnancy was recorded on birth

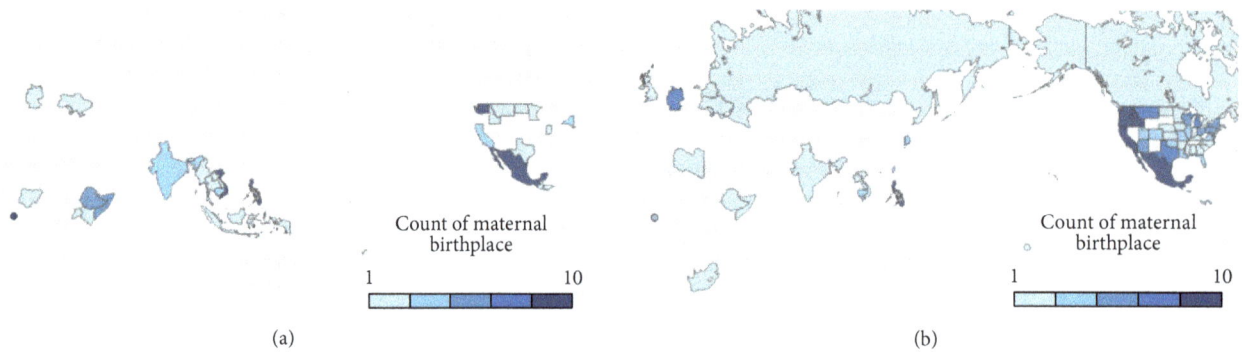

FIGURE 2: (a) Distribution of maternal birthplace for women with TB diagnosis. (b) Distribution of maternal birthplace for women without TB diagnosis.

certificates beginning in 1988; however, prepregnancy weight was only available after 1992.

2.1. Statistical Analysis. We performed simple descriptive analyses comparing the frequency and distribution of the identified potential confounders between the exposure groups. Unadjusted risk estimates (uRR) for SGA, LBW, and preterm birth were compared between mothers with and without TB using multinomial logistic regression with the risk estimate converted to relative risk ratios (using mlogit, rrr command in STATA). Given our limited sample size and the high proportion of missing data for some factors, only potential confounders that changed the relative risk of our prespecified adverse infant outcomes by more than 10%, with less than <10% missing data, were included in our final multinomial logistic regression model. Adjusted relative risks (aRR) were calculated using multinomial logistic regression models adjusted for maternal age and income as continuous variables and parity and maternal country of origin as categorical variables with risk estimates converted to relative risk ratios. Relative risk estimates were reported with 95% confidence intervals (CI) and significance level was an alpha of 0.05. STATA (StataCorp, version 12, College Station, TX, USA) was used for all statistical analysis.

3. Results

Women with delivery hospitalization discharge TB-associated diagnosis were generally similar to the unexposed group with regard to maternal age and BMI (Table 1). Women with TB were less likely to be white (20.5 versus 79.4%), to graduate from high school (40.7 versus 82.9%), or to smoke during pregnancy (6.4 versus 15.8%), compared to women without TB. A larger proportion of women with TB were foreign-born (78.4 versus 16.8%), lived in urban areas (80.7 versus 74.7%), were single (36.6 versus 28.8%), had 2 or more previous pregnancies (35.1 versus 22.9%), and had gestational diabetes (6.0 versus 3.7%). Median census tract income among women with TB was lower than those without TB. Women with TB were more likely to have had either inadequate prenatal care (attending < 80% of the generally recommended number of prenatal visits) or were more likely

to have experienced pregnancies with more intensive prenatal care visitation schedules (≥110%) than women without TB, who were most likely to have had the recommended prenatal care utilization. Among the 105 foreign-born women with TB, the majority were from Mexico (36.6%), followed by the Philippines (6.7%) and Vietnam (6.7%) (Figure 2).

Table 2 shows the unadjusted relative risks (uRR) for maternal TB exposure and adverse infant outcomes. Infants born to women with TB diagnosis at delivery were 2.64 times more likely to be LBW compared to infants born to women without TB (95% CI: 1.34–5.20). Similarly, infants born to women with TB were 1.95 times more likely to be SGA (95% CI: 1.11–3.41). Infants born to mothers with maternal TB had similar risk of preterm birth compared to those born to mothers without TB (RR 1.74, 95% CI: 0.89–3.43). After adjusting for maternal age, income, parity, and maternal country of origin, the risk of LBW remained increased (aRR 3.74 95% CI 1.40–10.00) for infants born to women with TB compared to those without TB. The risk of SGA remained similarly elevated (aRR 1.96 95% CI: 0.91–4.22) but no longer statistically significant. The risk of prematurity was attenuated but remained similar between infants born to women with and without TB (aRR 1.01 95% CI 0.39–2.58).

One infant born to a mother in our exposed cohort had a TB-associated diagnosis on readmission data within the first 24 months following birth; there were none in the unexposed cohort (data not shown). Two children in the exposed cohort and none in the unexposed cohort had an ICD-9 diagnosis code of "other congenital infections specific to the perinatal period" at their delivery admission or one of their readmissions during the first 24 months of life. This ICD-9 code includes TB, herpes simplex virus, listeriosis, malaria, and toxoplasmosis diagnoses. There was one fetal death reported in both the exposed and unexposed cohorts.

4. Discussion

In this population-based retrospective cohort study we found that maternal TB, as identified by maternal delivery discharge diagnosis ICD-9 codes, was significantly associated with low birth weight, with a trend toward an association with small

TABLE 1: Characteristics of women with and without tuberculosis-associated ICD-9 diagnosis during delivery hospitalization, Washington State, 1987–2012.

Maternal characteristic	% Missing	Maternal TB (N = 134) n^* (%)	No maternal TB (N = 536) n^* (%)
Age (years)	0		
<20		14 (10.5)	54 (10.1)
20–29		80 (59.7)	294 (54.9)
≥30		40 (29.9)	188 (35.1)
Median age (IQR)		26 (22–31)	27 (23–32)
Ethnicity	2.2		
White		27 (20.5)	415 (79.4)
Black		14 (10.6)	13 (2.5)
Asian		33 (25.0)	28 (5.4)
Hispanic		52 (39.4)	47 (9.0)
Native American		6 (4.6)	18 (3.4)
Other non-white		0 (0)	2 (0.4)
Education	34.8		
<High school graduate		51 (59.3)	60 (17.1)
High school graduate		35 (40.7)	291 (82.9)
Median year of education (IQR)		10 (9–12)	13 (12–16)
Urban residence§	10.3	96 (80.7)	360 (74.7)
Income (dollars)‡	8.1		
<35,000		63 (52.5)	209 (42.1)
35,000–49,999		48 (40.0)	174 (35.1)
≥50,000		9 (7.5)	113 (22.8)
Median income (in thousands) (IQR)		34 (26–40)	37 (31–48)
Single marital status	0.2	49 (36.6)	154 (28.8)
Foreign born	0	105 (78.4)	90 (16.8)
Maternal country of origin¶	1.5		
Low-income		53 (40.5)	235 (44.4)
Middle-income		32 (24.4)	173 (32.7)
High-income		46 (35.1)	121 (22.9)
Parity	1.5		
0		53 (40.5)	235 (44.4)
1		32 (24.4)	173 (32.7)
≥2		46 (35.1)	121 (22.9)
Prenatal care utilization†	11.2		
<80% PNC visits		53 (46.9)	157 (32.6)
80–109% PNC visits		36 (31.9)	248 (51.5)
≥110% PNC visits		24 (21.2)	77 (16.0)
Body mass index (BMI)#	72.5		
BMI < 18.5 underweight		0 (0)	4 (2.6)
BMI 18.5–24.9 normal		18 (56.3)	76 (50.0)
BMI 25.0–29.9 overweight		8 (25.0)	38 (25.0)
BMI ≥ 30.0 obese class I–III		6 (18.8)	34 (22.4)
Median BMI (IQR)		23.6 (20.7–27.9)	24.8 (22.2–29.4)
Weight gain in pregnancy (lbs)**	28.7		
Loss or no gain		0 (0)	2 (0.5)
1–9.9		6 (6.7)	12 (3.1)
10–19.9		17 (18.9)	40 (10.3)
20–39.9		48 (53.3)	205 (52.8)
>40		19 (21.1)	129 (33.3)
Median pregnancy weight gain (IQR)		26 (19–37)	33 (25–40)

Table 1: Continued.

Maternal characteristic	% Missing	Maternal TB ($N = 134$) n^* (%)	No maternal TB ($N = 536$) n^* (%)
Gestational diabetes	0	8 (6.0)	20 (3.7)
Smoked during pregnancy	5.5	8 (6.4)	80 (15.8)

*Numbers may not add up to totals because of missing data.
§Estimated by linking birth certificates to census tract records from U.S. Census Bureau 2000.
‡Estimated by linking birth certificates to census tract records from U.S. Census Bureau 2000, median income per census tract.
¶Per World Bank gross national income index classifications. Lower-middle and upper-middle income countries are categorized together as middle-income.
†Kotelchuck index classifies prenatal care based on birth certificate data on date prenatal care was initiated and number of prenatal visits.
$^#$BMI was not available on the birth certificate before 2003.
**Weight gain during pregnancy was recorded on birth certificates from 1988 on, however pre-pregnancy weight was only available after 1992.

Table 2: Risk of small for gestational age, low birth weight, and prematurity for infants born to women with tuberculosis-associated ICD-9 diagnosis during delivery hospitalization, Washington State, 1987–2012.

Outcome	Maternal TB ($N = 134$) n (%)	No maternal TB ($N = 536$) n (%)	Unadjusted RR uRR	(95% CI)	Adjusted RR§ aRR	(95% CI)
Birth weight (grams)						
LBW (<2,500)	15 (11.9)	24 (4.5)	**2.64**	(1.34–5.20)	**3.74**	(1.40–10.00)
Typical (2,500–3,999)	105 (78.4)	443 (82.7)	1.00	Referent	1.00	Referent
Macrosomia (≥4,000)	14 (10.5)	69 (12.9)	0.86	(0.46–1.58)	1.39	(0.59–3.30)
Weight for gestational age*						
SGA (<10%)	21 (15.8)	47 (8.9)	**1.95**	(1.11–3.41)	1.96	(0.91–4.22)
Typical (10–90%)	100 (75.2)	436 (82.4)	1.00	Referent	1.00	Referent
LGA (>90%)	12 (9.0)	46 (8.7)	1.13	(0.58–2.23)	1.69	(0.63–4.55)
Gestational age (weeks)*						
<37 (preterm)	13 (9.8)	32 (6.0)	1.74	(0.89–3.43)	1.01	(0.39–2.58)
37–41	112 (84.9)	481 (90.9)	1.00	Referent	1.00	Referent
≥42 (postterm)	7 (5.3)	16 (3.0)	1.91	(0.54–6.74)	1.91	(0.53–6.75)

*Numbers may not add up to totals due to missing data.
§Model adjusted for maternal age, income, parity, and maternal country of origin World Bank gross national income index category.

for gestational age, but not prematurity, in a low TB-burden setting.

Our findings are similar to prior longitudinal studies of maternal TB and adverse infant outcomes. In a retrospective cohort study evaluating infant outcomes associated with TB in pregnancy in Taiwan (a high TB burden setting), Lin et al. reported that infants born to mothers with TB were 1.35 (95% CI: 1.01–1.81) times as likely to be LBW and 1.22 (95% CI: 1.00–1.49) times as likely to be SGA compared to infants born to mothers without TB [17]. Similar to the current study, no association was found with prematurity (RR 0.97, 95% CI: 0.72–1.30). Lower mean birth weights and increased risk of LBW among infants born to mothers with TB compared to those born to others without TB have been reported in a retrospective single-hospital based cohort study in Mexico (mean birth weight 2,859 versus 3,099 grams; RR of LBW 2.2 (95% CI 1.1–4.9)) [16]. Similarly, a small case control study in three inner-city hospitals in the UK found that 24 infants born to women with TB had a mean birth weight of 2,735 grams, which was significantly lower than the mean weight of 3,135 grams ($p = 0.03$) of infants of mothers without TB

[18]. Finally, in an obstetric specialty clinic in India, infants born to women with TB were 2.1 times as likely to be born LBW (95% CI: 1.4–3.1) and 2.6 times as likely to be born SGA (95% CI: 1.4–4.6) [19].

We identified very few cases of infant TB in our study. Although we do not have specific maternal TB diagnosis and treatment information, it is likely that, in Washington State, once the diagnosis of maternal TB is made, the mother would have been initiated on therapy, significantly decreasing the risk of transmission of TB to the infant. Conversely, an infant TB diagnosis may have been made in the outpatient setting which would not have been captured by the inpatient diagnoses codes unless the infant was hospitalized. However, in our setting, gastric aspirates (one of the more common means for making infant TB diagnosis) often require hospitalization. Without medical record confirmation, it is difficult to assess congenital TB since the ICD-9 code used to identify congenital TB is used for a multitude of congenital infections in the perinatal period including TB, herpes simplex, listeriosis, and toxoplasmosis (however, in our study only two children were identified with this composite code).

The few prevalence estimates of TB in pregnancy in low burden settings vary widely and are primarily facility or hospital based [7, 10, 14, 18, 21–23]. Maternal TB is thought to be uncommon in the US; however, pregnancy status is not routinely collected or reported for either state or national TB estimates, and there is a gap in the literature for population-based studies of the risks of adverse neonatal outcomes in low TB prevalence settings. Our study is the first population-based study to our knowledge that evaluates the risk of adverse infant outcomes associated with maternal TB reflecting recent US TB epidemiologic trends while accounting for maternal country of origin. This investigation contributes to the understanding that adverse infant outcomes may be associated with maternal TB even in a low burden setting and can be used to inform targeted interventions in Washington, in the US, or in other low prevalence settings.

In the present study, TB in pregnancy is higher among women born outside of the United States and among women with lower educational attainment and income. Clinicians should be aware of at risk populations and the importance of diagnosing and treating TB during pregnancy. The US Centers for Disease Control and Prevention recommends that TB treatment should be initiated during pregnancy because the risk of untreated TB is a greater hazard for both the mother and infant [28]. Although we do not know the TB screening status of the patients in this study, pregnancy has been associated with missed opportunities for TB prevention [7, 29]. Universal screening of high risk obstetric patients for latent TB could identify a high proportion of women who are eligible for latent TB therapy [30]. Cost-effectiveness modelling estimates antenatal provision of isoniazid preventive therapy is potentially less costly with reduced maternal TB-associated case-fatality compared to postnatal TB prevention strategies [31]. Our findings reinforce the need for intrapartum support of mothers diagnosed with TB and sustained public health surveillance of maternal TB to minimize the likelihood of delivering LBW and potentially SGA infants.

Strengths of our study include using a large population-based cohort spanning 25 years. Utilizing an electronic repository of maternally linked birth outcome data allowed us to estimate the risk of adverse infant outcomes associated with maternal TB diagnosis. Given that the TB incidence in Washington State is similar to the US incidence in general, Washington State risk estimates of neonatal outcomes may also reflect current US TB epidemiology and aid in the characterization of poor infant outcomes associated with maternal TB in low burden settings.

There were some limitations with our approach. Ascertainment of both our exposure (maternal TB) and outcomes of interest (SGA, LBW, and prematurity) were based on data from the Washington State Birth Events Records Database (BERD) and Comprehensive Hospital Abstract Reporting System (CHARS). As with any large public database system, there may be issues with either misreporting or miscoding of information. In an evaluation of Washington State birth certificate and hospital discharge data, there was substantial underreporting of maternal conditional and pregnancy complications on birth certificates; however, hospital discharge data was found to be more accurate [32]. The combination of birth certificate and hospital discharge data, in the linked BERD and CHARS database, yields higher "true positives" than either data source alone [32]. The number of women in Washington with a TB diagnosis recorded on hospital discharge records was low; we cannot exclude the possibility of underdiagnosis or underreporting of maternal TB. Additionally, women are not routinely tested for TB during prenatal care visits and a woman who is asymptomatic or has atypical symptoms for TB may not be diagnosed [33]. There is no specific data element on the birth certificate for TB; rather we are relying on clinicians to report TB diagnosis in the hospital discharge records. The clinician may be unaware of the mother's TB status or may choose not to report TB on a discharge record for delivery. Our study is also limited by the lack of specific clinical information regarding date or method of TB diagnosis, as well as treatment. The risk of developing TB is higher among people living with HIV [34]. Washington birth certificate captures information on maternal HIV infection; but this sensitive data was not available for analysis. However, in Washington, the prevalence of HIV among new TB patients is low at 2.6% [35]. Therefore, we do not anticipate our lack of HIV data to alter our risk estimates.

In our cohort, the majority of mothers with TB were foreign-born, consistent with trends in both Washington State and the US in general. Despite a significant decrease in TB incidence in the general US population since 1993, the decrease among foreign-born persons has been much smaller, with the case rate among foreign-born persons approximately 13 times higher than among US-born (15.6 versus 1.2 per 100,000) [35]. The increased risk of adverse infant outcomes associated with maternal TB in our study could reflect an increased risk of SGA and prematurity of infants born to foreign-born mothers. In order to address this potential confounder directly, we adjusted our risk estimates of adverse infant outcomes by maternal country of origin (as categorized by World Bank gross national income index). However, residual confounding may remain. Although maternal country of origin may be an important driver of poor infant outcomes, there is a growing body of literature suggesting that infants born to foreign-born mothers may in fact have better birth outcomes compared to ethnically similar US-born mothers [36–40]. In the few comparable studies in the literature (i.e., Taiwan [17] and India [19]) the association between maternal TB and adverse infant outcomes was similar, suggesting that the difference between foreign-born and US-born mothers in our study is less likely to be influencing our results regarding neonatal outcomes.

In the current study, we adjusted for a number of factors, including maternal age, income, parity, and maternal country of origin. Missing data for a number of factors (maternal education, BMI, and weight gain during pregnancy) was substantial, limiting the ability to completely adjust for these factors. Therefore, it is possible that the relationship between maternal TB status and adverse infant outcomes in our study may be due to unmeasured or residual confounding. Future studies using larger population-based estimates may be needed to assess the importance of the factors more fully.

5. Conclusion

Our study found a substantially increased risk of LBW and a nonsignificant trend towards increased risk of SGA among infants born to mothers with TB diagnosis even in a low burden setting, suggesting that maternal TB remains an important risk factor for adverse infant outcomes. This highlights the importance of close clinical follow-up of pregnant women with TB and their infants. Women from high-incidence countries may warrant increased vigilance for latent TB screening and treatment to prevent adverse maternal and infant outcomes associated with maternal TB.

Further research regarding both the risk of TB in pregnancy and the risk of neonatal adverse outcomes associated with maternal TB is warranted, including detailed case ascertainment. Efforts could be aided by the addition of pregnancy status to TB surveillance efforts. A better understanding of mothers at risk for TB and the adverse infant outcomes associated with maternal TB may inform potential targeted interventions in other low prevalence settings.

Ethical Approval

This study was deemed exempt from ethical approval by the Human Research Review Section of the Washington Department of Social and Health Services (exemption E-041014-H, April 11, 2014) as it does not involve human subjects.

Disclosure

Preliminary data was presented at the 18th Annual Conference of the International Union Against Tuberculosis and Lung Disease-North America Region, Vancouver, BC, February 28–March 2, 2015.

Disclaimer

The funding sources had no involvement in study design, data collection, analysis or interpretation of data, writing of the report, or the decision to submit the article for publication.

Conflict of Interests

The authors report no conflict of interests.

Authors' Contribution

All authors (Sylvia M. LaCourse, Sharon A. Greene, Elizabeth E. Dawson-Hahn, and Stephen E. Hawes) contributed to the conception, planning, implementation, analysis, and writing of this work and accept responsibility for the paper as published.

Acknowledgments

This work was supported by the US National Institutes Health (NIH) STD/AIDS Research Training Grant [T32 AI007140 to Sylvia M. LaCourse] and the Ruth L. Kirschstein NRSA Training Award [T32HP10002 to Elizabeth E. Dawson-Hahn]. The authors would like to thank the Washington State Department of Health, for data access, and Mr. Bill O'Brien, Department of Epidemiology, University of Washington, for conducting the data linkages and for programming assistance. They also thank the Kizazi working group (University of Washington Global Center for Integrated Health of Women, Adolescents, and Children (Global WACh)) for their support during the preparation of this paper.

References

[1] J. S. Mathad and A. Gupta, "Tuberculosis in pregnant and postpartum women: epidemiology, management, and research gaps," *Clinical Infectious Diseases*, vol. 55, no. 11, pp. 1532–1549, 2012.

[2] H. Getahun, D. Sculier, C. Sismanidis, M. Grzemska, and M. Raviglione, "Prevention, diagnosis, and treatment of tuberculosis in children and mothers: evidence for action for maternal, neonatal, and child health services," *The Journal of Infectious Diseases*, vol. 205, supplement 2, pp. S216–S227, 2012.

[3] Centers for Disease Control and Prevention, "TB Incidence in the United States, 1953–2013," 2013, http://www.cdc.gov/tb/statistics/tbcases.htm.

[4] Washington State Department of Health, *Tuberculosis: Data and Reports*, Washington State Department of Health, 2014, http://www.doh.wa.gov/YouandYourFamily/IllnessandDisease/Tuberculosis/DataReports.aspx.

[5] N. Singh and J. R. Perfect, "Immune reconstitution syndrome and exacerbation of infections after pregnancy," *Clinical Infectious Diseases*, vol. 45, no. 9, pp. 1192–1199, 2007.

[6] D. Zenner, M. E. Kruijshaar, N. Andrews, and I. Abubakar, "Risk of tuberculosis in pregnancy: a national, primary care-based cohort and self-controlled case series study," *American Journal of Respiratory and Critical Care Medicine*, vol. 185, no. 7, pp. 779–784, 2012.

[7] N. Jana, S. Barik, N. Arora, and A. K. Singh, "Tuberculosis in pregnancy: the challenges for South Asian countries," *Journal of Obstetrics and Gynaecology Research*, vol. 38, no. 9, pp. 1125–1136, 2012.

[8] A. Gupta, A. Chandrasekhar, N. Gupte et al., "Symptom screening among HIV-infected pregnant women is acceptable and has high negative predictive value for active tuberculosis," *Clinical Infectious Diseases*, vol. 53, no. 10, pp. 1015–1018, 2011.

[9] C. J. Hoffmann, E. Variava, M. Rakgokong et al., "High prevalence of pulmonary tuberculosis but low sensitivity of symptom screening among HIV-infected pregnant women in South Africa," *PLoS ONE*, vol. 8, no. 4, Article ID e62211, 2013.

[10] M. Llewelyn, I. Cropley, R. J. Wilkinson, and R. N. Davidson, "Tuberculosis diagnosed during pregnancy: a prospective study from London," *Thorax*, vol. 55, no. 2, pp. 129–132, 2000.

[11] N. Jana, K. Vasishta, S. C. Saha, and K. Ghosh, "Obstetrical outcomes among women with extrapulmonary tuberculosis," *The New England Journal of Medicine*, vol. 341, no. 9, pp. 645–649, 1999.

[12] H. Bishara, M. Lidji, O. Vinitsky, and D. Weiler-Ravell, "Indolent pneumonia in a pregnant recent immigrant from Ethiopia: think TB," *Primary Care Respiratory Journal*, vol. 23, no. 1, pp. 102–105, 2014.

Risk of Adverse Infant Outcomes Associated with Maternal Tuberculosis in a Low Burden Setting...

211

[13] J. Sugarman, C. Colvin, A. C. Moran, and O. Oxlade, "Tuberculosis in pregnancy: an estimate of the global burden of disease," *The Lancet Global Health*, vol. 2, no. 12, pp. e710–e716, 2014.

[14] A. Kothari, N. Mahadevan, and J. Girling, "Tuberculosis and pregnancy—results of a study in a high prevalence area in London," *European Journal of Obstetrics Gynecology and Reproductive Biology*, vol. 126, no. 1, pp. 48–55, 2006.

[15] T. Pillay, M. Khan, J. Moodley, M. Adhikari, and H. Coovadia, "Perinatal tuberculosis and HIV-1: considerations for resource-limited settings," *The Lancet Infectious Diseases*, vol. 4, no. 3, pp. 155–165, 2004.

[16] R. Figueroa-Damian and J. L. Arredondo-Garcia, "Neonatal outcome of children born to women with tuberculosis," *Archives of Medical Research*, vol. 32, no. 1, pp. 66–69, 2001.

[17] H.-C. Lin, H.-C. Lin, and S.-F. Chen, "Increased risk of low birthweight and small for gestational age infants among women with tuberculosis," *BJOG*, vol. 117, no. 5, pp. 585–590, 2010.

[18] B. Asuquo, A. D. Vellore, G. Walters, S. Manney, L. Mignini, and H. Kunst, "A case-control study of the risk of adverse perinatal outcomes due to tuberculosis during pregnancy," *Journal of Obstetrics & Gynaecology*, vol. 32, no. 7, pp. 635–638, 2012.

[19] N. Jana, K. Vasishta, S. K. Jindal, B. Khunnu, and K. Ghosh, "Perinatal outcome in pregnancies complicated by pulmonary tuberculosis," *International Journal of Gynecology and Obstetrics*, vol. 44, no. 2, pp. 119–124, 1994.

[20] S. N. Tripathy and S. N. Tripathy, "Tuberculosis and pregnancy," *International Journal of Gynecology and Obstetrics*, vol. 80, no. 3, pp. 247–253, 2003.

[21] Centers for Disease Control and Prevention, "Tuberculosis among pregnant women—New York city, 1985–1992," *Morbidity and Mortality Weekly Report (MMWR)*, vol. 42, no. 31, pp. 611–612, 1993.

[22] J. T. Good Jr., M. D. Iseman, P. T. Davidson, S. Lakshminarayan, and S. A. Sahn, "Tuberculosis in association with pregnancy," *American Journal of Obstetrics and Gynecology*, vol. 140, no. 5, pp. 492–498, 1981.

[23] N. Schwartz, S. A. Wagner, S. M. Keeler, J. Mierlak, D. E. Seubert, and A. B. Caughey, "Universal tuberculosis screening in pregnancy," *American Journal of Perinatology*, vol. 26, no. 6, pp. 447–451, 2009.

[24] A. A. Herman, B. J. McCarthy, J. M. Bakewell et al., "Data linkage methods used in maternally-linked birth and infant death surveillance data sets from the United States (Georgia, Missouri, Utah and Washington state), Israel, Norway, Scotland and Western Australia," *Paediatric and Perinatal Epidemiology*, vol. 11, supplement 1, pp. 5–22, 1997.

[25] S. Lipsky, T. R. Easterling, V. L. Holt, and C. W. Critchlow, "Detecting small for gestational age infants: the development of a population-based reference for Washington State," *American Journal of Perinatology*, vol. 22, no. 8, pp. 405–412, 2005.

[26] M. Kotelchuck, "An evaluation of the kessner adequacy of prenatal care index and a proposed adequacy of prenatal care utilization index," *American Journal of Public Health*, vol. 84, no. 9, pp. 1414–1420, 1994.

[27] The World Bank Group, *Country and Lending Groups*, 2015, http://data.worldbank.org/about/country-and-lending-groups#High_income.

[28] Centers for Disease Control and Prevention, "Treatment of tuberculosis," *MMWR Recommendations and Reports*, vol. 52, pp. 1–77, 2003.

[29] M. E. Slopen, F. Laraque, A. S. Piatek, and S. D. Ahuja, "Missed opportunities for tuberculosis prevention in New York City, 2003," *Journal of Public Health Management and Practice*, vol. 17, no. 5, pp. 421–426, 2011.

[30] S. Mamishi, B. Pourakbari, M. Teymuri et al., "Diagnostic accuracy of IL-2 for the diagnosis of latent tuberculosis: a systematic review and meta-analysis," *European Journal of Clinical Microbiology and Infectious Diseases*, vol. 33, no. 12, pp. 2111–2119, 2014.

[31] K. A. Boggess, E. R. Myers, and C. D. Hamilton, "Antepartum or postpartum isoniazid treatment of latent tuberculosis infection," *Obstetrics and Gynecology*, vol. 96, no. 5, pp. 757–762, 2000.

[32] M. T. Lydon-Rochelle, V. L. Holt, V. Cárdenas et al., "The reporting of pre-existing maternal medical conditions and complications of pregnancy on birth certificates and in hospital discharge data," *American Journal of Obstetrics & Gynecology*, vol. 193, no. 1, pp. 125–134, 2005.

[33] E. J. Carter and S. Mates, "Tuberculosis during pregnancy: the Rhode Island experience, 1987 to 1991," *Chest*, vol. 106, no. 5, pp. 1466–1470, 1994.

[34] World Health Organization, "Global Tuberculosis Report 2014," 2014, http://www.who.int/tb/publications/global_report/en/.

[35] Centers for Disease Control, *Reported Tuberculosis in the United States, 2014*, 2014, http://www.cdc.gov/tb/statistics/reports/2013/pdf/report2013.pdf.

[36] C. Margerison-Zilko, "The contribution of maternal birth cohort to term small for gestational age in the United States 1989–2010: an age, period, and cohort analysis," *Paediatric and Perinatal Epidemiology*, vol. 28, no. 4, pp. 312–321, 2014.

[37] I. T. Elo, Z. Vang, and J. F. Culhane, "Variation in birth outcomes by mother's country of birth among non-Hispanic black women in the United States," *Maternal and Child Health Journal*, vol. 18, no. 10, pp. 2371–2381, 2014.

[38] T. L. Osypuk, L. M. Bates, and D. Acevedo-Garcia, "Another Mexican birthweight paradox? The role of residential enclaves and neighborhood poverty in the birthweight of Mexican-origin infants," *Social Science and Medicine*, vol. 70, no. 4, pp. 550–560, 2010.

[39] G. K. Singh and M. Y. Stella, "Adverse pregnancy outcomes: differences between US- and foreign-born women in major US racial and ethnic groups," *American Journal of Public Health*, vol. 86, no. 6, pp. 837–843, 1996.

[40] C. Qin and J. B. Gould, "Maternal nativity status and birth outcomes in Asian immigrants," *Journal of Immigrant and Minority Health*, vol. 12, no. 5, pp. 798–805, 2010.

Permissions

List of Contributors

Beryne Odeny
Department of Global Health, University of Washington, Seattle, WA 98104, USA

Jillian Pintye
Department of Global Health, University of Washington, Seattle, WA 98104, USA
Department of Nursing, University of Washington, Seattle, WA 98195, USA

Agnes Langat, Abraham Katana and Lucy Nganga
United States Centers for Disease Control and Prevention (CDC), Nairobi 00202, Kenya

Benson Singa
Center for Microbiology Research and Center for Clinical Research, Kenya Medical Research Institute, Nairobi 00202, Kenya

John Kinuthia
Department of Global Health, University of Washington, Seattle, WA 98104, USA
Department of Obstetrics & Gynecology, Kenyatta National Hospital, Nairobi 00202, Kenya

Grace John-Stewart
Department of Global Health, University of Washington, Seattle, WA 98104, USA
Department of Medicine, University of Washington, Seattle, WA 98195, USA
Department of Epidemiology, University of Washington, Seattle, WA 98195, USA

Christine J. McGrath
Department of Global Health, University of Washington, Seattle, WA 98104, USA
University of Texas Medical Branch, Galveston, TX 77555, USA

Huma Farid
Department of Obstetrics and Gynecology, Beth Israel Deaconess Medical Center, Boston, MA 02215, USA
Department of Obstetrics, Gynecology and Reproductive Biology, Harvard Medical School, Boston, MA 02115, USA

Trevin C. Lau
Department of Obstetrics, Gynecology and Reproductive Biology, Harvard Medical School, Boston, MA 02115, USA
Vincent Department of Obstetrics and Gynecology, Massachusetts General Hospital, Boston, MA 02114, USA

Anatte E. Karmon and Aaron K. Styer
Department of Obstetrics, Gynecology and Reproductive Biology, Harvard Medical School, Boston, MA 02115, USA
Vincent Department of Obstetrics and Gynecology, Massachusetts General Hospital, Boston, MA 02114, USA
Vincent Reproductive Medicine and IVF, Massachusetts General Hospital, Boston, MA 02114, USA

Matthew K. Hoffman
Department of Obstetrics & Gynecology, Christiana Care Health System, Newark, DE, USA

Mrutyunjaya B. Bellad, Umesh S. Charantimath, Avinash Kavi, Jyoti M. Nagmoti, Mahantesh B. Nagmoti, Shivaprasad S. Goudar Amit P. Revankar and M. S. Ganachari
KLE University Jawaharlal Nehru Medical College, Belgaum, Karnataka, India

Ashalata A. Mallapur, Geetanjali M. Katageri, Umesh Y. Ramadurg and Sheshidhar G. Bannale
S. Nijalingappa Medical College and HSK Hospital and Research Centre, Bagalkot, Karnataka, India

Richard J. Derman
Thomas Jefferson University, Philadelphia, PA, USA

Jodie Dionne-Odom, Nicole J. Rembert, Comfort Enah and Alan T. N. Tita
University of Alabama at Birmingham, Birmingham, AL 35294, USA

Samuel Tancho, Thomas K. Welty and Pius M. Tih and Rahel Mbah
Cameroon Baptist Convention Health Services (CBCHS), P.O. Box 1, Nkwen, Bamenda, Cameroon

Gregory E. Halle-Ekane
University of Buea, P.O. Box 12, Buea, Cameroon

Samsiya Ona and Khady Diouf
Department of Obstetrics and Gynecology, Brigham and Women's Hospital, 75 Francis Street, Boston, MA 02115, USA

Rose L. Molina
Department of Obstetrics and Gynecology, Beth Israel Deaconess Medical Center, 330 Brookline Avenue, Boston, MA 02215, USA
Division of Women's Health, Brigham and Women's Hospital, 1620 Tremont Street, OBC-34, Boston, MA 02120, USA

Catarina Marques
Maternidade Dr. Alfredo da Costa, Rua Viriato, 1069-089 Lisboa, Portugal

Cristina Guerreiro
Fetal Maternal Department, Maternidade Dr. Alfredo da Costa, Lisbon, Portugal

Sérgio Reis Soares
Instituto Valenciano de Infertilidade (IVI-Lisboa), Lisbon, Portugal

Jonathan Faro, Gerald Riddle and Sebastian Faro
TheWoman's Hospital of Texas, 7400 Fannin Suite 930, Houston, TX 77054, USA

Malika Mitchell, Yuh-Jue Chen and Sarah Kamal
The University of Texas Health Science Center at Houston, Medical College, Houston, TX 77054, USA

Sasha Herbst de Cortina
Division of Infectious Diseases, Department of Medicine, University of California Los Angeles, 10833 Le Conte Avenue, Los Angeles, CA 90095, USA

Claire C. Bristow
Division of Global Public Health, Department of Medicine, University of California San Diego, 9500 Gilman Drive 0507, La Jolla, CA 92093, USA

Dvora Joseph Davey
Department of Epidemiology, Fielding School of Public Health, University of California Los Angeles, 640 Charles E. Young Drive S., Los Angeles, CA 90024, USA

Jeffrey D. Klausner
Division of Infectious Diseases, Department of Medicine, University of California Los Angeles, 10833 Le Conte Avenue, Los Angeles, CA 90095, USA
Department of Epidemiology, Fielding School of Public Health, University of California Los Angeles, 640 Charles E. Young Drive S., Los Angeles, CA 90024, USA

Jennifer H. Tang
UNC Project-Malawi, Kamuzu Central Hospital, 100 Mzimba Road, Private Bag Box A-104, Lilongwe, Malawi University ofNorth Carolina School of Medicine,Department ofObstetrics&Gynecology, University of North Carolina at Chapel Hill, 101 Manning Drive, CB No. 7570, Chapel Hill, NC 27599 7570, USA

Jamie W. Krashin
University ofNorth Carolina School of Medicine,Department ofObstetrics & Gynecology, University of North Carolina at Chapel Hill, 101 Manning Drive, CB No. 7570, Chapel Hill, NC 27599 7570, USA

Wingston Ng'ambi, Linly Mlundira, Thom Chaweza and Bernadette Samala
The Lighthouse Trust, Kamuzu Central Hospital, 100 Mzimba Road, Lilongwe, Malawi

LeaMariaMargareta Ambühl, Ulrik Baandrup and Suzette Sørensen
Center for Clinical Research, North Denmark Regional Hospital and Department of Clinical Medicine, Aalborg University, Bispensgade 37, 9800 Hjørring, Denmark

Karen Dybkær
Department of Hematology, Aalborg University Hospital, Søndre Skovvej 15, 9000 Aalborg, Denmark

Jan Blaakær and Niels Uldbjerg
Department of Obstetrics and Gynecology, Aarhus University Hospital, Palle Juul-Jensens Boulevard 99, 8200 Aarhus N, Denmark

Jordan E. Cates, Daniel Westreich and Andrew Edmonds
Department of Epidemiology,The University of North Carolina at Chapel Hill, Chapel Hill, NC 27599, USA

Rodney L. Wright
Department of Obstetrics & Gynecology andWomen's Health, Albert Einstein College of Medicine, Montefiore Medical Center, Bronx, NY 10467, USA

Howard Minkoff
Department of Obstetrics & Gynecology, Maimonides Medical Center, Brooklyn, NY 11219, USA

Christine Colie
Department of Obstetrics & Gynecology, Georgetown University,Washington, DC 20007, USA

Ruth M. Greenblatt
Departments of Clinical Pharmacy, Medicine Epidemiology and Biostatistics, University of California, San Francisco, San Francisco, CA 94143, USA

Helen E. Cejtin
Department of Obstetrics and Gynecology, John H. Stroger Hospital of Cook County, Chicago, IL 60612, USA

Roksana Karim
Department of Preventive Medicine, Keck School of Medicine, University of Southern California, Los Angeles, CA 90032, USA

Lisa B. Haddad
Department of Gynecology and Obstetrics, Emory University School of Medicine, Atlanta, GA 30322, USA

Mirjam-Colette Kempf
Schools of Nursing and Public Health, Department of Health Behavior, University of Alabama at Birmingham, Birmingham, AL 35294, USA

Elizabeth T. Golub
Department of Epidemiology, Johns Hopkins Bloomberg School of Public Health, Baltimore, MD 21205, USA

Philip A. Chan, Ashley Robinette, Madeline Montgomery, Alexi Almonte, Susan Cu-Uvin, John R. Lonks, Erna M. Kojic and Erica J. Hardy
Division of Infectious Diseases, Department of Medicine,Warren Alpert Medical School, Brown University, Providence, RI 02903, USA

Kimberle C. Chapin
Department of Pathology, Rhode Island Hospital, Providence, RI 02903, USA

Lauren M. Stark and Michael L. Power
Research Department, American College of Obstetricians and Gynecologists, 409 12th Street SW,Washington, DC 20024, USA

Mark Turrentine
Department of Obstetrics & Gynecology, Kelsey-Seybold Clinic, 1111 Augusta Drive, Houston, TX 77057, USA

Renee Samelson
Division of Maternal Fetal Medicine, Department of Obstetrics & Gynecology, Albany Medical Center, 391 Myrtle Avenue, Suite 2, Albany, NY 12208, USA

Maryam M. Siddiqui
The University of Chicago Medicine, 5841 S. Maryland Avenue, MC 2050, Chicago, IL 60637, USA

Michael J. Paglia and Emmie R. Strassberg
Department of Maternal-Fetal Medicine, Geisinger Health System, 100 N Academy Avenue, Danville, PA 17822, USA

Elizabeth Kelly
Department of Obstetrics & Gynecology, Albany Medical Center, 391 Myrtle Avenue, 2nd floor, MC 74, Albany, NY 12208, USA

Katie L.Murtough and Jay Schulkin
American College of Obstetricians and Gynecologists, 409 12th Street SW,Washington, DC 20024, USA

Mark P. Lachiewicz
Department of Gynecology and Obstetrics, Emory University School of Medicine, 1639 Pierce Drive, 4th Floor WMB, Atlanta, GA 30322, USA

Laura J.Moulton and Oluwatosin Jaiyeoba
Cleveland Clinic Foundation,Women's Health Institute, Cleveland, OH, USA

Gweneth B. Lazenby
Department of Obstetrics and Gynecology, Medical University of South Carolina, 96 Jonathan Lucas Street, Suite 624, Charleston, SC 29425, USA

Okeoma Mmeje
Department of Obstetrics and Gynecology, University of Michigan, L4100Women's Hospital, 1500 East Medical Center Drive, Ann Arbor, MI 48109, USA

Barbra M. Fisher and Adriana Weinberg
Department of Pediatrics, University of Colorado Anschutz Medical Campus, 12700 E. 19th Box B168, Aurora, CO 80045, USA

Erika K. Aaron and Maria Keating
Department of Medicine, Drexel University, 1427 Vine Street, 2nd Floor, Philadelphia, PA 19102, USA

Amneris E. Luque
Department of Medicine, University of Rochester, 601 Elmwood Avenue, Box 689, Rochester, NY 14642, USA

Denise Willers
Department of Obstetrics and Gynecology,Washington University, 4921 Parkview Place, St. Louis, MO 63110, USA

Deborah Cohan
Department of Obstetrics and Gynecology, University of California, 350 Parnassus Avenue No. 908, San Francisco, CA 94117, USA

Deborah Money
Department of Obstetrics and Gynecology, University of British Columbia, 1190 Hornby Street, 4th Floor, Vancouver, BC, Canada V6Z 2K5

Ashwini Bhalerao-Gandhi
P. D. Hinduja Hospital and Medical Research Centre, Veer Savarkar Marg, Mahim, Mumbai 400016, India

Pankdeep Chhabra and Saurabh Arya
Sanofi Pasteur India Pvt. Ltd., 54/A, Mathuradas Vasanji Road, Andheri East, Mumbai 400093, India

James Mark Simmerman
Sanofi PasteurThailand, 87/2 CRC Tower, 23rd Floor, Wireless Road, Bangkok 10330, Thailand

Cora-Ann McElwain and Jay Schulkin
Department of Research, American College of Obstetricians and Gynecologists, 409 12th Street SW,Washington, DC 20024, USA

Katherine M. Jones
Department of Research, American College of Obstetricians and Gynecologists, 409 12th Street SW,Washington, DC 20024, USA
Department of Psychology, American University, 4400 Massachusetts Avenue NW,Washington, DC 20016, USA

Sarah Carroll and Debra Hawks
Practice Division, American College of Obstetricians and Gynecologists, 409 12th Street SW,Washington, DC 20024, USA

Christiana Smith, Emily Barr, Suzanne Paul and Elizabeth J. McFarland
1Division of InfectiousDiseases,Department of Pediatrics,University of Colorado School ofMedicine and Children'sHospital Colorado, Aurora, CO 80045, USA

AdrianaWeinberg
Division of InfectiousDiseases,Department of Pediatrics,University of Colorado School ofMedicine and Children'sHospital Colorado, Aurora, CO 80045, USA
Department of Medicine, University of Colorado School of Medicine, Aurora, CO 80045, USA
Department of Pathology, University of Colorado School of Medicine, Aurora, CO 80045, USA

Jeri E. Forster
Department of Biostatistics and Informatics, Colorado School of Public Health, Aurora, CO 80045, USA

Myron J. Levin
Division of InfectiousDiseases,Department of Pediatrics,University of Colorado School ofMedicine and Children'sHospital Colorado, Aurora, CO 80045, USA
Department of Medicine, University of Colorado School of Medicine, Aurora, CO 80045, USA

Jill Davies
Department of Obstetrics and Gynecology, University of Colorado School of Medicine, Aurora, CO 80045, USA
Denver Health Medical Center, Denver, CO 80204, USA

Jennifer Pappas and Kay Kinzie
Children's Hospital Colorado, Aurora, CO 80045, USA

Bassam H. Rimawi
School of Medicine, Department of Gynecology and Obstetrics, Division of Maternal Fetal Medicine and Reproductive Infectious Diseases, Emory University, 550 Peachtree Street, Atlanta, GA 30308, USA

Lisa Haddad
School of Medicine, Department of Gynecology and Obstetrics, Division of Family Planning, Emory University, 550 Peachtree Street, Atlanta, GA 30308, USA

Martina L. Badell
School of Medicine, Department of Gynecology and Obstetrics, Division of Maternal Fetal Medicine, Emory University, 550 Peachtree Street, Atlanta, GA 30308, USA

Rana Chakraborty
School of Medicine, Department of Pediatrics, Division of Infectious Diseases, Emory University, 2015 Uppergate Drive, NE, Atlanta, GA 30322, USA

Alison R. Migliori and Patricia Lauro
Department of Pathology & Laboratory Medicine,Women & Infants Hospital of Rhode Island, Providence, RI, USA

C. James Sung and Halit Pinar
Department of Pathology & Laboratory Medicine,Women & Infants Hospital of Rhode Island, Providence, RI, USA
Department of Pathology & Laboratory Medicine,Warren Alpert Medical School of Brown University, Providence, RI, USA

Mai He
Department of Pathology & Laboratory Medicine,Women & Infants Hospital of Rhode Island, Providence, RI, USA
Department of Pathology & Laboratory Medicine,Warren Alpert Medical School of Brown University, Providence, RI, USA
Department of Pathology and Immunology,Washington University School of Medicine, St Louis, MO, USA

Milton W. Musaba
Mbale Regional Referral & Teaching Hospital, P.O. Box 921, Mbale, Uganda

Mike N. Kagawa and Paul Kiondo
School of Medicine, College of Health Sciences, Makerere University, P.O. Box 7072, Kampala, Uganda

Charles Kiggundu
Mulago National Referral & Teaching Hospital, P.O. Box 7051, Kampala, Uganda

Julius Wandabwa
Faculty of Health Sciences, BusitemaUniversity, P.O. Box 1460, Mbale, Uganda

Gilles Faron, Leonardo Gucciardo and Walter Foulon
Department of Obstetrics and Prenatal Medicine, Universitair Ziekenhuis Brussel, 101 Laarbeeklaan, Jette, 1090 Brussels, Belgium

Ellen Vancutsem and Anne Naessens
Department of Microbiology, UZ Brussel, 101 Laarbeeklaan, Jette, 1090 Brussels, Belgium

Ronald Buyl
Department of Biostatistics and Medical Informatics, Faculty of Medicine and Pharmacy, Vrije Universiteit Brussel, 101 Laarbeeklaan, Jette, 1090 Brussels, Belgium

Sylvia M. LaCourse
Department of Medicine, Division of Allergy and Infectious Diseases, University ofWashington, Seattle,WA 98104, USA

Sharon A. Greene and Stephen E. Hawes
Department of Epidemiology, University ofWashington, Seattle,WA 98195, USA

Elizabeth E. Dawson-Hahn
Department of Pediatrics, University ofWashington, Seattle,WA 98121, USA

Sam Phiri
The Lighthouse Trust, Kamuzu Central Hospital, 100 Mzimba Road, Lilongwe, Malawi
University ofNorth Carolina School of Medicine,Department ofMedicine, Chapel Hill,NC 27599-3368, USA

Hannock Tweya
The Lighthouse Trust, Kamuzu Central Hospital, 100 Mzimba Road, Lilongwe, Malawi
The International Union against Tuberculosis and Lung Disease, 75006 Paris, France

Mina C. Hosseinipour
UNC Project-Malawi, Kamuzu Central Hospital, 100 Mzimba Road, Private Bag Box A-104, Lilongwe, Malawi
University ofNorth Carolina School of Medicine,Department ofMedicine, Chapel Hill,NC 27599-3368, USA

Lisa B. Haddad
Emory University School of Medicine,Department of Gynecology and Obstetrics, Emory University, 49 Jesse Hill Jr. Drive, Atlanta, GA 30303, USA

Index

www.ingramcontent.com/pod-product-compliance
Lightning Source LLC
Chambersburg PA
CBHW070153240326
41458CB00126B/4542